D0722043

LACTATION

LACT

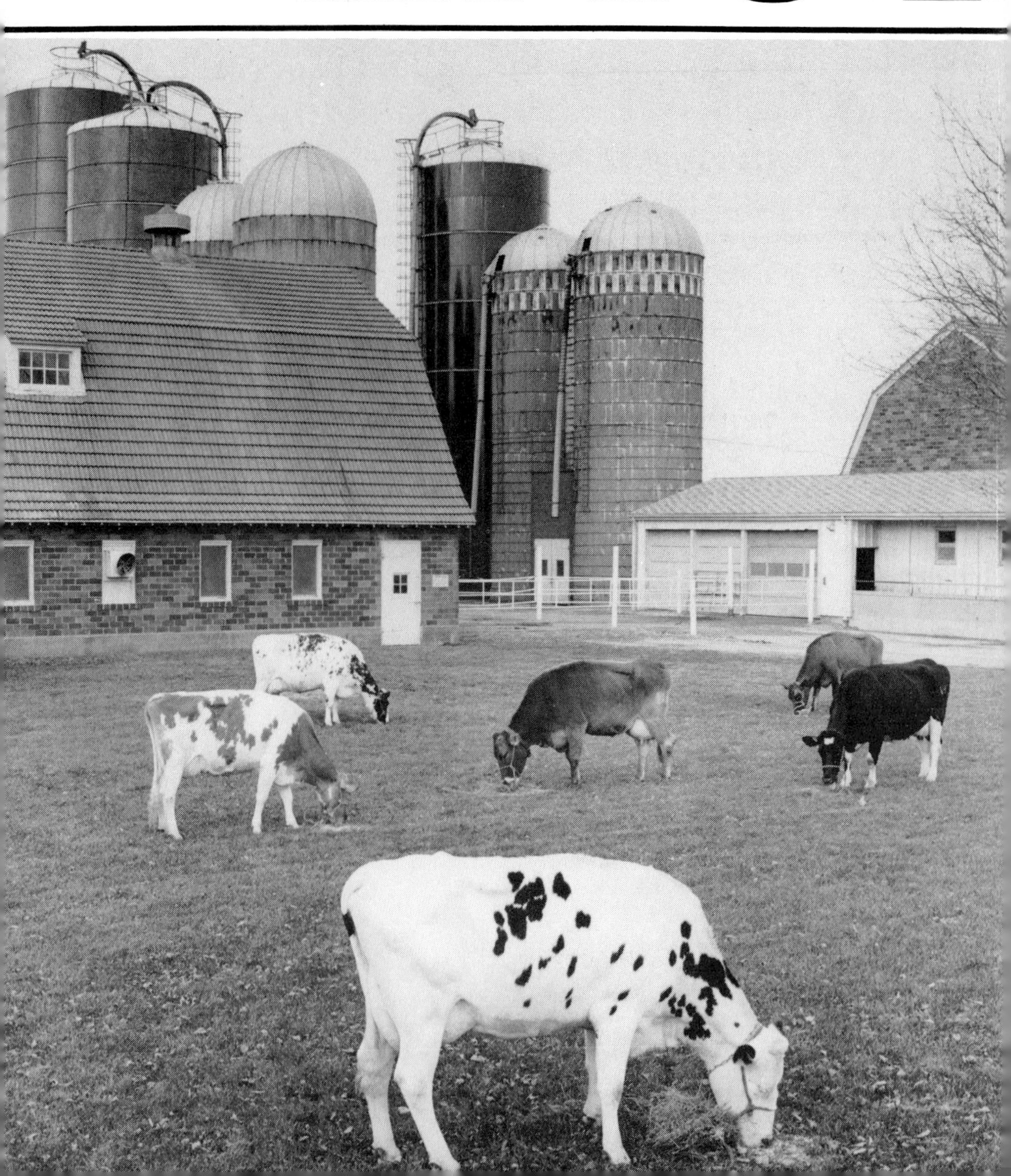

ATION

EDITED BY **BRUCE L. LARSON**

WRITTEN BY **RALPH R. ANDERSON**
Professor, Department of Dairy Science
University of Missouri, Columbia

ROBERT J. COLLIER
Associate Professor, Department of Dairy Science
University of Florida, Gainesville

ALBERT J. GUIDRY
Research Animal Scientist, Animal Sciences Institute
United States Department of Agriculture, Beltsville, Md.

C. WILLIAM HEALD
Professor, Department of Dairy and Animal Science
Pennsylvania State University, University Park

ROBERT JENNESS
Professor, Department of Biochemistry
University of Minnesota, St. Paul

BRUCE L. LARSON
Professor, Department of Dairy Science
University of Illinois, Urbana

H. ALLEN TUCKER
Professor, Department of Animal Science
Michigan State University, East Lansing

PUBLISHED BY **THE IOWA STATE UNIVERSITY PRESS / AMES**

Composed and printed by
The Iowa State University Press
Ames, Iowa 50010

First edition, 1985

TITLE PAGE: Dairy farm, University of Illinois, Urbana

Library of Congress Cataloging in Publication Data
Main entry under title:

Lactation.

Includes bibliographies and index.
1. Lactation. 2. Dairy cattle. 3. Milk. I. Larson, Bruce L. (Bruce Linder), 1927–
II. Anderson, Ralph R. [DNLM: 1. Dairying. 2. Lactation. SF 768 L151]
QP246.L3 1985 599.73′58 85–58
ISBN 0–8138–1063–9

C O N T E N T S

3. NUTRITIONAL, METABOLIC, AND ENVIRONMENTAL ASPECTS OF LACTATION by Robert J. Collier

5. BIOCHEMICAL AND NUTRITIONAL ASPECTS OF MILK AND COLOSTRUM by Robert Jenness

6. MILK COLLECTION by C. William Heald

7. MASTITIS AND THE IMMUNE SYSTEM OF THE MAMMARY GLAND by Albert J. Guidry

PREFACE

THE NEED ARISES periodically for a new or revised book on lactation that can serve as a textbook and general lactation reference book at the college level. The small demand compared to texts for other, more popular, college courses helps make it difficult to keep even a current one available. It now has been over 12 yr since G. H. Schmidt authored the *Biology of Lactation* (W. H. Freeman 1971). In the three previous decades, the five editions of *Secretion of Milk* (Iowa State University Press) filled the need. The first edition was authored by D. W. Espe in 1938 and the last by V. R. Smith in 1959. All the above books are now out of print, as well as out of date.

Lactation is a heterogeneous field embracing a host of complex biological areas. Rapid advances in the biological and chemical sciences have made it increasingly difficult for any one person to be knowledgeable in all aspects. Furthermore, the results of many decades of lactation research have made it difficult to reference properly all the studies that have gone into the development of the many concepts now generally accepted. Specialized extensive review articles on detailed aspects exist, as well as the complex four-volume, multiauthored reference books *Lactation: A Comprehensive Treatise* (Academic) edited by B. L. Larson and V. R. Smith (Vols. 1–3, 1974) and B. L. Larson (Vol. 4, 1978). While these have provided sources of detailed reference information, they are much too intricate and expensive to serve as a general textbook. The greatest current need perceived by instructors of lactation courses primarily concerned with dairy animals has been for an up-to-date book of concepts and summarized data that can be used as a classroom text.

The seven authors who have prepared this book have done so with that objective. All the authors are deeply involved in their respective areas and collectively have brought information together with individual insights that could not be accomplished by a single author. There are no reference citations in the text; specific items are not referenced unless acknowledged for copyright purposes (figures and tables). Each chapter is followed by references to more comprehensive sources.

It has been assumed that the user will have a background knowledge of basic chemistry and biology, as well as some more specific training in one or more biological disciplines, such as biochemistry, physiology, and nutrition, typical of an advanced undergraduate or early graduate student in an applied science curriculum. Basic discipline textbooks should be consulted if difficulties are encountered.

The chapter authors deserve collective thanks for their cooperation in the preparation of this book. Not all duplication has been eliminated, but that left is needed mainly for continuity in understanding within a chapter. Special appreciation is due to Helen M. Hegarty for her handling of the technical editing details with the manuscripts and the preparation of the subject index.

BRUCE L. LARSON

LACTATION

CHAPTER 1

MAMMARY GLAND

RALPH R. ANDERSON

1.1: INTRODUCTION

1.1-1: Phylogeny. The mammary gland is unique among glands of the body, not because it is exocrine or because it is a skin gland, but because it fills a unique function in transferring food from parent to offspring in a form that may be utilized by immature neonates. Fishes, amphibia, reptiles, and birds fulfill the requirement of nutrient transfer by producing eggs sufficiently large to have energy available to the embryo as it matures and eventually hatches. Such offspring are sufficiently mature at hatching to utilize food in the environment. Generally, this requires a highly mature digestive system. In a few instances, birds have overcome this problem by semidigesting food and regurgitating it for the offspring or, as in the case of pigeons, have developed highly specialized cells in the lining of their crop, which are regurgitated for assimilation by the rapidly growing offspring.

Mammals have taken a different course in adapting to more harsh, and generally colder, environmental conditions than are normally tolerated by the fishes, amphibia, reptiles, and birds. They are characterized by hair on the surfaces of their bodies as a means of trapping body heat and have developed a mechanism for transferring nutrients via a skin gland. Both these adaptations have proven to be highly successful in enabling the class Mammalia to spread its life forms to all but the coldest parts of the Earth. Mammals exist in terrestrial forms in sizes as small as the shrew (15 gm body weight) to the elephant (several thousand kg). Aquatic forms, such as whales, may reach body weights as much as ten times that of the elephant.

Adaptive features, such as four strong limbs, enabling terrestrial forms rapid locomotion, or strong flippers for outstanding speed and maneuverability in water, are extremely important in providing various mammals with specializations necessary for survival in certain environments. However, the one mechanism common to these complex forms of life (relative to fishes, amphibia, reptiles, and birds) is success of reproduction via the transfer of milk from mother to offspring. Viviparity is important to the success of the class Mammalia but is not unique to mammals, as may be demonstrated in a number of species of fishes and reptiles. The reptiles are dependent upon a warm, tranquil environment for survival and are not nearly as adaptable to harsh environmental changes as are the mammals that nurse their young to provide the offspring with protection, body warmth, and nutrient transfer in the form of milk.

Mammals are unique in the characteristic of body hair and nutrient transfer in the form of milk. But are they so different from reptiles and birds that links in relationships among these classes cannot be established? Many lines of evidence can be pointed out to show the similarities. For instance, two species of primitive mammals still exist, which represent many extinct species that were egg layers. These two remaining examples are the duckbill platypus (*Ornithorhynchus anatinus*) and the echidna (spiny anteater, *Tachyglossus aculeatus*). The duckbill platypus lays one or two leathery eggs in the spring and warms them periodically for approximately 12 days. The young are born very immature and are barely able to crawl onto the mother's abdomen, while she lies supine. An area of the abdomen contains long tubules that comprise the mammary system. Milk is synthesized in the epithelial cells of the tubular lining in response to prolactin, which is secreted when the eggs hatch. The offspring nuzzle the abdominal areas, releasing oxytocin from the neurohypophysis in the mother's pituitary gland. Myoepithelial cells surrounding the tubules contract in response to oxytocin, and milk is forced onto the hair of the abdomen. With its ducklike bill, the young platypus laps up the milk and grows very well. The mammary apparatus of the echidna is similar except the beginning development of a marsupium, or pouch, is evident. This device becomes much more developed in the Didelphidae, a suborder of mammals in which the length of gestation is short because there is no true placental attachment; the young need a pouch for protection while suckling because they are so tiny and immature when born.

Reptiles, which presently exist on earth, have no structures that may be suggestive as precursors to mammary apparati in mammals. Fossil evidence of reptiles, with mouth parts that suggest a function in suckling, have been interpreted by some to indicate a possible link with mammals and the suckling phenomenon by the offspring. However, no soft-tissue structures in present-day reptiles show any resemblance to a primitive mammalian mammary apparatus.

1.1-2: Ontogeny. Stages in the embryonic development (ontogeny) of many vertebrates, characteristically, are similar in their early stages. This evidence is based on the axiom that ontogeny recapitulates phylogeny. Indeed, only the most expert investigators are able to differentiate the embryo of a cow from a horse, a pig from a bear, or a rat from a cat. In rapid succession, the fertilized egg (zygote) goes from 2 cells, to 4, to 8, to 16 (a morula), a blastula, a gastrula, and finally a neurula with somites. Interestingly enough, primordial thickening of the ventrolateral aspect of the ectoderm appears very early in embryonic life, even before the embryo is readily identified as one of its own species. Serial changes in the thickened area of the ectoderm (skin) are identified as the mammary band, mammary streak, mammary line, mammary crest, mammary hillock, and mammary bud (Fig. 1.1).

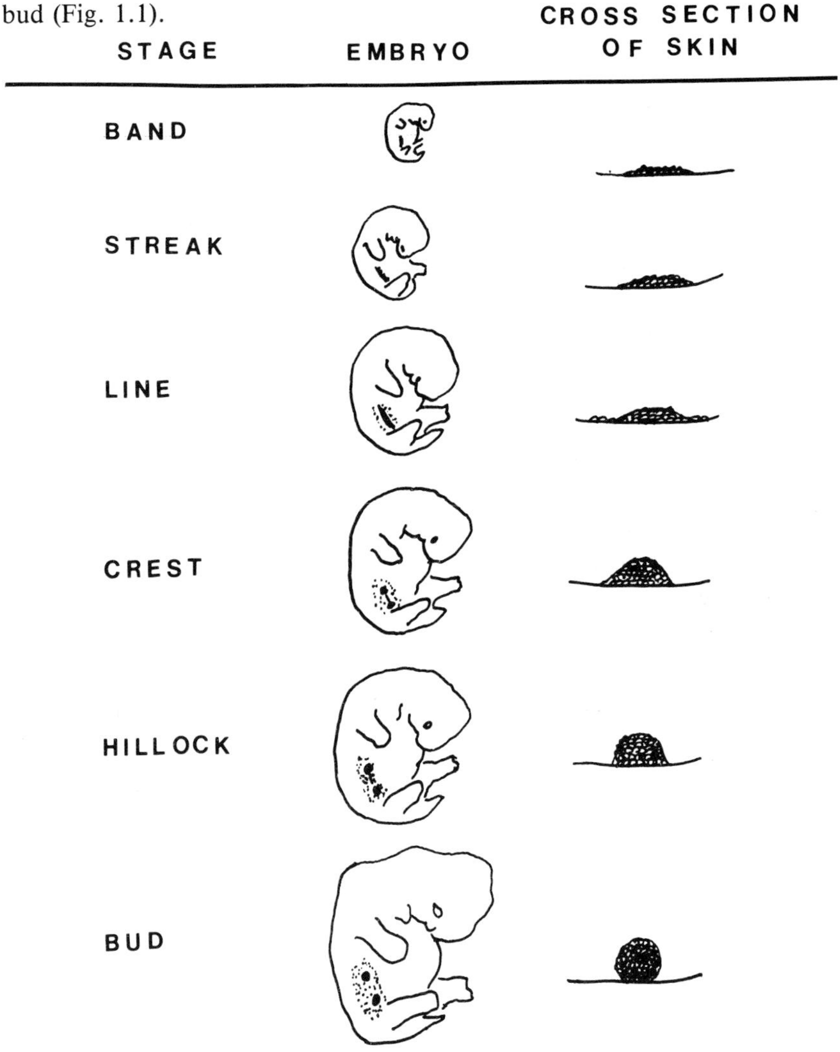

STAGE
EMBRYO
CROSS SECTION OF SKIN
BAND
STREAK
LINE
CREST
HILLOCK
BUD

Fig. 1.1. Developmental stages, from the band through the bud, of the mammary apparatus in the embryo.

Mammary band. At this stage, the skin on each side of the embryo's underside (ventral aspect) thickens along a faint line from a point near the front limb bud to a point near the hind limb bud.

Mammary streak. This area thickens until it becomes a distinct line along each side of the ventral midline between the limb buds (primordial structures of forelegs and hind legs).

Mammary line. As the embryo enlarges, it goes through rapid stages of differentiation. Although the change from mammary streak to mammary line is subtle, a definite orientation of epithelial cells proliferating along a straight line in a confined area is apparent.

Mammary crest. In certain areas along the line, cells proliferate rapidly, while other cells along the line do not. Where the rapid proliferation occurs, a mammary teat and gland will eventuate.

Mammary hillock. Rapid proliferation of the cells that make up the crest results in a hemisphere of epithelial cells, which grows into and crowds the mesodermal area within. At this stage, the mesoderm is called mesenchyme; it lacks a readily defined organization of individual cells.

Mammary bud. Complete proliferation along the line of cells, which become hemispherical in shape, results later in a sphere, known as a bud; it is from the ball of epithelial cells that the structures in the mature gland responsible for milk secretion arise. The sequence of progressions in primordial mammary development in the cow embryo occur from day 32 to 43 (Table 1.1).

Table 1.1. Embryonic development of the mammary apparatus in cattle, pigs, and humans

	Cattle		Pigs		Humans	
Stage of Development	Age of embryos, days	Crown-rump length of embryo, mm	Age of embryos, days	Crown-rump length of embryo, mm	Age of embryos, days	Crown-rump length of embryo, mm
Mammary band	32	14	21	10	35	6
Mammary streak	34	16	22	12	36	8
Mammary line	35	17	23	15	37	10
Mammary crest	37	19	25	18	40	13
Mammary hillock	40	21	26	20	42	15
Mammary bud	43	25	28	22	49	20

Embryonic differentiation of the bud continues to the fetal stage. The bud symbolizes an important differentiation and transitional stage in mammary gland development and, coincidentally, occurs when the embryo has differentiated sufficiently so the species that it represents begins to be recognizable. At this stage, a change in nomenclature from embryo to fetus is appropriate. The bud is the main structure from which all mammary glands arise, regardless of species. We will return to the subject of mammary development in fetal life and later stages after we look at the various ways by which mammary glands are measured.

1.2: INDICES OF MAMMARY GROWTH AND DIFFERENTIATION

In all research, methods of measuring that which the researcher is interested in studying must be developed. The mammary gland has been measured in many ways by various techniques, each of which has limitations. Measurements are either qualitative or quantitative; both are necessary to gain information about the gland and to find ways of increasing milk production. Some of the various ways to measure the mammary gland are listed.

1.2-1: Macromeasures. The palpation method has been used for many years as a means to evaluate udder development in heifer calves and yearlings. Generally, it has been used subjectively in comparing animals of the same age. Attempts have been made to measure the fatty pad, using calipers, and/or teat length and teat spread, using a ruler. These measurements are subject to large errors and are limited in value.

When the animals are lactating, caliper and ruler measurements are more reliable than in younger animals. Dimensions used to study mammary development at this time have been length, width, circumference, height from floor, length of teats, diameter of teats, angle of udder, width of rear attachment, and others.

Attempts to measure udder volume have included these measures as well as techniques such as water displacement, plaster casts, and sonorays; none have been very satisfactory.

1.2-2: Histological. Mammary gland tissues are very soft and, therefore, not as easily studied as some other tissues, such as muscle. However, many excellent studies have been done using the microscope as the primary tool to relate structure and function.

1.2-2a: Light microscopy. Microscopes using light as the means to differentiate structures have been available to researchers for many years. Two types have been used primarily: the dissecting microscope with the ability to magnify 10–100 times, and the standard light microscope with the ability to magnify up to several thousand times.

Dissecting microscopes enable the researcher to identify relatively large features of mammary glands, such as the gland cistern, large ducts and clusters of alveoli, lobules, and lobes. This technique has been used very effectively in studying mammary gland growth qualitatively and semiquantitatively (Fig. 1.2). The main limitation is that it may be used only with glands that are relatively thin, such as those of mice, rats, hamsters, and rabbits; it is not very effective in studying mammary glands of cattle, goats, or sheep.

Standard light microscopes have the advantage of exposing the intricate microstructures of the udder, that is, alveoli and individual epithelial cells. Both qualitative and quantitative data may be gathered by studying

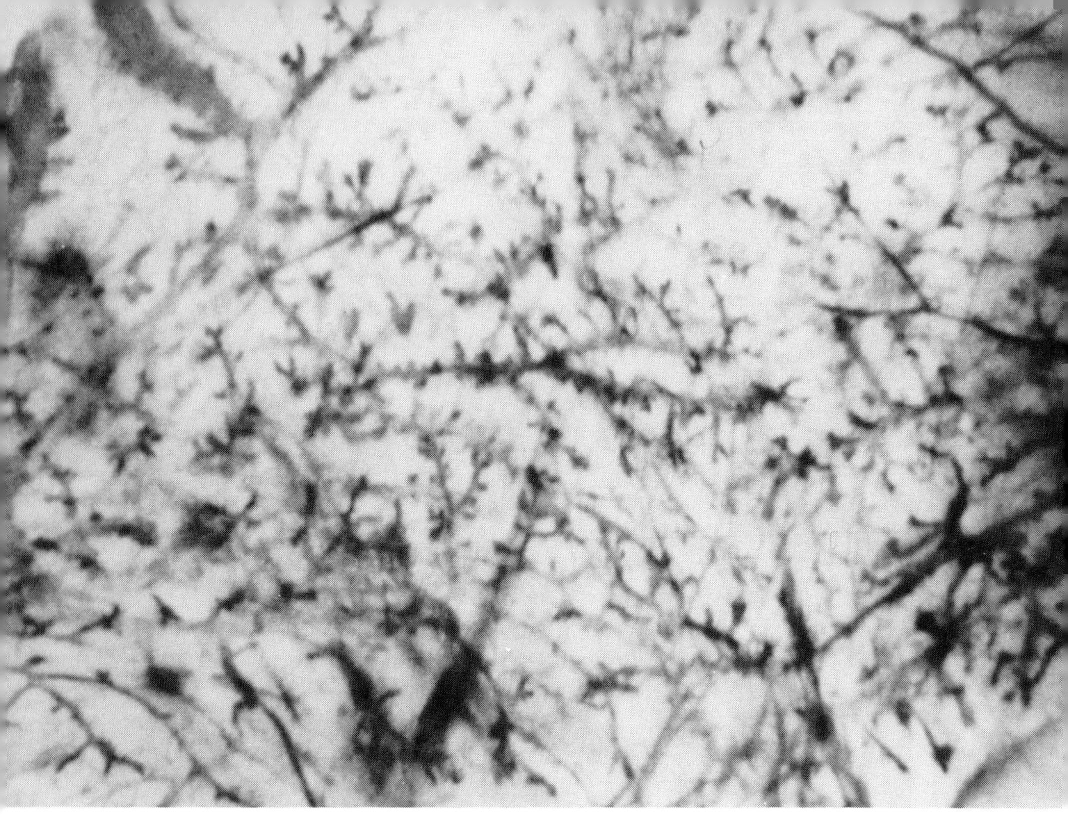

Fig. 1.2. A whole mount of a mammary gland from a rat showing ducts and end buds (stained with hematoxylin; ×10 magnification). (From Wright and Anderson 1982)

microscopically thin sections of the gland. These sections may be cut to as thin as 2 μm, considerably thinner than a mammary gland epithelial cell. By using various staining techniques, eosin and hematoxylin being the most common, various intra- and intercellular structures may be identified (Fig. 1.3).

1.2-2b: Electron microscopy. The electron microscope became available to a limited number of researchers shortly after World War II; its use is limited because it is so expensive. Whereas the light microscope allows us to see structures as small as 1 μm, the transmission electron microscope enables us to see objects as small as 1 nm, enabling the differentiation of many structures inside the cell not differentiated by the light microscope. Great progress in cell physiology has been made using the electron microscope. Examples of transmission electron microscope slides may be seen in Figures 4.4–4.7 and Figure 4.12.

A more recent adaptation of the electron microscope is the scanning electron microscope, which is particularly effective in showing surfaces of living cells, such as spermatozoa and alveoli of the mammary gland.

1.2-3: Cytology. Histology is the study of tissues; cytology is the study of cells. Through studies of the mammary gland, investigators have appreciated the cooperative interactions of groups of cells to enable a particular function, such as milk synthesis, to proceed. An example is the requirement of the alveolar structure to be maintained as a unit in order to have normal milk synthesis occur. However, the basic unit of the alveolus is the individual epithelial secretory cell. In order to study cells, numerous techniques have been employed to measure components of the cell, such as nucleus, endoplasmic reticulum, mitochondrion, lysosome, Golgi apparatus, secretory vesicle, and cell membrane.

Among the approaches used to study the structures and functions of cells are (1) light microscopy, (2) electron microscopy, (3) immunofluores-

Fig. 1.3. A histological section of a goat mammary gland in late pregnancy. Note large connective tissue septa between lobes and smaller amount of connective tissue around lobules and alveoli, composed of secretory epithelia (stained with hematoxylin-eosin; ×66 magnification).

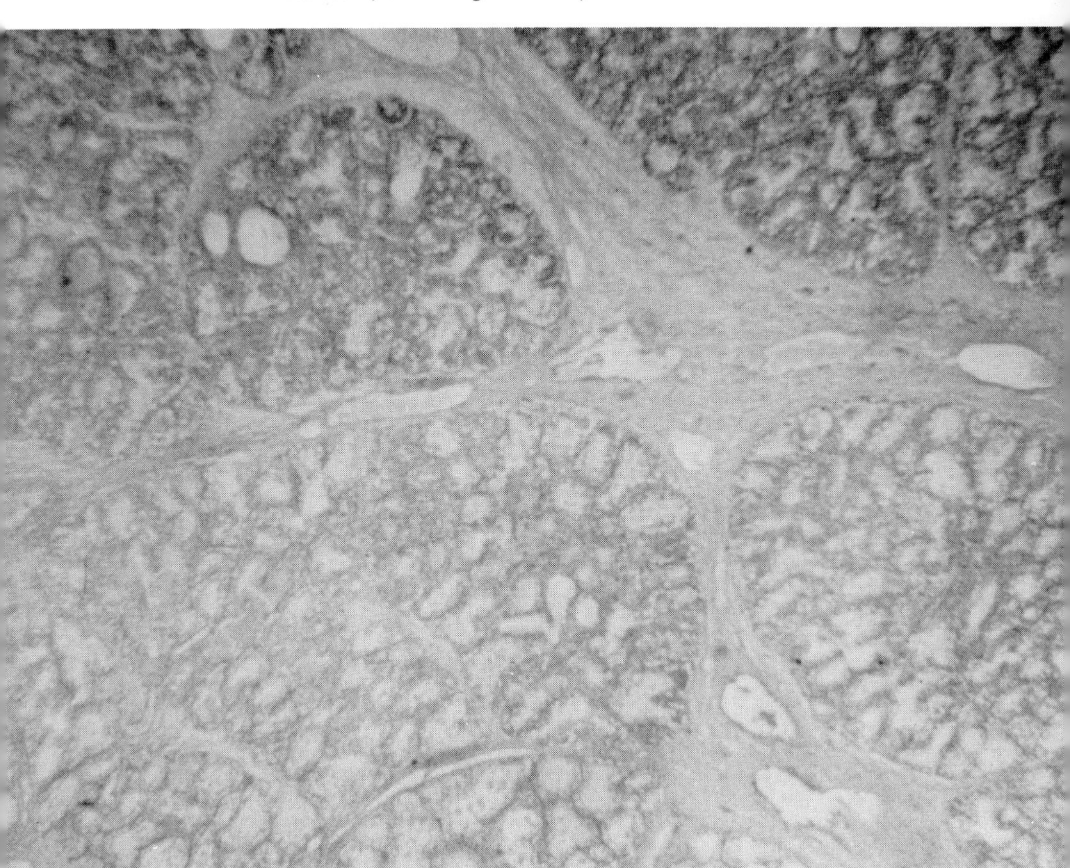

cent tagging, (4) radioisotope labeling, (5) sucrose gradient centrifugation, (6) gel filtration, and others.

1.2-4: In vivo techniques to measure mammary glands. Earlier in this chapter we mentioned macromeasures of the mammary gland, including calipers, rulers, water displacement, plaster casts, and sonoray. The advantage of these methods is that the animal need not be sacrificed to obtain data; the disadvantage is the data are limited in value. The researcher must obtain more complete data to understand the inner workings of the gland by sacrificing the animal at specified times in the stages of development. Small laboratory animals, such as mice and rats, primarily have been used for this purpose. Because the knowledge to be gained from these animals is limited, others had to be studied, including hamsters, guinea pigs, rabbits, goats, sheep, pigs, and cattle. The gland is removed from the animal and weighed; this is the wet weight. In the case of the cow, goat, or sheep, the udder is trimmed to remove the skin, teats, supramammary lymph nodes, extra fat, large blood vessels, and milk, if any. Remaining tissue is weighed and designated trimmed wet weight.

Water and lipids are extracted from the trimmed mammary tissue using hot ethanol and then hot ether. The remaining white-colored tissue, made up of protein (75–80%) and nucleic acids (DNA and RNA), is dried completely and weighed and is known as dried fat-free tissue (DFFT). Aliquots of DFFT are used to measure DNA, RNA, and hydroxyproline by elaborate time-consuming chemical procedures. Protein is measured by a colorimetric dye-binding technique. DNA is hydrolyzed and the deoxyribose measured colorimetrically by complexing it with para-nitrophenylhydrazine. RNA is hydrolyzed by a different procedure and the ribose measured colorimetrically using orcinol as the color-complexing agent. Hydroxyproline is a specific and significant amino acid component of the complex protein collagen. Since collagen is the primary component of mammary gland connective tissue, the measurement of hydroxyproline enables the researcher to determine connective tissue of the mammary in toto and as a percent of the total; the remainder is an estimate of parenchymal tissue. Many mammary glands are 80% parenchyma and 20% stroma during the lactation phase. An example of the information accumulated using these measures is shown in Figure 1.4.

1.2-5: In vitro techniques for mammary gland evaluation. Mammary glands grow much better in the intact animal than they do in the test tube. The goal of the researcher is to try to understand why this is so and, while in the process of doing so, develop in vitro techniques that enable the stimulation of growth comparable to that observed in vivo.

Tissue cultures of mammary gland have not been very successful, mainly because epithelial cells die quickly and fibroblasts do not. The result

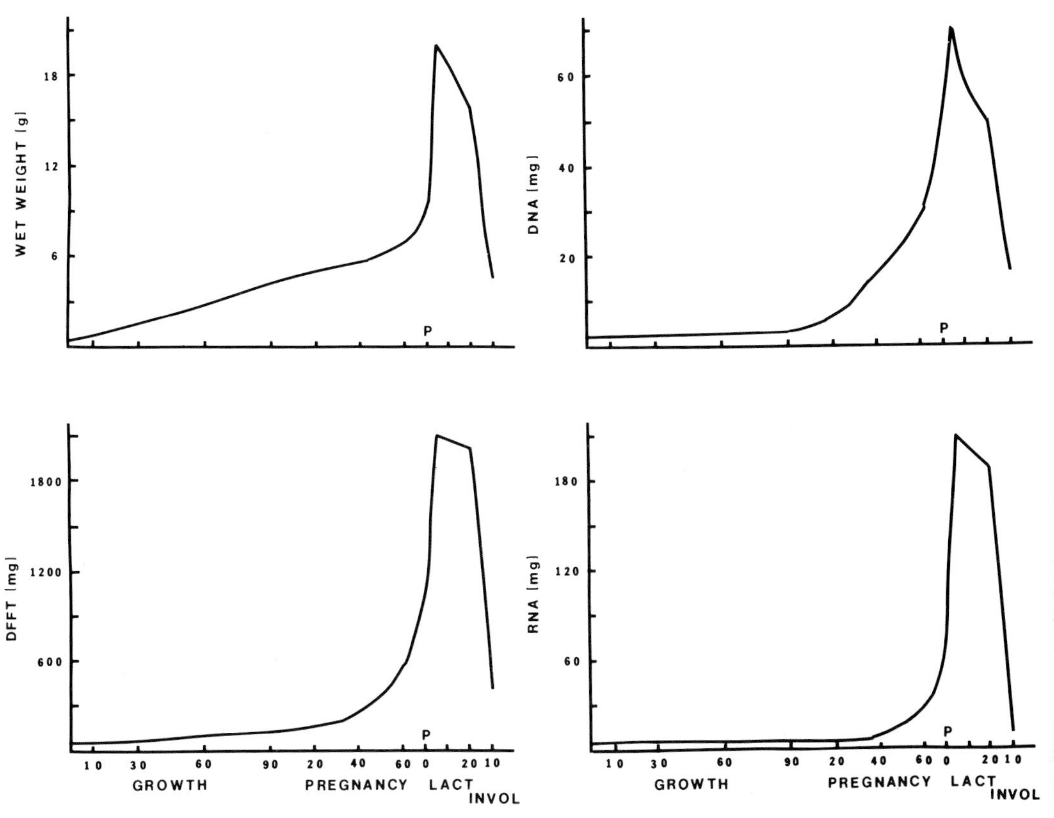

Fig. 1.4. Mammary growth in guinea pigs during the growth phase, pregnancy, lactation (*LACT*), and involution (*INVOL*). *P* designates parturition. Indices of mammary development include wet weight, DFFT, DNA, and RNA.

is an abnormal tissue that is valuable only as a tool to study fibroblasts and connective tissue components.

Limited success in mammary tissue cultures has been achieved mainly with fetal tissue. A significant finding from this work is that an immature mammary epithelial cell does not acquire the competency to synthesize milk until it achieves a final cell division from a mother cell into two daughter cells. This competency may be held in check by high levels of progesterone. When certain hormones (a combination of insulin, prolactin, and cortisol) are added to the medium in which the tissue is immersed, initiation of milk synthesis may take place in the epithelial cells of an intact alveolus.

The culturing of individual epithelial cells or myoepithelial cells has not met with any degree of success to date, while fibroblasts are relatively easy to culture. A new technique using collagen layers, upon which the epithelial cells may adhere, is a promising development. It appears that a mammary gland secretory cell, and perhaps a myoepithelial cell as well, cannot survive and multiply in the absence of a material that mimics the basal lamina, which the collagen layer does in this case.

1.3: DIVISIONS OF MAMMARY GLAND DEVELOPMENT, FUNCTION (LACTATION), AND DECLINE (INVOLUTION)

1.3-1: Introduction. As stated earlier in this chapter, differentiation of cells destined to develop into a functional mammary apparatus occurs very early in embryonic development. In rapid succession, these stages are known as the band, streak, line, crest, hillock, and bud. Maturation of the bud generally coincides with the embryo becoming a fetus. The term fetus is reserved for placental mammals (Eutheria), because other suborders of mammals undergo a decisive change at approximately the same stage in their development, which does not parallel the continued uterine nourishment. In the case of egg-laying mammals (Protheria), the incubation period terminates at approximately the same stage of development that embryos change to fetuses in the eutherians. Similarly, the mammals commonly referred to as marsupials (Metatheria) terminate pregnancy at this stage. No true placental attachment has occurred in these species; the young crawl from the uterus to the mammary apparatus on the mother's abdomen. This is frequently associated with a pouch, or marsupium, but not always.

1.3-2: Stages of development in fetuses

1.3-2a: Primary sprout(s). The mammary bud of the cow's udder is represented by the end of the teat in the area of the streak canal. As soon as the group of cells has reached a spherical shape, new differentiation occurs. Some cells in the sphere are programmed to break out of the sphere to form a branch called a primary sprout. This primordial structure is destined to become an opening in the teat by which milk exits the gland to the outside of the body; these openings are known as galactophores. Variations in numbers of galactophores per teat, or nipple, are considerable in the class Mammalia. Cows, goats, sheep, mice, rats, and guinea pigs have 1 opening per teat, horses have 2, pigs 3, rabbits 6, dogs 10, and humans 15–25. Each galactophore is predetermined by a primary sprout growing from the mammary bud. For example, the human fetus has at least 15 primary sprouts proliferating from each bud.

Several species of mammals are characterized by the lack of teats, or nipples, in the male: mouse, rat, horse, and beaver. Others probably exist but have not been described. In these species, the male mammary apparatus grows normally to the stage of the primary sprout. In the rat and mouse, at least, a surge of testosterone, presumably secreted by the fetal testes, causes a pinching-off (pycnosis) of the neck of the primary sprout, separating it from the mammary bud and resulting in the lack of teat formation. The part of the primary sprout retained in the fatty pad of the rodent is viable; many male rats and mice have been stimulated to form an extensive lobule-alveolar apparatus in response to injections of estrogens and progesterone. Even milk synthesis has been demonstrated in these cases, but obviously the milk is trapped in situ.

1.3-2b: **Canalization of the primary sprout.** Proliferation of the primary sprout is rapid and, in a short time, the sprout is much larger than the bud from which it originated. Eventually, the epithelial cells comprising the center of the sprout can no longer be nourished and they die, just as the cells on the outside layer of skin die. The result is a canal in the center of the primary sprout, which eventually becomes the gland cistern at the proximal end of the sprout (toward the body of the cow) and the teat cistern at the distal end of the sprout.

1.3-2c: **Secondary sprouts.** Cells multiply and branch from the primary sprout when it reaches a certain size. These branches are called secondary sprouts and are the first structural features destined to become large milk ducts leading into the gland cistern at the time when the gland becomes functional.

1.3-2d: **Mammary fatty pad.** All stages of growth and differentiation, identified to this point, are representative of epithelial cells from ectoderm, which is the embryonic skin. Other layers of the early embryo are mesoderm and endoderm. The middle layer, or mesoderm, gives rise to connective tissues, such as areolar, fibrous, and elastic, and adipose tissue and blood. An early feature of mammary gland development is a layer of adipose cells around the mammary bud and subsequent epithelial cell structures of mammary differentiation. A necessary part of the successful progression of mammary gland growth is an adequately developed mammary fatty pad. Very early in fetal life, the female develops a more extensive fatty pad than the male. This is particularly true in species such as cattle, goats, and sheep, in which the mammary gland is in close proximity to the scrotum in the male. In such instances, the fatty pad has no room to proliferate in the male fetus, resulting in mammary development that is doomed to terminate at a primitive stage of development. Only primary ducts are seen in the mammary apparatus of male cattle, sheep, and goats. Attempts to grow the mammary glands of steers and bulls have met with failure; only the teat responds to any extent and, in steers given estrogen, the teat will extend 3 or 4 in. (7.5–10 cm), similar in length to a cycling heifer.

1.3-2e: **Median suspensory ligament.** The udder of the cow is divided into two distinct halves, separated by a prominent ligament that provides the primary support for the udder. The structure, known as the median suspensory ligament, is composed of elastic and fibrous connective tissues that arose from the mesoderm. Highly specialized cells known as fibroblasts are thought to produce the highly complex molecules of elastin and collagen making up the ligament. Approximately 6 mo into the pregnancy, a median suspensory ligament is discernible in the fetus. As the four glands grow in fetal life, the fatty pads become larger and, with them, the median suspensory ligament becomes more prominent. At birth, four distinct quarters are readily detectable by palpation in the heifer calf.

When the cow is mature and in production, the elastin is prominent in this supportive structure, allowing absorption of the shock created when the cow walks and moves while lying down. Two excellent views of the median suspensory ligament are provided in Figures 1.5 and 1.6. All other supportive structures surrounding the parenchyma have been dissected away.

Other supportive structures, composed of extracellular components making up connective tissues that support the udder, are the lateral suspensory ligaments and lamellar plates that extend from them to intersperse the parenchyma. These structures contain more collagen than elastin and, thus, provide support in the absence of much elasticity. Figures 1.7 and 1.8 show

Fig. 1.5. Side view of the median suspensory ligament (*a*) that supports the cow's udder and its contents. (From Swett et al. 1942)

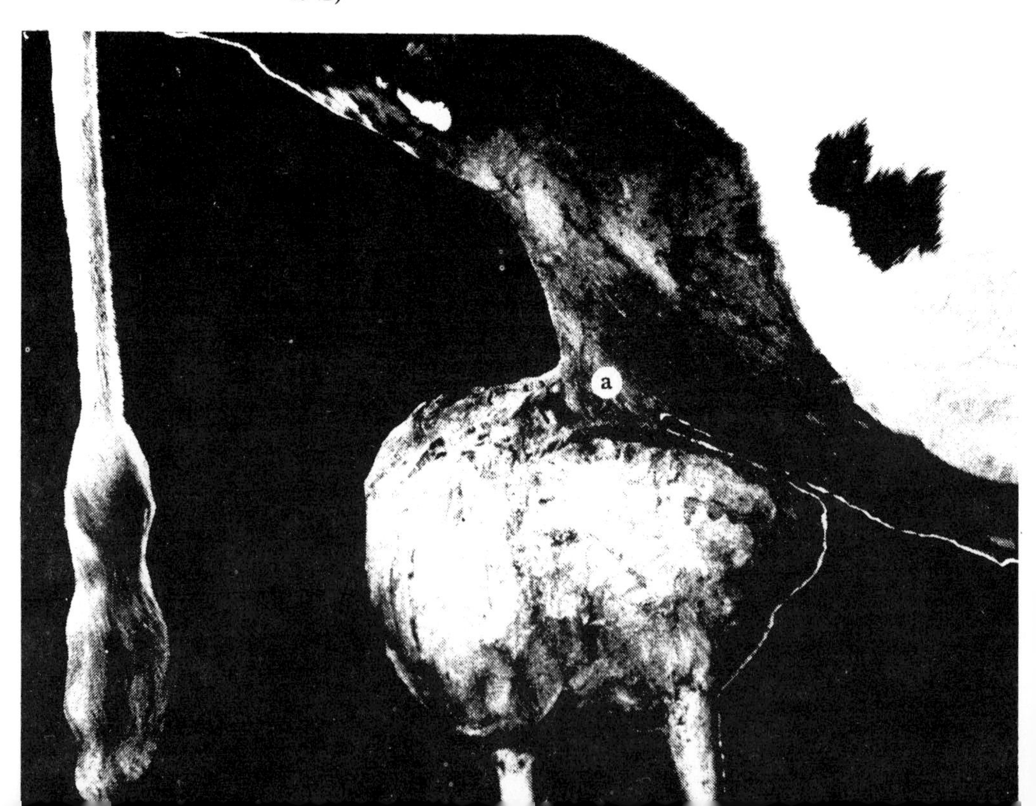

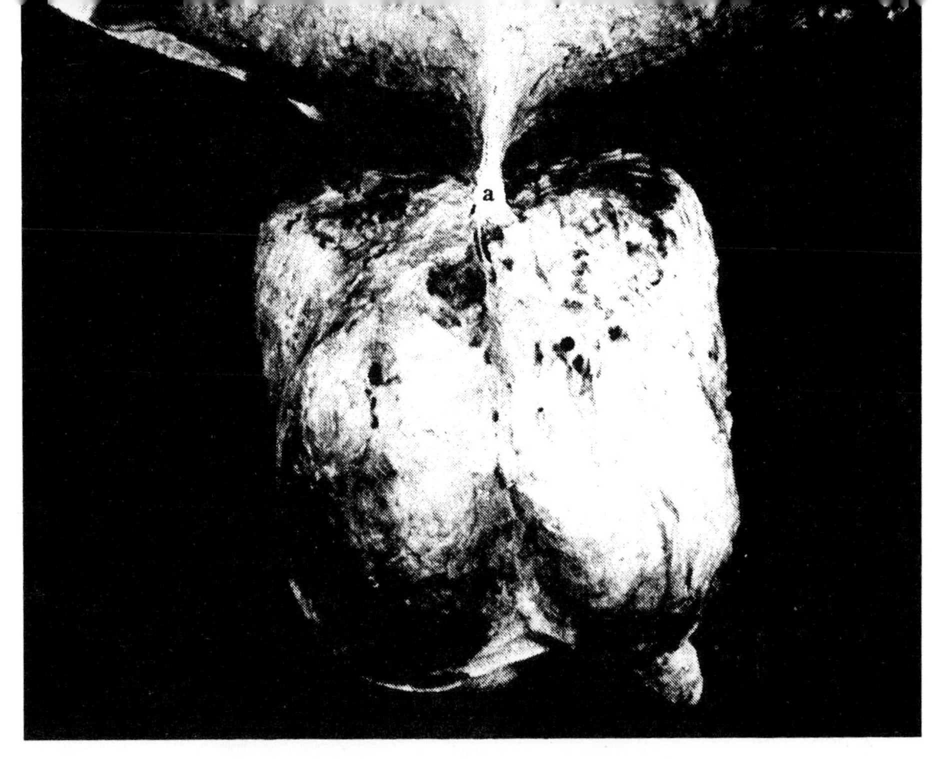

Fig. 1.6. Rear view of the median suspensory ligament (*a*) that provides the major support for the cow's udder. (From Swett et al. 1942)

Fig. 1.7. Lateral suspensory ligaments (*a*) of a cow's udder. (From Swett et al. 1942)

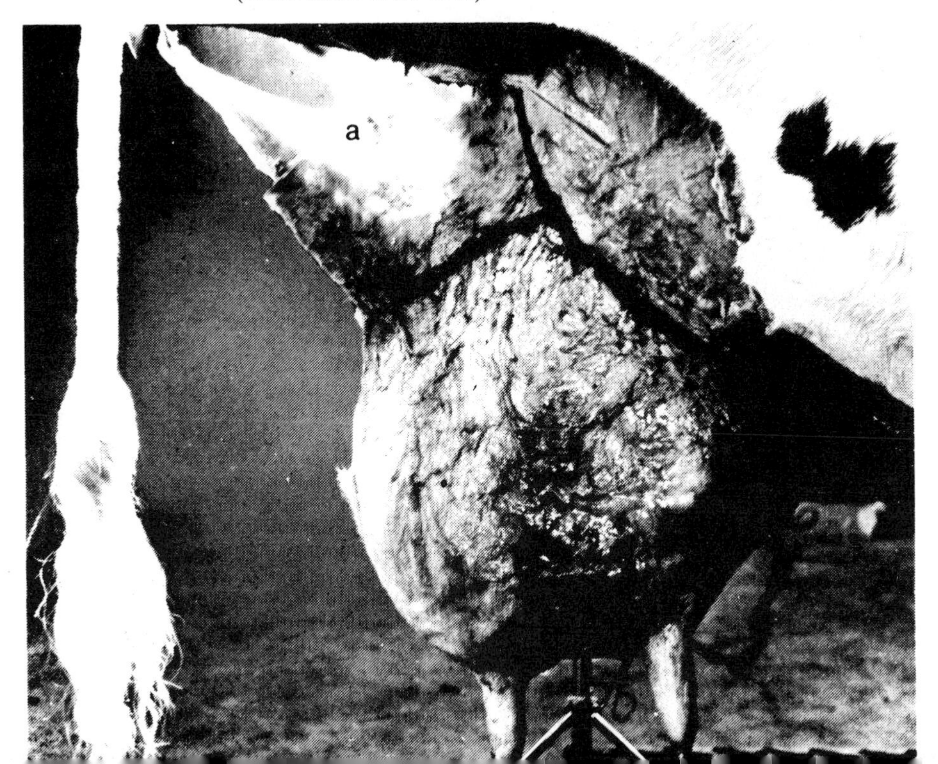

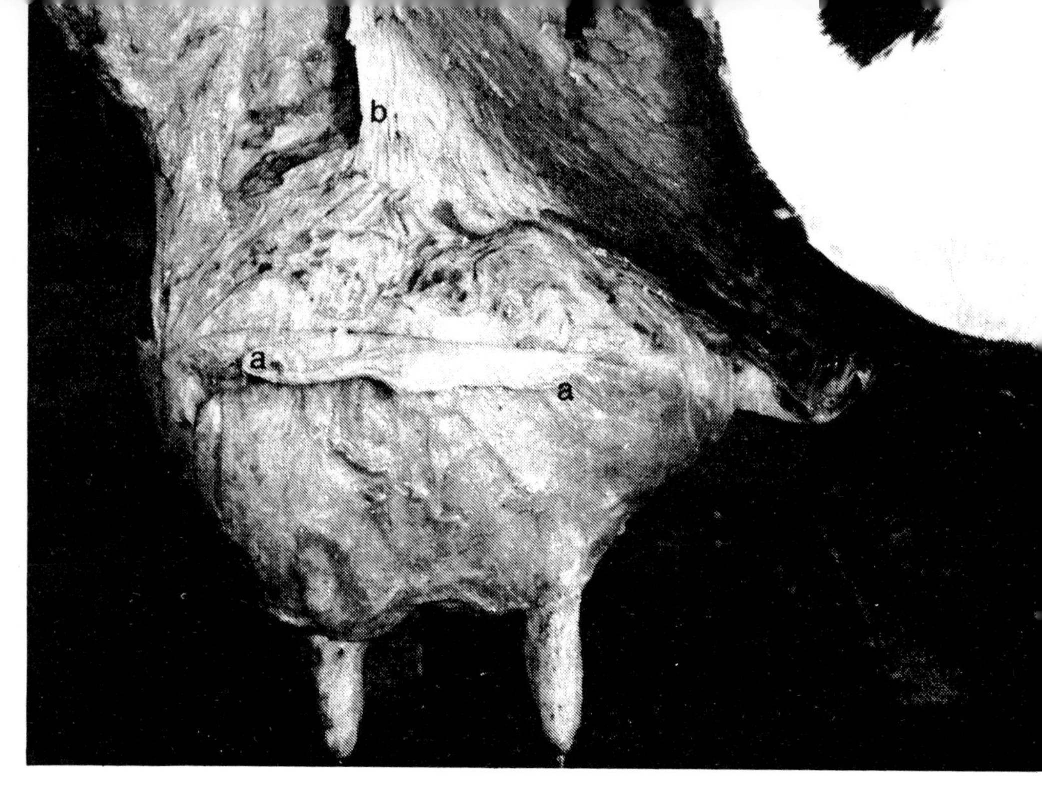

Fig. 1.8. Lateral suspensory ligaments (*a*) of a cow's udder, peeled away to expose the median suspensory ligament (*b*). (From Swett et al. 1942)

the lateral suspensory ligaments of the udder after the skin has been dissected away.

Skin provides the udder with protection (Fig. 1.9) but little support. Any break in the skin of the udder or teats results in mammary infection, which is difficult to control.

Most eutherian mammals in the northern hemisphere adapt their reproductive activities to survival of the offspring. Fetal life of eutherians continues until the offspring are mature enough to survive the environment characteristic of the species. The newborn are exposed to temperatures that will allow survival, such as those in spring and summer; few have their offspring in the middle of winter. Some mammals, such as rabbits, mice, and rats, are born very immature and helpless. Others, such as cattle, sheep, and goats, are mature enough to accompany the mother on her journeys within hours after birth. In rabbits, mice, and rats, the mammary gland has developed little beyond the teat, teat cistern, gland cistern, and primary milk ducts; branching of ducts has not occurred. In ungulates (hooved animals), the development has progressed only slightly more. The fatty pad is prominent and a few secondary ducts may have branched from the primary ducts. In the case of those that have an udder (all ungulates are considered to be in this category), the structure of the udder is evident, including the teats, fatty pads, and halves separated by the median suspensory ligament. Differentiation of mammary development in cattle during fetal life is shown in Figure 1.10.

1.3-3: Progression of mammary growth after birth

1.3-3a: Birth to puberty. Growth of the mammary apparatus from birth to puberty is not exceptional. The rate of growth is the same as the rest of the body and, therefore, is referred to as an isometric growth rate. The mammary gland may be considered a skin gland that responds to female sex hormones, which are in extremely low levels in the female during the years of rapid skeletal growth from birth to puberty. The length of this part of the mammal's life varies greatly from species to species. For example, it is only 25–30 days in guinea pigs, 40 days in rats, 6–8 mo in dairy cattle, and 10–12 yr in humans.

1.3-3b: Puberty. Sexual activity is preceded by several hormonal changes in the body. The female releases follicle-stimulating hormone (FSH) and luteinizing hormone (LH), in a cyclic pattern, from the anterior pituitary gland. These hormones stimulate the ovaries to synthesize and release female sex steroid hormones, estrogens and progestins. The primary estrogen is estradiol; the predominant progestin is progesterone. The part

Fig. 1.9. A suspended udder of a cow showing the skin covering of the udder and four teats.

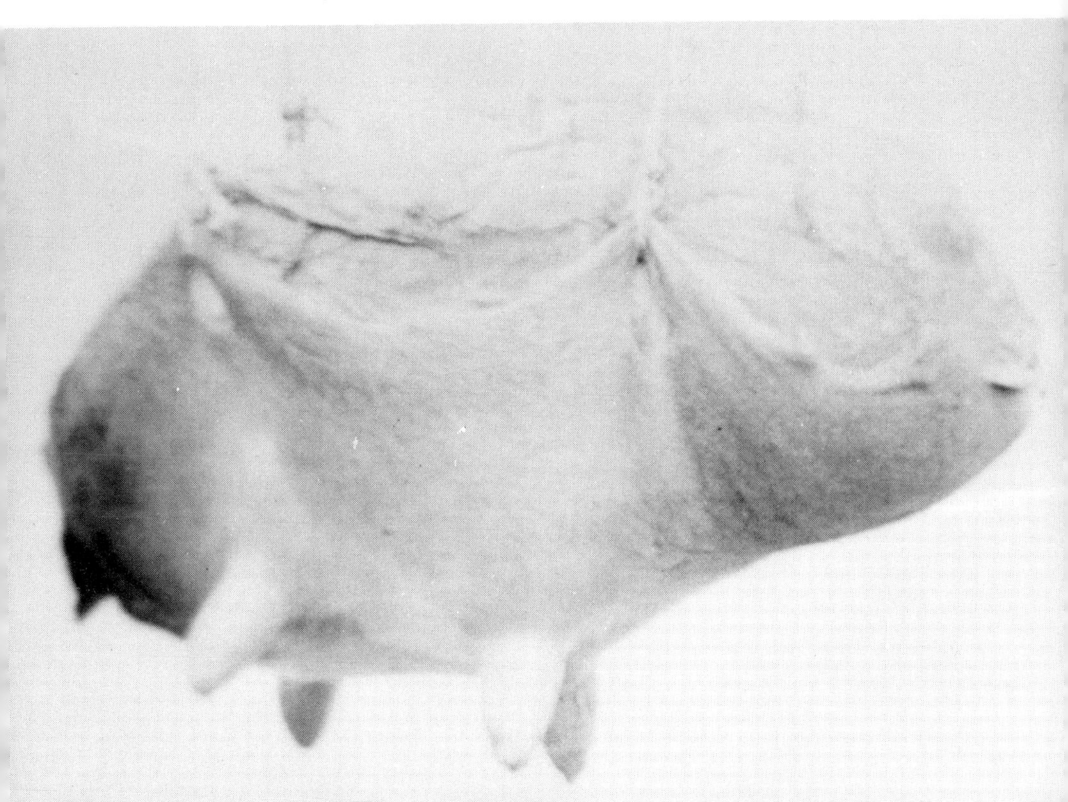

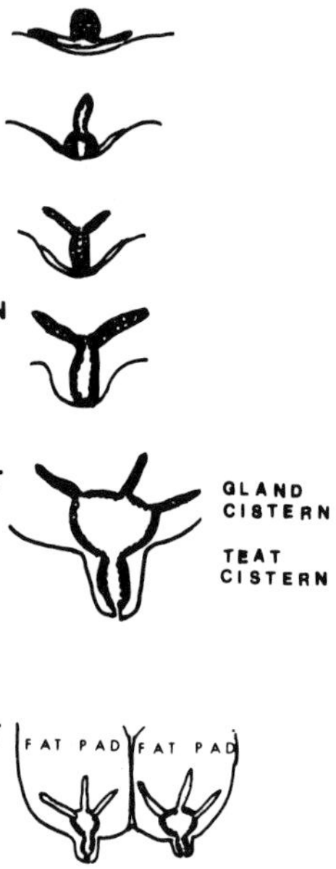

STAGE		TIME OF DEVELOPMENT, DAY OF GESTATION	CROWN-RUMP LENGTH OF FETUS, MM
EARLY TEAT FORMATION		65	80
PRIMARY SPROUT		80	120
SECONDARY SPROUTS		90	160
CANALIZATION OF PRIMARY SPROUT		100	190
DEVELOPMENT OF GLAND AND TEAT CISTERNS	GLAND CISTERN	110	230
	TEAT CISTERN	130	300
DEVELOPMENT OF MEDIAN SUSPENSORY LIGAMENT	FAT PAD FAT PAD	180	480

Fig. 1.10. Mammary development during fetal life in cattle.

of the ovarian cycle characterized by follicular growth is dominated by estrogen, while the part characterized as the luteal phase of the cycle, when the corpus luteum develops, is dominated by progesterone. With each cycle, a surge of estrogen stimulates mammary gland proliferation. The growth is mainly that of the ducts lengthening and branching. Estrogen, by itself, does not stimulate duct growth very well. This action occurs in synergism with the anterior pituitary (adenohypophysial) hormones, prolactin and somatotropin (growth hormone). Some branching, lengthening, and thickening of ducts occurs in response to estrogen.

Mammals that demonstrate short cycles are mice, rats, and hamsters. The phase of the cycle that is functional in these animals experiencing 4- to 6-day cycles is the follicular phase. The luteal phase does not occur in the absence of coitus or other stimuli to cause release of prolactin, which is luteotropic in these species. With each recurring estrous cycle, the mammary gland is stimulated by estrogen from the ovary in synergism with prolactin and somatotropin from the pituitary gland. The result is a lengthening and branching of ducts with no sign of end buds or alveoli until the animal becomes pregnant or pseudopregnant.

In contrast to short-cycling species, those with long cycles (cattle, goats, sheep, hogs, horses, and humans) demonstrate functional corpora lutea, which secrete progesterone during the luteal phase of the cycle. Length of the follicular phase of the cycle is approximately 5 days in estrous-cycling species, while in species having a menstrual cycle, the follicular phase is much longer (14 days in humans). The luteal phase of the estrous cycle in cattle is 21 − 5, or 16 days; in the hog, it is similar; in sheep, it is 13 days; and in goats, 15 days. Horses are thought to have 21-day cycles and, thus, the luteal phase is 16 days in the mare. During this part of the cycle, progesterone is available to synergize with estrogen, prolactin, and somatotropin. During the first several cycles of the female's life, growth takes the form of duct lengthening, thickening, and branching. Eventually a differentiation into lobule alveoli takes place (Fig. 1.11).

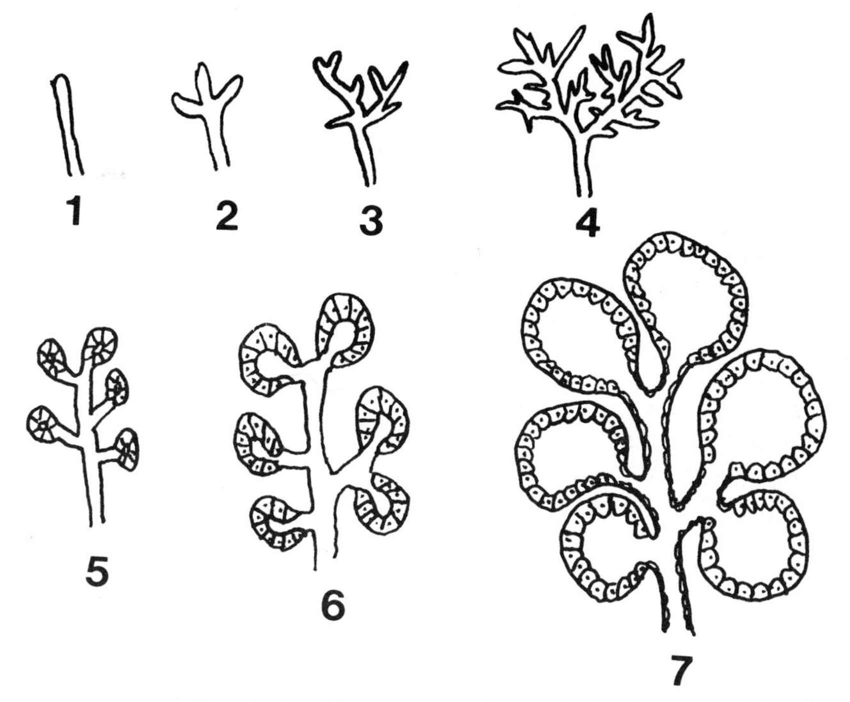

Fig. 1.11. Mammary gland growth is characterized by duct growth from a single duct (*1*), to branching (*2*), to more complex branching (*3*), to compound branching (*4*). End buds form on ends of ducts (*5*) and continue to enlarge in response to hormonal stimuli (stages *6* and *7*).

Heifers of dairy breeds frequently begin to show outward expressions of estrous cyclicity at 6 mo. If they have been on a reasonably good plane of nutrition, the skeletal frame is large enough to conceive at 15 mo, and at 24 mo they have their first calf. Frequently, the beef breeds show delayed puberty until over 1 yr of age. Research concerning the development of mammary glands in heifers is not extensive, but it may be inferred from data accumulated that heifers have a system of ducts in the mammary gland from birth to 18 mo. The ducts then begin to differentiate into alveoli at the endings. The lobule alveoli continue to increase in number and volume with each recurring estrous cycle. A peak is thought to be reached at 30–36 mo in the maximum amount of lobule-alveolar growth sustainable by estrous cycles alone.

1.3-3c: Pregnancy. The major portion of mammary gland growth occurs during pregnancy and is controlled primarily by hormones; pregnancy is the condition that fosters the maximal hormonal combinations for such development. This design is very logical because mammary gland growth should correspond to fetal growth, which would allow the newborn to have sufficient nourishment from its mother's milk to survive in the harsh environment outside the relatively ideal environs of the uterus.

Shortly after the ovum is fertilized, it signals the uterus, ovaries, and pituitary that it is viable and growing. Changes in hormonal levels are necessary for its survival; the ovary must secrete more estrogen and progesterone than it would normally, and the pituitary must secrete more prolactin and somatotropin than it would normally. These hormones not only enhance changes in the uterus that are conducive to survival of the implanting zygote, but they are hormones that stimulate the mammary gland to grow and differentiate in preparation for future milk production.

Growth of the mammary gland is slow at the beginning of pregnancy, but the rate of growth accelerates as the pregnancy advances. This rate is exponential and may be expressed as a mathematical equation for each species. In the mammary gland of the nonpregnant animal, a fairly prominent fatty pad exists. The adipose cells of this pad are slowly eroded away and gradually replaced with ducts, lobule alveoli, blood vessels, lymph vessels, and connective tissue structures of collagen and elastin. Extension of the ducts and alveoli into all areas of the fatty pad requires long periods of time in some species; it is generally synchronized with the length of gestation for that particular species. For example, the cow has a gestation length of approximately 280 days. Figure 1.12 shows a sagittal section of an udder of a cow 8 mo pregnant. Hematoxylin stain reveals the extent of lobule-alveolar growth into the fatty pad. Mammary growth, in terms of ductal and lobule-alveolar proliferation, continues for the entire 9 mo, and there may be cellular division of secretory cells in the early part of lactation.

Research using the infusion of dye via the teat canal (streak canal, galactophore, portal) shows the quarters of the mammary gland are completely separated from each other by a connective tissue septum (Fig. 1.13). Although an anastomosis of blood from quarter to quarter and half to half exists, this is not the case with secretory cells of the lobule-alveolar structures.

Hormones unique to the pregnant female include pregnant mare serum gonadotropin (PMSG) and human chorionic gonadotropin (HCG). In the case of PMSG, the hormone is secreted into the blood from the placenta and acts in a follicle-stimulating capacity. New follicles are transformed into new corpora lutea, which produce estrogen and progesterone. The additional amounts of sex hormones are needed for growth and maintenance of the uterus and the mammary glands. The PMSG disappears after 150 days of a 335-day gestation. It is not needed during the last one-half of pregnancy in the mare because the placenta matures and differentiates sufficiently, producing the estrogen and progesterone needed to maintain the conceptus and stimulate udder growth.

HCG appears in the blood and urine of the pregnant human approximately 16 days after ovulation. It acts as a luteotropin, that is, it maintains the corpus luteum of the ovary and stimulates it to a higher level of steroid

Fig. 1.12. A sagittal section of the udder of a cow 8 mo pregnant. Lobule alveoli have penetrated deep into the mammary fatty pad. (From Hammond 1927)

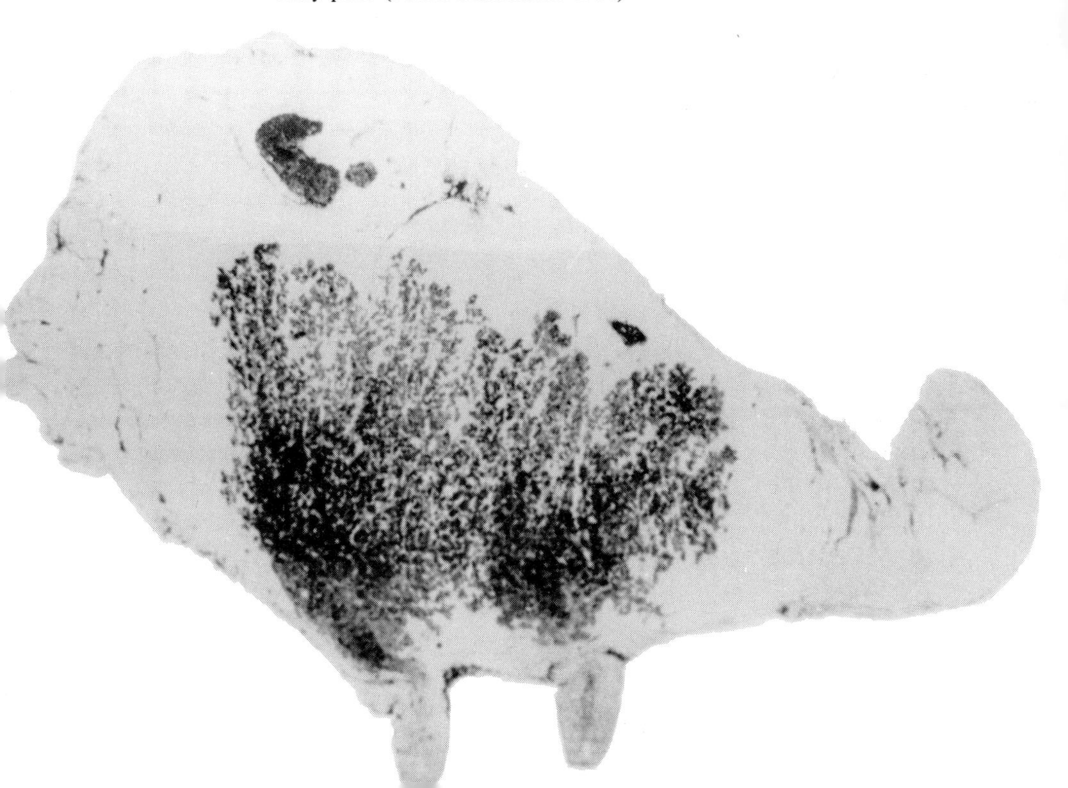

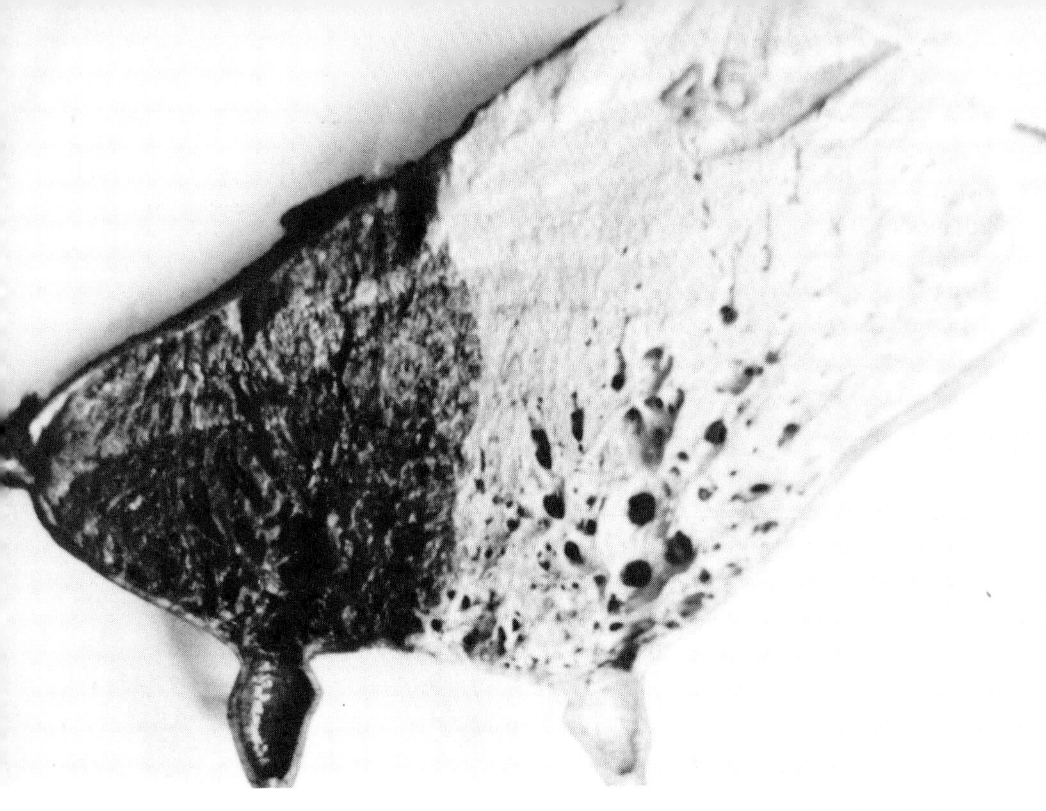

Fig. 1.13. Longitudinal section of a cow's udder in which a dark-colored dye was infused via the teat canal into the fore quarter. The structure dividing front and rear quarters is the connective tissue septum.

hormone production than it would have otherwise. The HCG disappears from the blood and urine at approximately 160 days of gestation, after which time the placenta produces the estrogen and progesterone required for uterine maintenance and mammary growth (from 160 days to term, about 270 days in humans).

A third hormone of pregnancy is placental lactogen. This hormone has properties and a chemical makeup similar to prolactin and somatotropin. It is a protein hormone of 25,000–35,000 daltons. It differs chemically from PMSG and HCG in that they are glycoproteins, while placental lactogen is a protein without a carbohydrate component. Placental lactogen synergizes with estrogens and progesterone to grow the mammary gland and, perhaps, the uterus, placenta, and fetus; its origin is the fetal placenta. A fourth hormone, which is in much higher titer in the blood during pregnancy than any other time in the life of the female, is relaxin. This hormone is known to have an action upon connective tissues of the pelvis and the pubic symphysis, allowing these to soften and stretch, causing the birth canal to enlarge. Similarly, the cervix is softened to accommodate the passage of the fetus through the birth canal. We believe that relaxin rearranges connective tissue elements of the mammary gland in a way similar to its action on connective tissue of the cervix and pubic symphysis. It is probably in low titers in the nonpregnant animal, although not well documented, in addition to being present in high titers during pregnancy. Relaxin is thought to have a role in stimulating synthesis of collagen IV, a prominent protein of the basement membrane. This structure is a necessary prerequisite to multiplication of epithelial cells at the ends of milk ducts. Thus, relaxin is another hormone making up the complex of hormones required for optimal mammogenesis.

1.3-3d: Early lactation. Mammary gland growth in lactation has been measured using indices such as mammary wet weight, DFFT, and DNA, which in many species continue to increase into early lactation. In the rat and mouse, the maximum is reached at or near day 10 of lactation. In the rabbit, it is day 15, while in the guinea pig and the goat, it is approximately day 5. Relatively little postparturient mammary gland growth was found in studies of mammary glands from hamsters and sheep.

Growth of the mammary gland has been shown to be exponential in cattle, goats, and guinea pigs (Fig. 1.14); cell numbers increase at an increasing rate. Since this continues at least to parturition, the process cannot be halted abruptly. The result is a continuation of mammary epithelial cell division into early lactation. Increases in mammary DNA, from parturition to days 2–5 of lactation, are particularly dramatic in rats, guinea pigs, and rabbits. If suckling by the young is not permitted in these species, the great increases in DNA during the few days after parturition will not occur. This

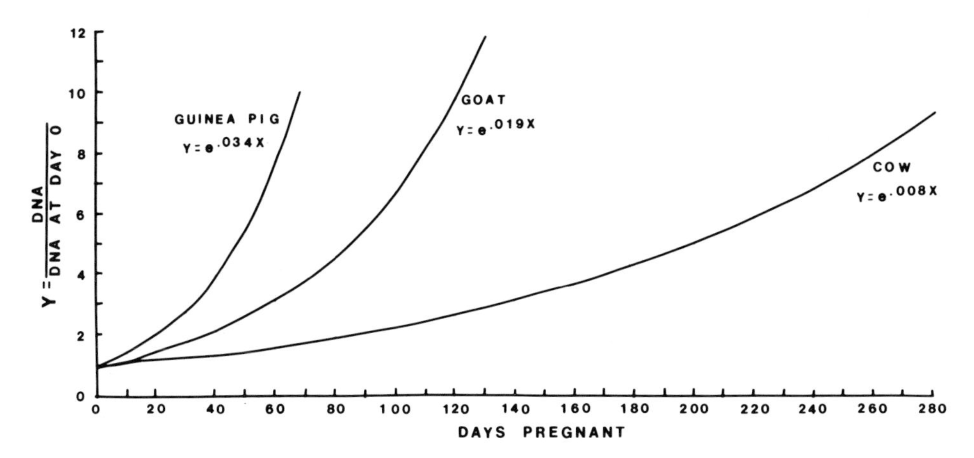

Fig. 1.14. Mammary DNA increases at an exponential rate during pregnancy. The rate of growth is inversely proportional to the length of gestation.

suggests that the phenomena of suckling and milk removal are important signals, which cause a widespread mammary gland mitosis during the first few days of lactation in these species.

1.3-3e: Declining lactation. To a certain degree, the amount of milk produced by a mammary gland is dependent on the number of cells in the gland secreting milk. Other very important factors are precursors from the blood to supply the building blocks for milk synthesis, hormones to stimulate the secretory cells that allow the optimal use of precursors, and frequent milk removal to assure the most efficient use of precursors and hormones. If the secretory cells are important controllers of the quantity of milk, why do they disappear or involute or regress? Nature operates so that a calf has its mother's milk for about 6 mo, if it is to have a good chance to survive and grow into a strong adult. Optimal milk production in the cow is reached at approximately 45 days, at which point the calf is beginning to supplement its diet with green grass, hay, and grain. For the remaining 4½ mo, the milk provides essential amino acids to ensure the best possible assimilation and utilization of all food consumed. To be in condition for the next pregnancy, the mother must stop lactating before the end of the year.

Humans have imposed upon the dairy cow a demand to continue high milk production for 10 mo, rather than 6 mo. The animals that fulfill these needs best are those that have high peak milk production and good persistency. In order to be persistent, the cows have mammary gland epithelial cells, which either do not disappear very rapidly or are replaced by cell division and replacement. The factors involved in high persistency are controlled by genetic mechanisms because this trait is highly heritable. However, the physiological mechanisms by which the genes operate are not understood. Recent research suggests that milk production decreases before cell numbers decrease, possibly indicating persistency of milk production is controlled by factors other than cell numbers.

1.3-3f: Dry period. Involution of mammary secretory cells accelerates when milk removal is stopped, building intramammary pressure to the extent that continual milk synthesis cannot occur. The precursors are prevented from moving into the secretory cells because pressure is greater from the lumen of the alveolus than it is from blood pressure. The alveoli farthest from the gland cistern break apart first, and the involution progresses from those extremes to the ones closer to the gland cistern. The space previously occupied by the degenerating alveoli is replaced with adipose cells in a fatty-pad configuration. The extent to which alveoli degenerate varies with species and is governed by the ability of the estrous cycle hormones to maintain lobule-alveolar structures. Since the rat has short 5-day cycles without a luteal phase, the entire lobule-alveolar system disappears after a normal pregnancy and lactation. Species experiencing long cycles with a functional luteal phase are able to retain some of the alveolar structure.

1.3-3g: Recurring pregnancies and lactation. Dairy cows are subjected to somewhat severe reproductive stress because they are expected to be pregnant and lactating during 7 mo of the year. Conception should be approximately 85 days into lactation in order to maintain a 12-mo calving interval. They should lactate 10 mo and be dry 2 mo. Few other mammals are required to do this. Some (the mare and the wild cottontail rabbit) may be pregnant and lactating at the same time. The mare does not have an exceedingly heavy lactation stress because she provides milk for only one offspring. The dairy cow, on the other hand, provides enough milk for ten calves when it is lactating and pregnant simultaneously. The cottontail rabbit rivals the dairy cow by becoming pregnant immediately after parturition and being pregnant and lactating for approximately 18 days. It then weans its young for a much needed dry period of 8–10 days before it goes through parturition again. This is repeated four to six times in a season; cottontails rarely survive long enough to repeat this beyond two seasons. Dairy cattle survive long enough to repeat this 4 times on the average, but some outstanding individuals have repeated the reproductive cycle 20 times, or seasons.

1.3-3h: Aging. Considering the reproductive pattern of cattle, their life expectancy is not surprising. They usually have the first calf when they are 2 yr old. Many cows survive 6–10 yr, but some survive and reproduce for 20 yr, or more. Dairy bulls have survived as studs until they were 17 yr old. Generally speaking, the life expectancy in mammals suggests that the female survives approximately 10% longer than the male; this is true in humans and appears to be true in most other mammals, such as mice, rats, gerbils, guinea pigs, dogs, and cats. Milk production records of dairy cows show that the peak is reached in the fifth lactation, when the animal is 7 or 8 yr old; the cow also reaches maximum skeletal size at this time. Milk production maintains a plateau for several years and then begins to decline beyond 12 yr of age. Mammary glands increase in size during the first to the fifth lactations. Since milk production depends on mammary size and hormonal stimuli, it is believed that the milk production pattern in recurring lactations is a reflection of the two phenomena. Just as a man loses his ability to function well as a baseball or football player beyond 40 yr of age, the cow slows in hormonal secretions to synthesize milk when she reaches and exceeds 12 yr (Fig. 1.15).

Recurring pregnancies and lactations result in increases of approximately 30% in milk production from the first to the fifth lactation. It is about 13% from the first to the second, 9% from second to third, 5% from third to fourth, and 3% from fourth to fifth. Part of the increase is due to maturation of the skeleton and an increase in body weight, which can

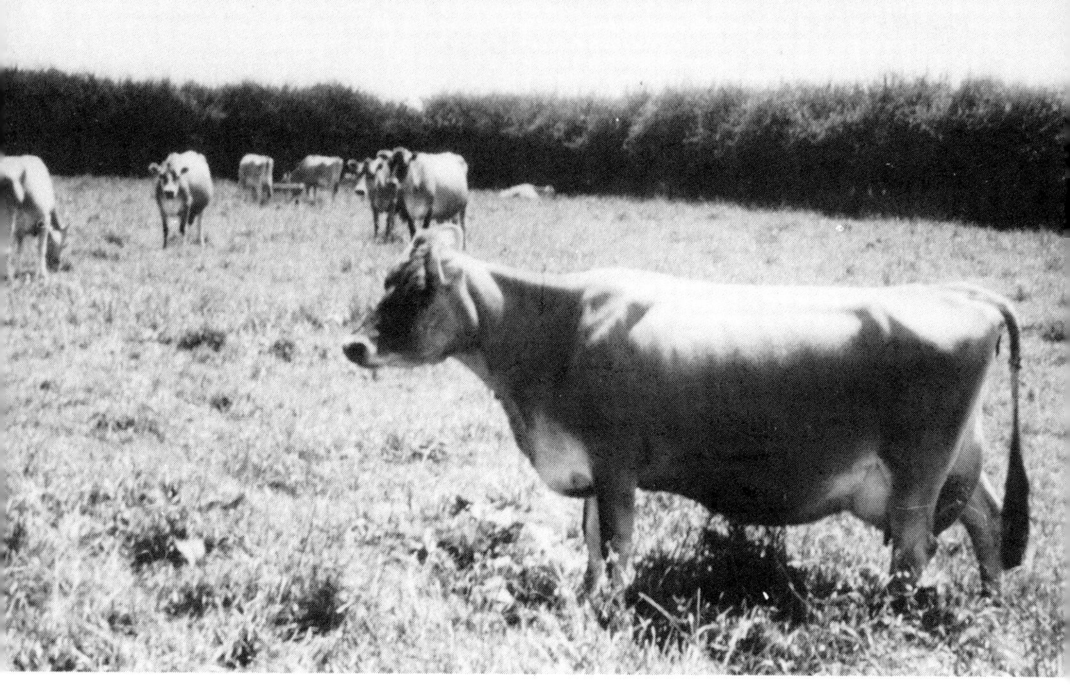

Fig. 1.15. This 14-yr-old Jersey cow in New Zealand exemplifies the advantage that longevity affords the dairy enterprise.

accommodate a larger udder; the other part is due to the effects of recurring pregnancies and lactations. Older studies in cows, based upon milk production data, suggested that 20% of the increase was due to increased body weight and 80% to the effects of recurring pregnancies and lactations. More recent data on DNA in mammary glands of guinea pigs suggest that 60% is due to increased body weight and 40% to the effects of pregnancy and lactation. A graphic presentation of increased mammary gland capacity, in terms of total size as well as increased numbers of secretory cells, is presented in Figure 1.16.

1.4: BLOOD SUPPLY TO AND FROM THE MAMMARY GLAND

1.4-1: Introduction. Mammary glands occupy various positions along the ventral side of the body and are almost always in pairs. Positions range from cervical, or neck, to thoracic, to abdominal, to inguinal. In rare cases, they are so far laterally as to be on the sides of the animal, such as in nutria and vizcachas. Even more rare is the crural position (on the inside of the thighs), as exemplified by the Cuban solenodon. In all cases, a rich blood supply must lead to the mammary glands, and at least one route must return venous blood to the heart.

1.4-2: Cow

1.4-2a: Arterial route to the udder. The cow has four inguinal mammary glands. These are furnished with arterial blood by vessels that pass through the paired inguinal rings, openings in the posterioventral area of the muscular layers, which protect the viscera.

A convenient approach to understanding the circulation of blood to a body tissue is to begin at the heart and trace the route from that point. The heart has four chambers consisting of the right atrium, or auricle, the right ventricle, the left atrium, and the left ventricle. Venous blood enters the right atrium via two large vessels; the anterior vena cava, carrying blood from the area of the head, and the posterior vena cava, carrying blood from the rear half of the body. From the right atrium, blood passes through the tricuspid valve to the right ventricle. This chamber contracts when the heart beats, pushing the blood through the pulmonary valve to the pulmonary artery. The blood courses through capillary beds in the lung, where carbon dioxide is eliminated into the air and oxygen is taken into the blood by the hemoglobin. The blood returns to the heart via the pulmonary vein. It is worth noting that the pulmonary vein is the only vein in the body that carries oxygenated blood. Blood enters the left atrium from the pulmonary vein, passes thorough the mitral valve, and enters the left ventricle, the highly muscularized part of the heart. With each heart beat,

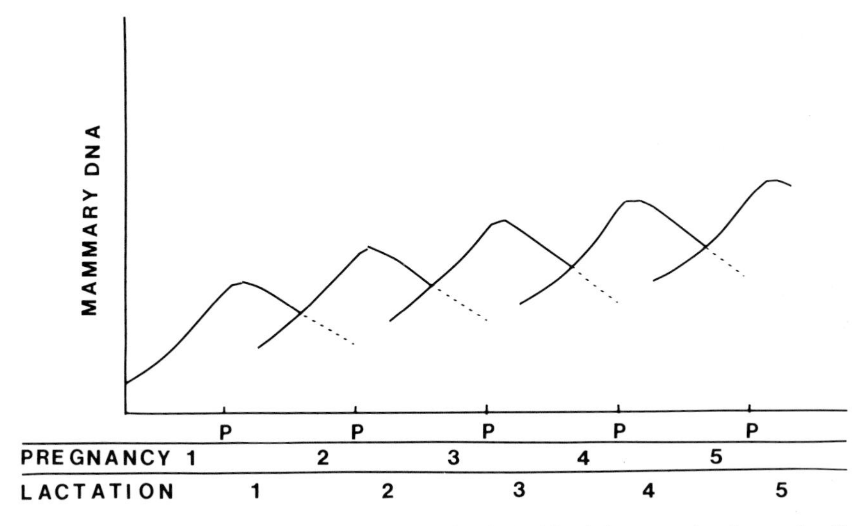

Fig. 1.16. Mammary glands (udders) increase in size and cell numbers (as indicated by increase in DNA) in each succeeding lactation for the first 5 lactations. New cells added during pregnancy do not synthesize milk until the succeeding lactation. *P* designates parturition.

blood is carried through the aortic valve to the aorta, which has considerable elasticity in its wall to accommodate the sudden changes in blood pressure as the heart beats. It divides into two branches shortly after leaving the heart, one coursing anteriorly and one posteriorly. The former is called the anterior dorsal aorta, and the latter is the posterior dorsal aorta. The posterior dorsal aorta passes through the diaphragm high on the dorsal side of the body near the vertebrae and spinal cord and becomes known as the abdominal posterior dorsal aorta. It then bifurcates to become the left common iliac artery and the right common iliac artery. After a short distance, a second bifurcation occurs; the two arteries on each side are known as the external iliac and internal iliac arteries. The internal iliac artery carries blood to the dorsoposterior areas of the body. The external iliac artery carries blood to the ventroposterior areas and gives rise to the femoral artery, which enters the hind leg. Shortly after it courses toward the leg, it has a branch known as the prepubic artery, the name referring to its close proximity to the anterior part of the pubic bone, a part of the pelvic girdle. The prepubic artery passes through the inguinal ring. As it exits this ring, it becomes known as the external pudic (external pudendal) artery. After a short distance in the upper part of the udder, it is known as the mammary artery. Soon after penetrating the mammary gland, it branches; the forward-coursing branch is called the cranial mammary artery, and the branch directed to the rear of the udder is known as the caudal mammary artery. Numerous branches from these vessels provide blood to all parts of the udder. The arteries in the teat are extensions of these and are known as the papillary arteries (Fig. 1.17). Arteries branch into smaller arterioles, which branch into metarterioles, the smallest blood vessels having three layers: an endothelial layer, a smooth muscle layer, and an outer connective tissue layer. Beyond these are the capillaries, which are composed of a single layer of endothelial cells. When blood is shunted from one type of tissue or organ to the other, such as when the animal is frightened, the smooth muscles of the arterioles in the mammary gland contract, shunting blood to other areas where the smooth muscles of the arterioles have dilated.

1.4-2b: Venous routes away from the udder. Only one route of paired blood vessels carries arterial blood to the udder of the cow. Two routes of venous blood carry the carbon dioxide and other products of metabolism back to the heart. Starting in the teat, many papillary veins course upward and join, making several large mammary veins that enter the venous circle, large veins resting above the parenchyma of the udder. Anterior extensions of these veins, the subcutaneous abdominal veins, are very prominent and turgid in lactating cows and have been called milk veins. Not visible are the paired external pudic veins, which arise from the venous circle approximately two-thirds the length of the udder from the

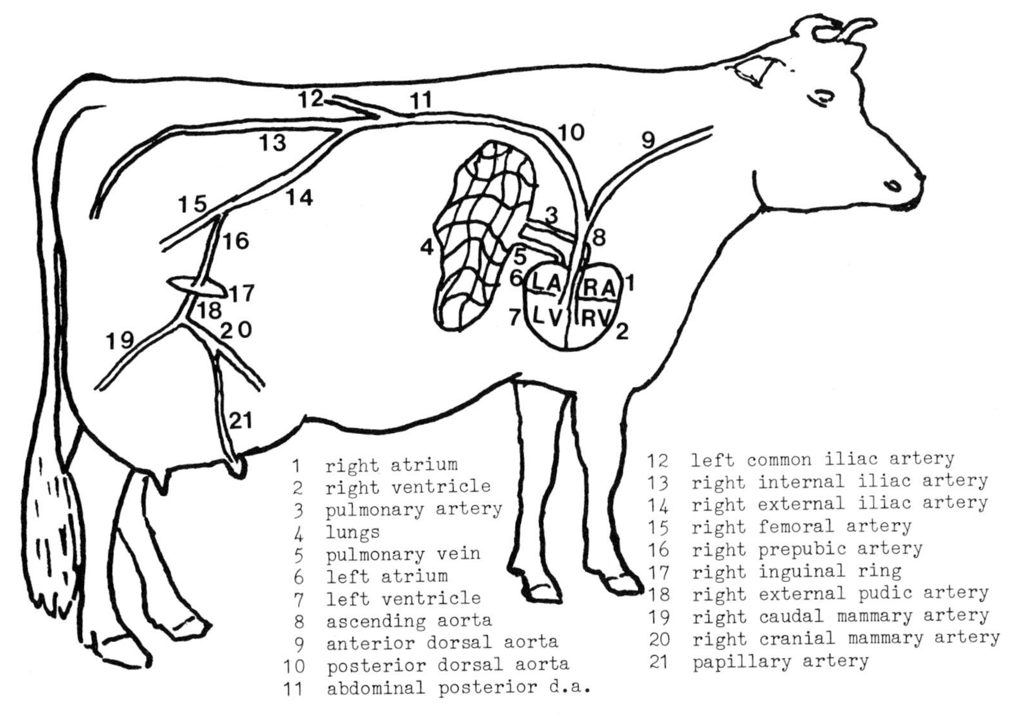

Fig. 1.17. Arterial blood system of the cow from the right atrium to the papillary artery.

most anterior point; these veins also are much larger in the lactating cow. Valves in the large veins direct blood from mammary veins to either the external pudic or subcutaneous abdominal veins. Experiments have demonstrated that two-thirds of the blood travels via the external pudic veins and one-third via the subcutaneous abdominal veins (Fig. 1.18).

External pudic veins (pudendal veins) pass through the inguinal rings. The nomenclature of veins returning to the heart is the same as the arteries, which they parallel. The external pudic veins become the prepubic veins; these lead into the femoral veins, which in turn become the external iliac veins, which become the common iliac veins beyond the juncture of the external and internal iliac veins. The common iliac veins join in the abdomen where the posterior dorsal aorta or abdominal aorta divides, forming two common iliac arteries. The vein running parallel with the artery is called the posterior vena cava, which terminates in the right atrium of the heart.

Subcutaneous abdominal veins (milk veins) abruptly reach a point where they seem to stop just behind the ribs. The enlarged vein at this juncture is known as the milk well. The vein penetrates the muscular ab-

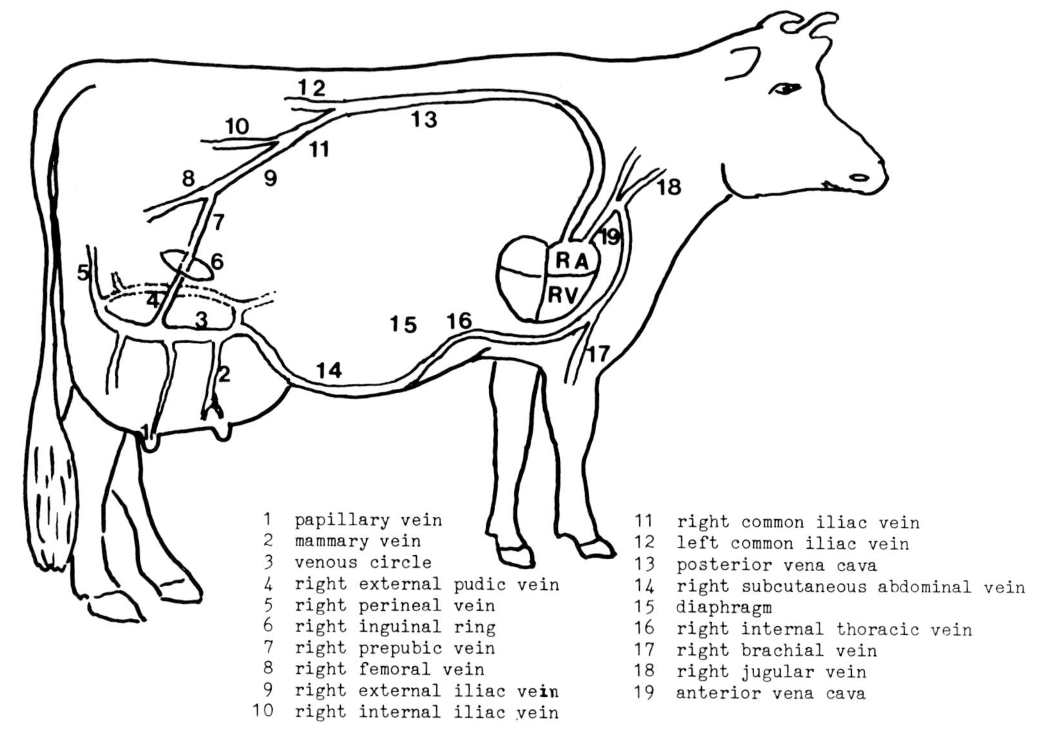

Fig. 1.18. Routes of venous blood from the udder of the cow to the heart.

dominal wall to become the internal abdominal vein, which turns forward and penetrates the diaphragm. On the other side of the diaphragm, it is known as the internal thoracic vein, until it joins with the brachial vein running upward from the foreleg. Moving down from the head and neck, the brachial vein unites with the jugular vein; the two veins fuse into the anterior vena cava, which terminates in the right atrium. The anterior and posterior vena cavae do not unite but enter the heart separately.

1.4-2c: Importance of blood to the udder. Although the scope of this chapter is not to discuss in detail the physiology of blood and the circulatory system, its importance cannot be overemphasized. The blood carries building blocks of metabolism to the udder and carries away the waste products of metabolism.

Blood pressure is maintained by heart beats, which number 60–80/min in the cow. Each beat accommodates a given volume of blood, known as the stroke volume. This amounts to approximately 0.7 l in a cow weighing 500 kg (multiplication of stroke volume times heart rate produces the minute volume); this may be extended to hourly or daily volume. Daily volume is approximately 71,000 l in the 500-kg cow. The ratio of blood required for each unit of milk produced has been estimated to be about 400:1. A cow producing 35 l milk/day would require 14,000 l blood to pass through the udder, or nearly 20% of the entire output by the heart.

Another important consideration is blood pressure; it may be 140 mm Hg in the aorta, but it drops to 25 mm in the capillaries of the udder. This pressure is the main driving force transferring nutrients from the blood to the milk-secreting epithelial cells of the alveolus. It also drives the blood through the venous system back to the heart. Practical considerations include problems of udder edema and the buildup of intramammary pressure. Myoepithelial cells contract to eliminate milk from the udder; they can raise the intramammary pressure to 60 mm Hg, or higher. As long as this pressure is maintained above 25 mm, milk synthesis is effectively stopped. This is why the system has been designed to allow intramammary pressure to remain high for no longer than 10 min during the time of milk harvest. Delays in removing milk from the udder for intervals in excess of 14 hr also would result in a slowing of milk synthetic rates and a drop in milk production.

1.5: LYMPHATIC SYSTEM

1.5-1: Introduction. The lymphatic system is designed to move fluids that bathe cells. These fluids collectively are called interstitial fluid, or extracellular fluid, excluding the vascular and cerebrospinal fluids. In order to assure their circulation, the body has a system of unique vessels (lymphatic system) to carry this material to the vascular system. In the mammary gland, a number of small lymphatic vessels begin as open tubes in widely scattered areas of the gland. These angle dorsally and posteriorly, terminating in the supramammary lymph nodes. There are two of these nodes located above the parenchyma approximately one-fifth of the length of the udder from the posterior end. Each node is slightly smaller than a fist. Interstitial fluid in the udder is moved into the lymph vessels and eventually passes through the supramammary lymph nodes.

1.5-2: Lymph transport to the blood. Lymph flows in one direction. To prevent backflow, the lymphatic vessels are equipped with one-way valves very similar to those in veins. Movement of the lymph in the vessels is slow because there is no pump, such as the heart, in the enclosed vascular system. Therefore, other forces are relied upon to move lymph. Among these forces are muscle movement, or exercise, breathing, the heart beating, and massaging. If the udder becomes edematous after parturition, massaging the udder in a direction toward the supramammary lymph node enhances the movement of lymph and reduces the swelling.

Once lymph passes beyond the supramammary lymph node, it travels via a vessel through the inguinal ring to the deep inguinal lymph node, external iliac lymph node, or prefemoral lymph node. These paired nodes then connect to more dorsally located internal iliac lymph nodes, which then connect to a single lumbar lymph trunk. This trunk and the intestinal lymph trunk, from the lacteals surrounding the intestines, join to create a cisterna chyli, an enlargement in the trunk. The forward extension of this, the thoracic lymph duct, proceeds cranially until it joins the anterior vena cava. At this junction, a valve regulates movement of lymph into the blood by opening and closing in concert with filling and emptying of the right atrium of the heart (Fig. 1.19).

1.5-3: Functions of lymph and lymph nodes. Lymph is a fluid similar to interstitial fluid, where the fluid first enters the lymph vessel. However, as lymph moves through the system, its composition changes, increasing in protein concentration as it moves along. When lymph from

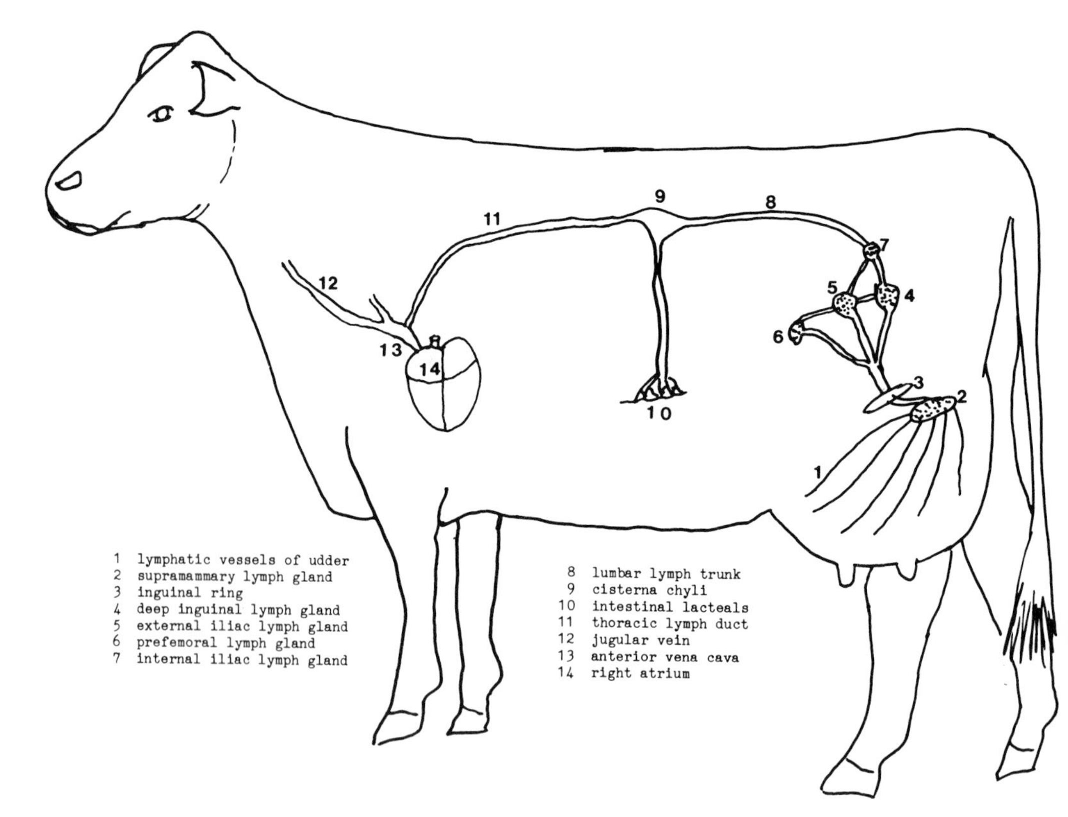

Fig. 1.19. Lymphatic system in the cow showing lymph flow from the udder to the anterior vena cava.

the lacteals mixes with lymph from other parts of the body, lipids are added in the form of chylomicra. These are spheres of triacylglycerols, approximately 1 μm in diameter, surrounded by a membrane with a configuration similar to a cell membrane. The chylomicra are an important source of glycerol and fatty acids for synthesis of milk fat by mammary secretory cells. In addition to supplying chylomicra, the lymph carries waste products away from active cells, immune bodies from lymph nodes, and dissipates heat from cells. The coagulating protein, fibrinogen, is also carried by the lymph.

1.6: NERVOUS SYSTEM

1.6-1: Introduction. Control of growth of epithelial secretory cells and the subsequent secretion of milk is almost exclusively hormonal and only minimally neural. However, the neural control of milk removal, or the inhibition of it, is considerable. The nervous system, which has an embryonic origin from the neural ectoderm, has sufficient complexity to induce a number of approaches that subdivide it into distinct parts. In order to understand the role of the nervous system in regulating the udder of the cow, we may divide it into a somatic nervous system, under voluntary control by the brain, and the autonomic system, or involuntary nervous system.

1.6-2: Autonomic nervous system. Certain nerves of the body allow an animal to function when conditions in the environment allow it to relax. At other times, the body must react quickly to conditions of stress or alarm. To carry out bodily functions such as urination, defecation, and sexual acts, the absence of stress or alarm from the environment is necessary. The parasympathetic part of the autonomic nervous system must be activated for such bodily functions to be fulfilled. The parasympathetic system includes parts of cranial nerves and sacral spinal nerves. Cranial nerves having parasympathetic functions are the third (oculomotor), seventh (facial), ninth (glossopharyngeal), and tenth (vagus). The third cranial nerve controls the iris, the seventh controls the lacrimal (tear) glands, the ninth controls the salivary glands, and the tenth controls the heart, lungs, digestive tract, and spleen. Sacral spinal nerves, numbers one, two, and three, innervate the urinary bladder, colon, and external genitalia. In most cases, the neurotransmitter substance associated with the parasympathetic nervous system is acetylcholine.

The sympathetic part of the autonomic nervous system comes into action when an animal is frightened, is fleeing, or is attacking (fright, flight, or fight). A series of ganglia along the sides of the vertebral column and connected to it by nerve fibers are the main part of the sympathetic nervous system. These ganglia send nerves to more peripherally located strategic ganglia, such as the cervical, splanchnic, celiac, and mesenteric ganglia. When the sympathetic nervous system is stimulated, it produces a number of changes that enable the animal to cope with an adverse situation, such as dilating pupils in the eye; increasing secretion of lacrimal glands of the eye; constricting blood flow to salivary glands; accelerating heart rate; expanding bronchioles in the lung; inhibiting blood flow to the stomach, duodenum, and pancreas; stimulating release of catecholamines from the adrenal medulla; dilating the urinary bladder; constricting the anal sphincter; constricting the cremaster muscle of the testes; and constricting blood flow to the udder. Postganglionic nerve endings of the sympathetic nervous system secrete epinephrine and norepinephrine, both of which act primarily on smooth muscles. Walls of arteries and arterioles are innervated with sympathetic nerves that secrete these catecholamines to constrict smooth muscles in the walls, resulting in a reduction in blood flow to the organ.

Nerves between the brain and udder include those from the first to fourth lumbar nerves and communications with the spinal ganglia. These nerves travel laterally and ventrally toward the udder. The nerve arising from the first lumbar nerve reaches the front of the udder but does not innervate the parenchyma. The second lumbar nerve joins, or anastomoses, with the third lumbar nerve, which fuses with the second and fourth lumbar nerves, giving rise to the inguinal nerve. This nerve passes through the inguinal ring to innervate all parts of the parenchyma of the udder and the skin. The inguinal nerve is made up of afferent and efferent components: the afferent part sends electrical signals to the spinal cord and brain, the efferent part sends signals from the brain and spinal cord to the udder via the ventral root ganglia (Fig. 1.20).

1.6-3: Neuroendocrine arc in milk removal. In cows, neural receptors are present in the skin of the teats and udder. These specialized nerve endings are responsive to touch by the calf or by the milker. Nerve impulses are carried via the afferent nerve fibers to the brain, which integrates the impulses into useful information. Areas of the brain most affected are the hypothalamus and pituitary. Training the nerve impulse from the udder involves the mammary nerves that coalesce to form the inguinal nerve. This courses through the inguinal ring to the second, third, and fourth lumbar nerves; the dorsal roots of these nerves carry the afferent messages to the brain via the spinal cord. Groups of nerve cell bodies in the hypothalamus are called nuclei. One group of these is located laterally and very close to the third ventricle; thus, they are called paraventricular nuclei. The cell bodies synthesize oxytocin, which trickles down the axon of the cell body to be stored at its end, located in the posterior lobe of the pituitary gland. When a signal reaches the cell body in the paraventricular nucleus, depolarization of the nerve cell membrane occurs. When this action termi-

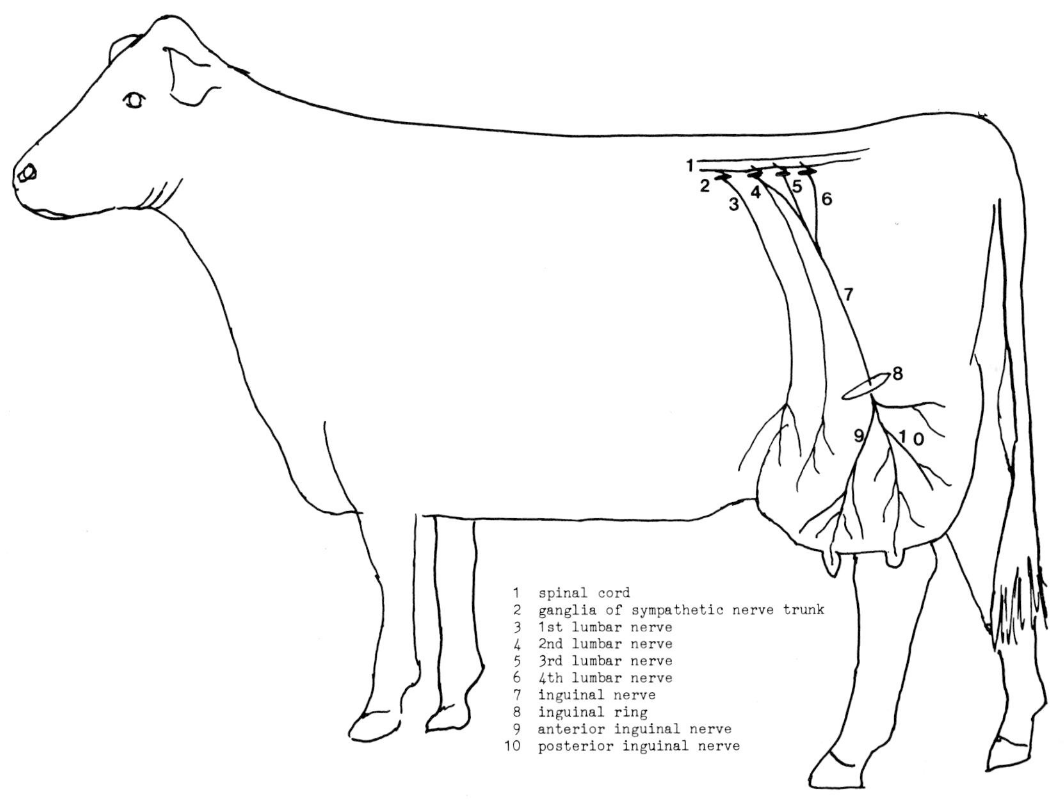

Fig. 1.20. Nerves of the udder having afferent and efferent components that connect to the spinal cord.

nates in the posterior lobe, the oxytocin is released from the axon by a process called exocytosis. The hormone is released into the perivascular space and diffuses between two endothelial cells into the blood. From here the oxytocin finds its way to all parts of the body, the most significant of which are the myoepithelial cells of the mammary gland. The time span for the sequences of this arc has been developed fairly accurately through research. Movement of electrical impulses along nerves is extremely rapid. For these to travel from the skin of the teat and udder to the nerve cell bodies of the paraventricular nuclei requires an elapsed time of a fraction of a second. Probably no more than a second or two are required for depolarization of the nerve cell membrane and contraction of the nerve cell's action, which enhances expulsion of oxytocin and neurophysin from the stored vesicles, movement of the oxytocin through the perivascular space, and interstitial fluid to the lumen of the capillary. From this point, the time for blood to circulate through the heart and lungs and back through the heart to the mammary gland cells is estimated to be 19–22 sec. Contraction of the myoepithelial cells to their maximum degree requires 6 sec. Filling the spaces in the enclosed milk storage system, including teat cistern, gland cistern, large milk ducts, and smaller ducts until a pressure of 60 mm Hg or higher is reached, may take another 20–30 sec. Therefore, a period of 45–60 sec should elapse after udder massage to allow for maximum intramammary pressure before milking machine teat cups are placed on the cow.

1.7: FUTURE DIRECTIONS IN STUDIES OF MAMMARY GROWTH AND DIFFERENTIATION

1.7-1: Epithelial secretory cells. Research has shown that ductal end buds proliferate into grapelike alveolar clusters. The mechanisms controlling this differentiation are not known except that hormonal combinations, including prolactin, progesterone, and somatotropin, will enhance this and will encourage complete extension of these structures into far extremes of the fatty pad. Another interesting problem is to understand the mechanism and the time at which a mother cell of the alveolus divides into two daughter cells before competence to synthesize milk is gained by the epithelial cell. This phenomenon occurs gradually throughout the latter part of pregnancy; at no time is there a sudden doubling of cell numbers in the mammary gland.

Epithelial cells of mammary gland origin are difficult to culture. Rapid progress is being made to overcome this problem, particularly in research concerning the interfacing of connective tissues and collagen types with epithelial cell growth.

1.7-2: Myoepithelial cells. Progress in many areas of research is slow compared to the life span of humans. As early as 1910, Ott and Scott found that a substance, which enhanced the harvest of milk, was secreted by the posterior pituitary gland. Not until 1940 was this action linked to a specialized cell of the mammary gland that contracted in response to increased intramammary pressure and, thus, aided in milk removal. The substance was chemically characterized in 1950, and anatomical evidence for the existence of a specialized mammary myoepithelial cell was presented about the same time. Since then, little progress has been made regarding the origin and function of this unique cell type. The contractile elements are assumed to respond like smooth muscle cells. The cell is thought to remain in place, while epithelial cells of the alveolus involute, but this is not certain. Alpha and beta receptors are thought to regulate contraction and relaxation in response to certain hormones and drugs, but this area of research is far from clarified. The myoepithelial cells are so important to the efficiency of the milking operation that a great deal more research is warranted.

1.7-3: Connective tissue, or stroma. A much neglected area of mammary gland research is the stroma, or structure, of the gland that provides support for the many parenchymal cells. Microscopic studies have shown bands of supportive structures in the gland that are arranged in well-organized units called lobules and lobes. In addition, units of support are the obvious ligaments, including the median suspensory ligament, the lateral suspensory ligament, and the lamellar plates. Only recently has research progress on these tissues increased because they are connective tissues, and humans are plagued with a variety of connective tissue diseases. Practical applications to the dairy cow are several. Udder attachments weaken and tear as a consequence of the great weight of a full udder. A wide variation in quality of udders exists; in part, this is due to differences in quantity of stroma. Udders respond to mastitic infections by walling off the area with connective tissue. Knowledge of the mechanisms by which connective tissues are produced and rearranged would help us control the connective tissue components of the mammary gland. In this category, we may include the less obvious but very important connective tissues, adipose tissue, and blood. Blood flow has long been known to be a limitation to milk synthesis, and the fatty pad has been alluded to previously as a limitation to proliferation of mammary epithelia.

1.7-4: Involution of the mammary gland. Research emphasis on mammary gland involution and regrowth has not been extensive. Milk production reaches a peak and then declines; involution of mammary cells and lack of replacing them is one suggestion as to the cause. An understanding of this phenomenon might enable us to maintain the level of milk production for much longer periods of time than are now possible. Involution of the mammary epithelia during the dry period seems obvious, yet little is known about this in the dairy cow. Although it has been studied in a few laboratory species, the mechanism of regrowth of mammary structures when pregnancy accompanies the postweaning period is not known. A postulate concerning growth of new structures that replace involuting structures in succeeding lactations has been presented in this chapter. Much more work needs to be done to expand this concept. Involution appears to be related to the different types of reproductive cycles of animals. Because rats do not have a functional luteal phase in their 5-day cycles, the mammary gland regresses almost completely to a duct system only. The normal-cycling cow does not experience involution to this extent, but cows that have reproductive difficulties may. Our attempts to stimulate mammary growth and subsequent lactation in problem breeder cows suggest that involution has reached a point of no return. Much additional research is needed if we are to return to profitability some of the purebred cows that are now discarded because of low production and breeding difficulties.

REFERENCES

Hammond J. 1927. The Physiology of Reproduction in the Cow. Cambridge: Cambridge Univ. Press.

Larson, B. L., ed. 1978. Lactation: A Comprehensive Treatise, vol. 4. New York: Academic.

Larson, B. L., and V. R. Smith, eds. 1974. Lactation: A Comprehensive Treatise, vols. 1–3. New York: Academic.

Schmidt, G. H. 1971. Biology of Lactation. San Francisco: Freeman.

Smith, V. R. 1959. Physiology of Lactation. 5th ed. Ames: Iowa State Univ. Press.

Swett, W. W., P. C. Underwood, C. A. Matthews, and R. R. Graves. 1942. Arrangement of the tissues by which the cow's udder is suspended. J. Agric. Res. 65:19–42.

Turner, C. W. 1952. The Mammary Gland, vol. 1. The Anatomy of the Udder of Cattle and Domestic Animals. Columbia, Mo.: Lucas Bros.

______. 1979. Harvesting Your Milk Crop. 4th ed. Oak Brook, Ill.: Babson Bros.

Wright, L. C., and R. R. Anderson. 1982. Effect of relaxin on mammary growth in the hypophesectomized rat. In Advances in Experimental Biology and Medicine, vol. 143, Relaxin, ed. R. R. Anderson, 348. New York: Plenum.

CHAPTER 2

ENDOCRINE AND NEURAL CONTROL OF THE MAMMARY GLAND

H. ALLEN TUCKER

2.1: INTRODUCTION

The endocrine and nervous systems integrate, control, and adjust body functions to meet changing metabolic and environmental needs of the animal. As a general rule, the endocrine system regulates relatively long-duration processes, whereas the nervous system is responsible for rapid (usually within milliseconds) control of body function. For example, mammary growth, lactogenesis, and lactation are long-duration processes involving days or months; thus, the endocrine system is the primary regulatory factor. The endocrine system is composed of a variety of specialized, ductless glands located in various parts of the body (Fig. 2.1). These glands synthesize organic chemicals (hormones) that are secreted into blood in response to a variety of internal and external stimuli. Hormones of importance to mammary function are given in Table 2.1.

Hormones are transported in the blood to their target cells, where they bind specifically with high affinity to receptor molecules (Fig. 2.2). Peptide hormones bind to specific protein receptors on the cell surface membrane and, by means of a transducer, most peptide hormones activate the adenylate cyclase system, which in turn converts adenosine triphosphate (ATP) to cyclic adenosine monophosphate (cAMP). The cAMP activates a protein kinase system composed of inhibitory and stimulatory subunits. Activation occurs when cAMP complexes with the inhibitory subunit, allowing activation of the enzyme. This leads to phosphorylation of proteins, an amplification process whereby a few molecules of hormone induce synthesis of many molecules of product. Examples of mammary cell responses include increased transportation of compounds across membranes, synthesis of

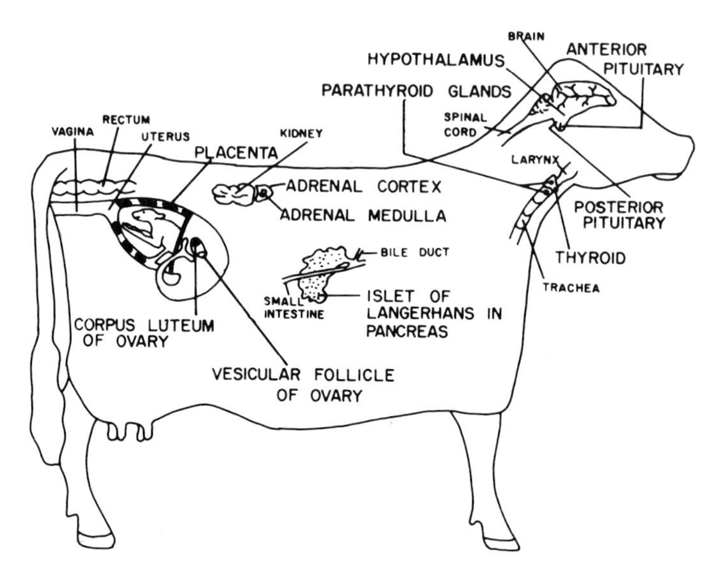

Fig. 2.1. Location of the major endocrine glands of the cow. (From Bath et al. 1978)

proteins in endoplasmic reticulum, synthesis of deoxyribonucleic acid (DNA) and ribonucleic acid (RNA), and differentiation of organelles. In contrast to most peptide hormones, prolactin inhibits the cAMP system. Steroid hormones enter target cells and bind to specific cytoplasmic receptors. The steroid hormone-receptor complex becomes activated and translocated to the nucleus, where it binds to chromatin acceptor sites. Inside the nucleus, the activated steroid-receptor complex induces transcriptional production of specific messenger RNA (mRNA) molecules that code production of new proteins. Thus, both steroid and peptide hormone-receptor complexes evoke a series of reactions, which result in a variety of biological responses typical for each particular hormone–target cell interaction.

The nervous system is composed of the central nervous system (brain and spinal cord), peripheral nerves, and autonomic nerves. The basic cell of the nervous system is the neuron, which conducts neural impulses from peripheral receptors in the mammary gland to the spinal cord. At this point, the impulse may be relayed via other neurons to the brain or directly back to an effector organ, which delivers an appropriate response. The autonomic nervous system is involuntary and composed of the sympathetic and parasympathetic systems; however, only the sympathetic system innervates the mammary gland. The primary effect of the sympathetic system on mammary function is to inhibit the milk ejection reflex, which suppresses the process of milk removal from the mammary gland.

2.2: NEUROENDOCRINE SYSTEM

The nervous and endocrine systems are functionally coordinated. For example, some neurons synthesize hormones, while some affect the nervous system, and the endocrine glands are frequently stimulated or inhibited by secretions of the nervous system. The organ central to the control of the

Table 2.1. Major hormones affecting mammary function

Endocrine Gland	Hormone Secreted	Major Function Associated with Mammary Gland
Anterior pituitary	Follicle-stimulating hormone (FSH)	Estrogen secretion
	Luteinizing hormone (LH)	Progesterone secretion
	Prolactin (PRL)	Mammary growth; initiation and maintenance of lactation
	Growth hormone (GH)	Stimulates milk production
	Thyroid-stimulating hormone (TSH)	Stimulates thyroid gland to secrete thyroxine, triiodothyronine
	Adrenocorticotropic hormone (ACTH)	Stimulates adrenal gland to secrete glucocorticoids
Posterior pituitary	Oxytocin	Milk ejection
Hypothalamus	Growth hormone–releasing hormone	Stimulates GH release
	Somatostatin	Inhibits GH release
	Thyrotropin-releasing hormone (TRH)	Stimulates TSH (also prolactin and GH) release
	Corticotropin-releasing factor	Stimulates ACTH release
	Prolactin-inhibiting factor (dopamine)	Inhibits prolactin release
Thyroid	Thyroxine; triiodothyronine	Stimulates oxygen consumption, protein synthesis, and milk yield
	Thyrocalcitonin	Calcium and phosphorus metabolism
Parathyroid	Parathyroid hormone	Calcium and phosphorus metabolism
Pancreas	Insulin	Glucose metabolism
Adrenal cortex	Glucocorticoids (cortisol, corticosterone)	Initiation and maintenance of lactation
	Mineralocorticoids (aldosterone)	Electrolyte and mineral metabolism
Adrenal medulla	Epinephrine and norepinephrine	Inhibition of milk ejection
Ovary	Estradiol	Mammary duct growth
	Progesterone	Mammary lobule-alveolar growth; inhibition of lactogenesis
Placenta	Estradiol	See ovary
	Progesterone (species dependent)	See ovary
	Placental lactogen	Mammary growth

neuroendocrine system is the hypothalamus, which regulates secretion from the anterior and posterior pituitary glands (Fig. 2.3).

The anterior pituitary gland receives no direct innervation; rather, it is controlled by secretions (hormones or factors) synthesized in the neurons of

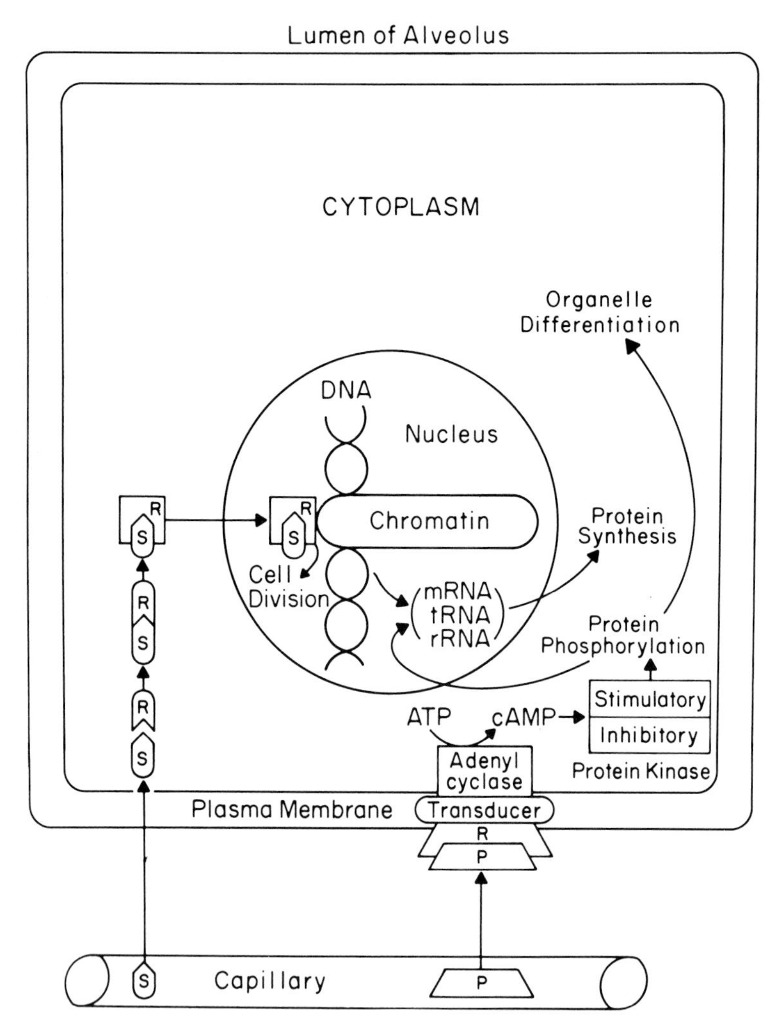

Fig. 2.2. Diagram of hormone binding in target cells. Steroid (*S*) and peptide (*P*) hormone binding and mechanism of action in the mammary parenchymal cell. *R* = receptor; *ATP* = adenosine triphosphate; *cAMP* = cyclic adenosine monophosphate; *DNA* = deoxyribonucleic acid; *mRNA* = messenger ribonucleic acid; *tRNA* = transfer ribonucleic acid; *rRNA* = ribosomal ribonucleic acid.

the hypothalamus. The hypothalamus secretes releasing or inhibiting hormones for each of the major anterior pituitary hormones. These hypothalamic hormones or factors are delivered to the anterior pituitary cells via a portal blood vessel system. The hypothalamus acts as a discrete amplifier

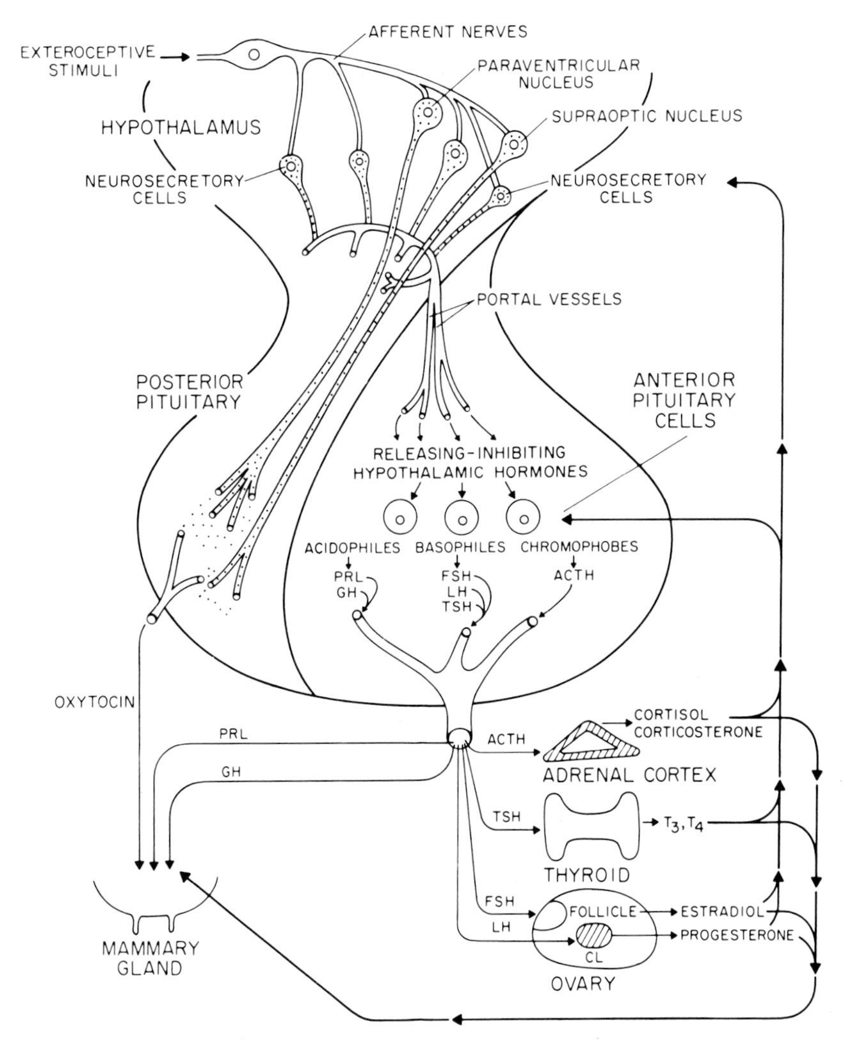

Fig. 2.3. Relationship of the hypothalamus, anterior and posterior pituitary glands, and target endocrine glands of importance to mammary function. *PRL* = prolactin; *GH* = growth hormone; *FSH* = follicle-stimulating hormone; *LH* = luteinizing hormone; *ACTH* = adrenocorticotropin hormone; *TSH* = thyroid-stimulating hormone; T_3 = triiodothyronine; T_4 = thyroxine.

of the hormonal and neural stimuli received from the internal and external environments (Fig.2.3).

Thyrotropin-releasing hormone (TRH) is a tripeptide hypothalamic hormone that has been isolated from hypothalamic tissue and has been synthesized in the laboratory; TRH causes release of thyroid-stimulating hormone (TSH). When TRH is administered to cattle and certain other species, prolactin and growth hormone (somatotropin) are released from the anterior pituitary. It is uncertain if TRH normally controls secretion of prolactin or growth hormone, two hormones implicated in several aspects of mammary function.

Secretion of prolactin is under dominant and chronic control of a hypothalamic-inhibiting factor. Thus, if the anterior pituitary is transplanted to a site remote from the hypothalamus, prolactin secretion increases, whereas secretion of other hormones diminishes. The bulk of the evidence suggests that the prolactin-inhibiting factor (PIF) from the hypothalamus is dopamine, although other putative factors, perhaps peptides, cannot be ruled out at this time. The hypothesis is that dopamine is released from neurons in the medial basal hypothalamus into portal vessels that deliver blood from the hypothalamus to the anterior pituitary (Fig. 2.3). The anterior pituitary gland contains receptors for dopamine, which, when activated, dramatically reduce synthesis and release of prolactin.

In addition to an inhibitory control system for prolactin secretion, there is evidence of a system that increases release of prolactin into blood. The hypothalamic factor most closely associated with release of prolactin is serotonin. Other hypothalamic factors that will acutely release prolactin into the blood include TRH, gamma amino butyric acid, and various endorphins. It is unknown which of these inhibiting or stimulating factors controls secretion of prolactin in response to the various stimuli associated with mammary gland function.

Secretion of growth hormone is inhibited by somatostatin, a tetradecapeptide; recently, a growth hormone–releasing hormone has been isolated. How these regulatory hormones control growth hormone in response to mammary function has yet to be established.

The interrelationships between the hypothalamus and secretion of hormones from the posterior pituitary are described in 2.9.

2.3: HORMONAL CONTROL OF MAMMARY GROWTH

Changes in secretion of certain hormones during the various reproductive states cause the mammary growth described in Chapter 1. Most mammary growth occurs only at certain times of the reproductive cycle: during puberty, pregnancy, and for a short period postpartum. The primary hormones known to stimulate mammary growth include estrogens, progestins, prolactin, growth hormone, and placental lactogen.

2.3-1: Ovarian steroids. The ovary secretes two primary steroid hormones, estradiol and progesterone (Table 2.1), which synergize to evoke mammary development during puberty and pregnancy, but not during the early postpartum period. For example, ovariectomy before puberty prevents the expected increases in mammary development at this stage. Ovariectomy followed by transplantation of the ovary to other parts of the body, or administration of various estrogens, restores normal increments in mammary growth. Meaningful data on mammary growth in response to ovariectomy during pregnancy is not possible because, depending on the species, either abortion occurs or the placenta secretes estrogens and progesterone, which maintain mammary growth increments. Ovariectomy on the day of parturition does not affect the normal increases in mammary development during the early stages of lactation, which suggests that the ovary is not essential for mammary growth during lactation.

2.3-1a: Administration of hormones. Injection, feeding, or implantation of either natural or synthetic estrogen into normal or gonadectomized animals primarily will stimulate mammary duct growth (Fig. 2.4). In some species, including cattle, an intermediate amount of lobule-alveolar development will be induced. However, the histological appearance of these alveoli is not normal since the lumina are frequently very large and papillomatous outgrowths are numerous.

Large numbers of alveoli must form in the mammary gland to secrete large quantities of milk. Normal lobule-alveolar mammary growth occurs when functional corpora lutea persist for long periods, as during gestation. Progesterone alone will induce formation of alveoli; however, estrogens plus progesterone synergize to produce lobule-alveolar development characteristic of pregnancy (Fig. 2.4c). The absolute quantities of estrogens and progesterone administered are of greater importance than the ratio of the hormones needed to induce lobule-alveolar development. To date, however, only in rats has a daily combination of estradiol (1 μg) and progesterone (2 mg) stimulated total mammary development equal to that found during normal gestation.

2.3-1b: Hormone concentrations in serum. Secretion of estradiol is greatest during proestrus and minimal during the luteal phase of estrus (Fig. 2.5). Thus, increased secretion of estrogens is related to rapid mammary growth at estrus. Progesterone secretion is greatest during the luteal phase of the estrous cycle and minimal during proestrus-estrus. The asynchrony between secretion patterns of these two hormones probably accounts for the failure to sustain large amounts of mammary growth during recurring estrous cycles.

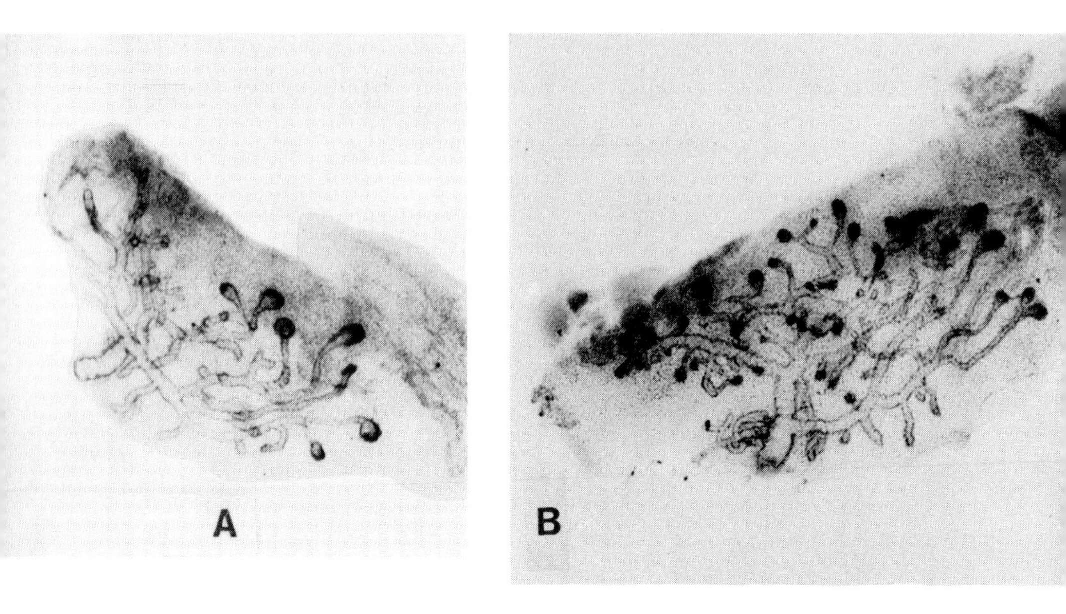

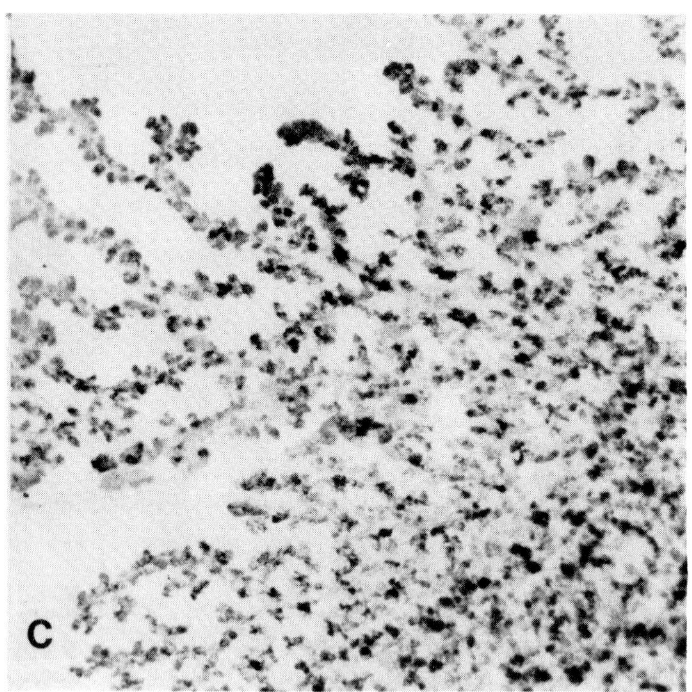

Fig. 2.4. Mammary development in mice. *A*. Mammary ducts at 3 wk of age before hormonal stimulation. *B*. Mammary duct development at 5 wk of age due to increased estrogen secretion. *C*. Mammary lobule-alveolar development at midpregnancy due to increased secretion of estrogen and progesterone. (Courtesy of Dr. Evelyn Rivera, Michigan State University)

In contrast, during pregnancy, secretion of estrogens and progestins is elevated simultaneously for a prolonged period (Fig. 2.5), which likely accounts for the sustained allometric growth observed during this physiological state.

2.3-1c: Mechanism of action. Estrogens and progesterone accelerate the rate of cell division in the mammary gland, especially in the terminal end buds. Progesterone also stimulates cell division along the duct walls. High-affinity binding sites (receptors) for these steroids are located in the mammary epithelial cell, as well as in adipose and connective tissue components of the mammary gland. Increasing numbers and/or affinities of the binding sites increase the biological response of a target tissue to a particular hormone. However, modulation of these receptors probably is restricted to the epithelial components of the mammary gland. Each steroid hormone traverses the basal membrane of the mammary epithelial cell and binds to a specific cytoplasmic protein receptor (Fig. 2.2). As a result of binding to

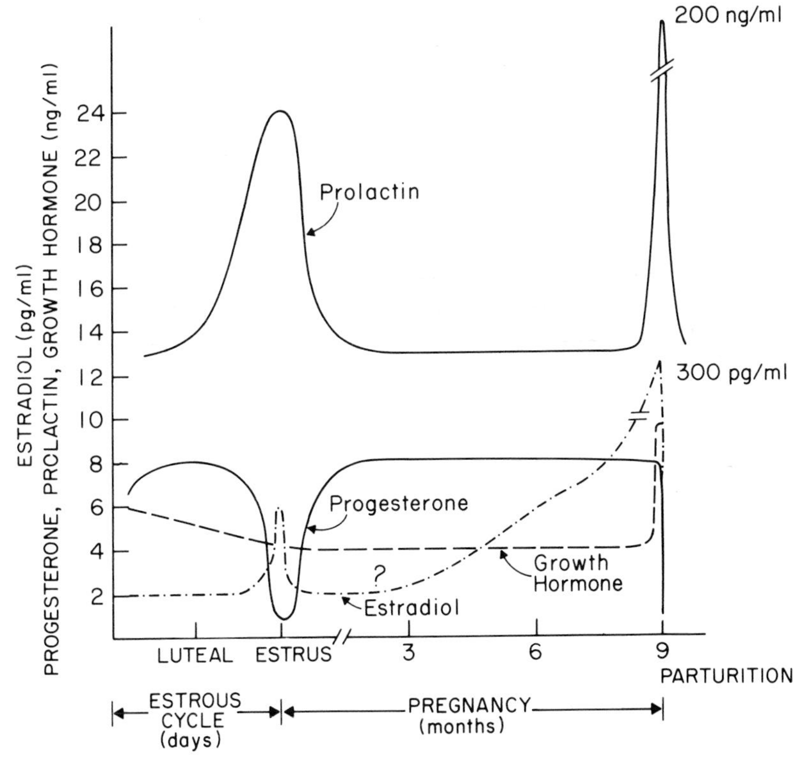

Fig. 2.5. Changes in concentrations of estradiol, progesterone, prolactin, and growth hormone in blood of cattle during the estrous cycle and pregnancy.

receptors, the mammary gland concentrates and retains the hormones against a large concentration gradient. A variety of estrogens are secreted into blood, and they bind to estrogen receptors in the mammary gland according to their individual biological activities. Nonestrogenic hormones do not bind to the estrogen receptor. Accordingly, progesterone binds to the progesterone receptor, but not to the estrogen receptor. However, progesterone also will bind to the glucocorticoid receptor; thus, progesterone binding is less specific than estrogen binding. The steroid hormone-receptor protein complex of the cytoplasm is translocated to the nucleus, where it binds to chromatin and stimulates cell division. There is some new evidence, however, that steroid hormones may not directly affect mitosis in the nucleus. Rather, they induce production of local factors in the mammary tissue, which in turn mediate cell division.

Estrogen receptors in mammary tissue initially appear coincident with onset of puberty, and receptor numbers increase with increasing tissue weight. Increasing concentrations of estrogens increase the synthesis of the estrogen receptor, provided the animal is sexually mature. Moreover, estrogen increases the shift of the receptor from the cytoplasm to the nucleus. Prolactin stimulates synthesis of the cytoplasmic estrogen receptor.

Progesterone receptors also have been detected in mammary tissue of virginal and pregnant animals. Estradiol increases the number of progesterone receptors in mammary tissue of virgin mice. This response likely contributes to the synergism observed between estradiol and progesterone on mammary growth before lactation. During lactation, estradiol has no effect on progesterone receptors. Indeed, during lactation, the progesterone receptor decreases and, in some species, is virtually absent. The relative absence of the progesterone receptor may account, in part, for the fact that administration of progesterone is without effect in the mammary gland during lactation.

2.3-2: Anterior pituitary peptides. The anterior pituitary secretes prolactin and growth hormone (Table 2.1), which are essential for mammary growth. For example, hypophysectomy of young animals produces mammary atrophy, which can be restored by administration of prolactin and growth hormone. Hypophysectomy during pregnancy of those species that secrete placental lactogen does not inhibit mammary growth because placental lactogen is an adequate replacement of the anterior pituitary hormones.

The other hormones of the anterior pituitary (TSH, adrenocorticotropic hormone [ACTH], follicle-stimulating hormone [FSH], and luteinizing hormone [LH]) do not directly affect mammary development. Rather, they affect mammary growth by stimulating secretion from their respective target endocrine glands (Fig. 2.3).

2.3-2a: **Administration of hormones.** Systemic injections of prolactin induce a marked lobule-alveolar development of the mammary gland (Fig. 2.6). These effects are probably mediated directly at the mammary gland, because localized injections of prolactin into the mammary gland induce an alveolar hyperplasia and secretion of milk only in those sectors into which they are injected.

In hypophysectomized-ovariectomized-adrenalectomized rats, administration of estradiol plus growth hormone induced some mammary duct growth; to obtain lobule-alveolar development required a combination of estradiol, progesterone, growth hormone, and prolactin. Maximal ductular and lobule-alveolar development, although less than that obtained in normal pregnancy, was achieved with the addition of glucocorticoids. In some strains of mice, growth hormone is interchangeable with prolactin in stimulating lobule-alveolar development. In hypophysectomized-ovariectomized ruminants (goats), mammary development comparable to mid-pregnancy was obtained with a combination of estrogen, progesterone,

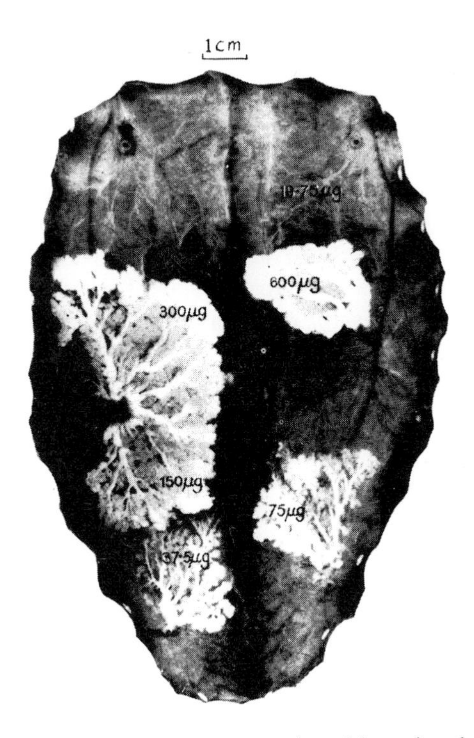

Fig. 2.6. Mammary growth and lactational responses of mammary tissue of pseudopregnant rabbits injected intraductally with various doses of prolactin. (From Bradley and Clarke 1956)

prolactin, growth hormone, and ACTH. Intact animals bearing heterotransplants of anterior pituitary tissue have increased development of the mammary gland, but the increment in mammary development is substantially less in ovariectomized animals. Therefore, synergism between pituitary hormones and ovarian steroids is essential to obtain maximal mammary development.

2.3-2b: Hormone concentrations in serum. Increased secretion of prolactin coincides with a small mammary growth spurt during proestrus-estrus (Fig. 2.5). Basal concentrations of prolactin do not change significantly during the greater portion of pregnancy when the mammary gland undergoes rapid development. The conclusion is that some prolactin is required for mammary growth but prolactin secretion is not limiting to the process.

In most species, concentrations of growth hormone do not change during the estrous cycle or pregnancy (Fig. 2.5). On the other hand, level of nutrition dramatically affects secretion of growth hormone; namely, high nutrient intakes are associated with reduced secretion of growth hormone. Since high planes of nutrition reduce mammary development in cattle, it has been speculated that reduced secretion of growth hormone may be associated with lowered mammary growth. It may be concluded that growth hormone is probably required, but not normally limiting for mammary development.

2.3-2c: Mechanism of action. Polypeptide hormones bind to protein receptors on the plasma membranes of cells and do not enter the cells as free hormone (Fig. 2.2). Most studies of the mechanisms whereby peptide hormones affect mammary growth have focused on prolactin receptors. The number of prolactin receptors per mammary cell is suppressed during gestation in rats and mice but increased in rabbits. These species differences may be associated with differences in secretion rates of placental lactogen (see 2.3-3), a peptide that binds to the prolactin receptor site. For example, rabbits possess no placental lactogen, whereas rats and mice have large quantities. Therefore, occupancy of the prolactin receptor by placental lactogen in rats and mice may mask measurements of prolactin receptors. Other mechanisms have been suggested whereby prolactin receptors in the mammary tissue are controlled. Since progesterone administration inhibits prolactin receptors, the suppressed numbers of prolactin receptors during gestation in rats and mice may be associated with increased secretion of progesterone. Conversely, estradiol administration to virginal rats increases the number of prolactin receptors in mammary glands; this response may explain the synergism between these two hormones.

2.3-3: Placental hormones. The placenta is an important source of mammogenic hormones (Table 2.1). There is a positive correlation between mammary development and the numbers and weights of the placentas of litter-bearing species. Maternal hormones are the primary sources of mammogenic hormones during early pregnancy, but after midpregnancy, the placenta becomes an important source of mammogenic hormones. In fact, hypophysectomy after midpregnancy does not affect subsequent mammary development. The placenta produces estrogens and, in some species (but not cattle), progesterone. In addition, placental lactogen, a polypeptide hormone unique to the placenta but possessing structural and immunological homologies with prolactin and growth hormone, is secreted in several species. Administration of saline extracts of rat placentas stimulates considerable mammogenesis in hypophysectomized-ovariectomized rats. In most species, secretion of placental lactogen from the fetal placenta to the maternal blood increases at midpregnancy and is maintained until parturition. Concentrations of placental lactogen in pregnant rats and mice are correlated positively with the number of fetuses, which are correlated with mammary development. In sheep and goats, greatest secretion of placental lactogen coincides with the most intense growth of the lobule-alveolar system during gestation. Placental lactogen binds competitively with prolactin and growth hormone at a common receptor site on the mammary gland membranes of laboratory species.

Cattle possess a placental lactogen with a molecular weight of approximately 32,000. Current evidence suggests that it is secreted primarily into fetal, not maternal, circulation. Thus, the relationship of placental lactogen to mammary function in cattle is unclear. The sire of the calf affects subsequent lactation in the dam. Presumably, this is a result of hormones secreted from the fetal placenta, one-half of which is derived genetically from the sire and the remainder from the dam. Indeed, there is evidence to suggest that secretion of estrogens from the conceptus may account partially for "sire-of-fetus" effects.

2.3-4: Adrenal steroids. The role of the adrenal steroids in mammogenesis is probably secondary to that of pituitary, ovarian, and placental hormones. For example, administration of glucocorticoids to immature animals induces ductular and lobule-alveolar development, but adrenalectomy inconsistently reduces subsequent mammary development. Administration of glucocorticoids during pregnancy increases mammary cell numbers, but glucocorticoid administration has a greater effect on metabolic activity of the cells.

2.3-5: Thyroid hormones. The thyroid gland is not essential for mammogenesis because thyroidectomized animals will conceive and lactate following parturition. Nevertheless, hypothyroidism retards ductal and lobule-alveolar development of the mammary gland. Conversely, low doses of thyroxine enhance the mammary growth effects of estrogen and progesterone, as well as mammary growth during gestation. Thus, the thyroid hormones probably are needed for maximal mammary development.

2.3-6: Other hormones and factors. Secretion of the parathyroid hormone has been implicated as a secondary factor in mammogenesis. Administration of parathyroid hormone, estrogen, and progesterone stimulated greater mammary development in ovariectomized-thyroid-parathyroidectomized rats than responses observed in similar rats given only estrogen and progesterone. It remains to be determined if parathyroid hormone limits normal mammogenesis.

When cultured in vitro, insulin has no effect on growth of mammary tissue derived from animals before the first pregnancy or during mammary involution. However, insulin is mitogenic in vitro when cultured with tissue from pregnant or lactating animals. Although insulin stimulates mitosis of the mammary parenchyma in vitro, it is not absolutely essential for mammary growth in vivo. For example, severely diabetic mice treated with estrogen and progesterone develop an extensive mammary lobule-alveolar system, but addition of insulin increases development still further. Insulin must be present in hypophysectomized animals to permit estrogen and progesterone stimulation of mammary development. The effects of insulin on mammary development are likely to be mediated through high-affinity binding sites for insulin, which are present at least during estrous cycles and pregnancy. Since insulin concentrations in serum decrease during gestation in cattle, it seems unlikely that insulin limits normal mammary gland development, at least in this species.

Relaxin, a protein hormone synthesized from the corpus luteum of the ovary, has little mammogenic activity per se. However, there is evidence that relaxin is capable of synergizing with anterior pituitary hormones and ovarian steroids to enhance mammogenesis in rats; its role in other species is unknown.

Postnatally, teats are absent in the males of several species, e.g., mice, rats, and horses. This aberration is associated with increased secretion of androgens from the fetal testis, which causes partial or complete destruction of the mammary bud during its embryological development. The stage when the bud is susceptible to androgens is very discrete; maximal susceptibility occurs on day 14 of fetal development in mice. The target tissue for the androgen is the mesenchyme into which the mammary bud grows. However, the response depends on the presence of the mammary epithelium, which induces formation of androgen receptors in the cells of adjacent mesenchyme, thereby controlling androgen sensitivity in the tissue.

In normal postnatal animals, injections of androgens stimulate duct growth in guinea pigs and lobule-alveolar development in rats. In hypophysectomized animals, on the other hand, androgens have no effect on mammogenesis, but androgens will synergize with exogenous growth hormone to stimulate lobule-alveolar development. In males with extensive mammary development, enhanced secretion of androgen may be involved.

In recent years, a number of factors have been identified that will stimulate growth of a number of tissues. Perhaps the most widely studied factor is epidermal growth factor, a peptide initially isolated from submaxillary glands. Epidermal growth factor induces mitosis of mammary cells cultured in vitro, and some have claimed that growth factors produced locally in the mammary tissue may mediate the effects of the well-established hormones on mammary development. During gestation, cAMP increases in mammary cells, and factors that increase cAMP (e.g., cholera toxin) also stimulate mammogenesis. Moreover, cholera toxin synergizes with epidermal growth factor and fibroblast growth factor to increase mammary mitosis in vitro. It seems reasonable to postulate that this area of knowledge will markedly expand in the future.

2.4: NEURAL CONTROL OF GROWTH

Removal of nerve impuse flow to and from the mammary gland does not interfere with mammary growth during pregnancy. During lactation, however, increasing suckling frequency or litter size will increase the number of mammary cells. Suckling retards mammary involution during lactation even if milk is not removed. In fact, maintenance of integrity of the mammary alveolar cells is more easily accomplished than maintenance of the synthetic capacity of the cells. The effects of the nervous system on mammary development are very likely mediated via release of hormones from the anterior pituitary gland. In other words, direct efferent neural connections to the mammary secretory cells are of no importance in mammary development.

2.5: HORMONAL CONTROL OF LACTOGENESIS

Lactogenesis is a process of differentiation whereby the mammary alveolar cells acquire the ability to secrete milk; it is conveniently defined as a two-stage mechanism. The first stage consists of cytologic and enzymatic differentiation of the alveolar cells and coincides with limited secretion of milk before parturition. The second stage begins with the copious secretion of all milk components shortly before parturition in most species and extends through several days postpartum. Although association of specific hormones with the two stages of lactogenesis has been difficult, the minimal requirement for lactogenesis consists of increased secretion of prolactin, ACTH (which stimulates secretion of glucocorticoids), and estrogens and the relative absence of progesterone.

2.5-1: Anterior pituitary peptides. Hypophysectomy of pregnant animals markedly suppresses subsequent lactation. Failure of lactation in hypophysectomized animals occurs despite the fact that the young are delivered normally. Administration of crude extracts of the anterior pituitary to normal animals initiates and maintains lactation. Thus, there is no doubt that secretions from the anterior pituitary are involved in lactogenesis.

2.5-1a: Administration of hormones. The first evidence that pituitary hormones are involved in lactogenesis came from studies in pseudopregnant rabbits. Injection of an aqueous extract of anterior pituitary glands into these rabbits initiated lactation. Tests using purified fractions of the anterior pituitary gland identified one fraction that stimulated growth of the pigeon crop sac mucosa and also induced a localized secretion when injected into individual galactophores of the mammary gland of pseudopregnant rabbits (Fig. 2.6). The active hormone was subsequently called prolactin.

Choice of rabbits as an experimental model was fortuitous because later research showed the mammary gland of this species to be much more sensitive to prolactin than mammary glands of other species. For example, injection of prolactin in normal pregnant rats and mice does not initiate lactation. This is probably associated with the fact that prolactin is luteotrophic in rats and mice, and when progesterone secretion is elevated, lactogenesis is inhibited.

One of the most dramatic bits of evidence demonstrating that prolactin plays a major role in lactogenesis came from a study of a hypophysectomized goat during lactation. As expected, hypophysectomy resulted in a rapid decrease in milk yields (Fig. 2.7). Administration of a synthetic glucocorticoid (dexamethasone), triiodothyronine, and growth hormone restored lactation to approximately 28% of normal. When prolactin was added to the mixture, milk yields were completely restored to prehypophysectomy levels.

Many studies show that addition of prolactin to media containing mammary gland explants from a variety of species, including cattle, will initiate secretion of several milk components. Thus, the effects of prolactin on lactation are undoubtedly exerted directly on mammary tissue.

Although exogenous growth hormone can be substituted for prolactin in certain strains of mice to cause lactogenesis, there is little evidence suggesting that it plays a major role in most species. Indeed, growth hormone failed to induce secretion of α-lactalbumin in bovine mammary tissue explants cultured in vitro. On the other hand, growth hormone of human origin has intrinsic lactogenic properties even though only 16% of the amino acid sequences are identical with human prolactin. Changes in secretion of human growth hormone during lactogenesis have not been reported; a definitive role for this hormone in lactogenesis has yet to be established.

ACTH is another anterior pituitary hormone that is important to lactogenesis. However, all of the effects of ACTH are mediated via secretion of glucocorticoids and will be discussed in 2.5-3.

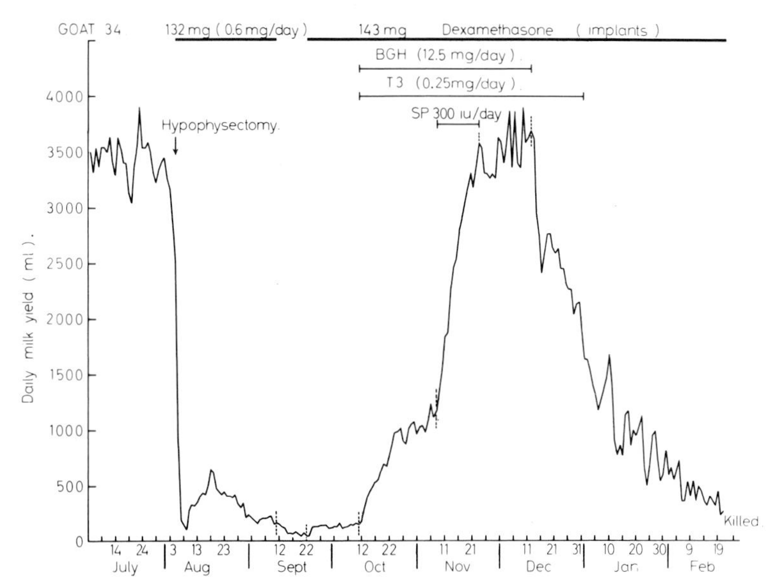

Fig. 2.7. Daily milk yield of a goat before and after hypophysectomy and during replacement therapy. *BGH* = bovine growth hormone; T_3 = triiodothyronine; *SP* = sheep prolactin. (From Cowie 1969)

2.5-1b: Hormone concentrations in serum. Although it is possible to induce secretion of milk with exogenous hormones, this does not necessarily mean they normally function in this capacity. Indeed, measurements of prolactin during pregnancy clearly show that the concentration of this hormone does not change in the serum of many species for the greater portion of gestation (Fig. 2.5). Moreover, the increases in mammary enzymatic activity and organelle differentiation during the first stage of lactogenesis is not associated with an alteration in basal concentrations of prolactin in serum. However, there is a major surge in secretion of prolactin immediately before parturition in several species (Fig. 2.8). This surge coincides with development of the second phase of lactogenesis. Moreover, suppression of the periparturient surge of prolactin by administration of ergot alkaloids inhibits subsequent milk secretion in monogastric species and partially reduces lactation in cattle (Fig. 2.9). This decreased milk yield in cattle is associated with decreased metabolic activity of the mammary cells. There is no effect on numbers of mammary cells.

In the absence of the parturition-induced surge of prolactin, mammary alveolar cells of cattle are less differentiated. If cows are given the ergot alkaloid plus exogenous prolactin in sufficient quantities to mimic the periparturient surge of prolactin, subsequent lactation is not reduced (Fig. 2.9);

thus, the periparturient surge of prolactin is essential for maximal lactogenesis.

Most studies of peptide hormone control of lactogenesis have focused on prolactin; however, prolactin is by no means the only hormone whose concentration changes during lactogenesis. For example, there is a surge in secretion of growth hormone that coincides with parturition (Fig. 2.8), but the importance, if any, of this increase for lactogenesis remains to be determined. ACTH (as reflected by increased concentrations of glucocorticoids) is also released during the periparturient period; these aspects will be discussed in 2.5-3b.

2.5-1c: Mechanism of action of prolactin. As previously discussed, changes in concentrations of hormones will be without effect if receptors in the mammary gland are not present to bind the hormone. Inactivation of the prolactin receptor, with antibodies against the receptor, blocks the abil-

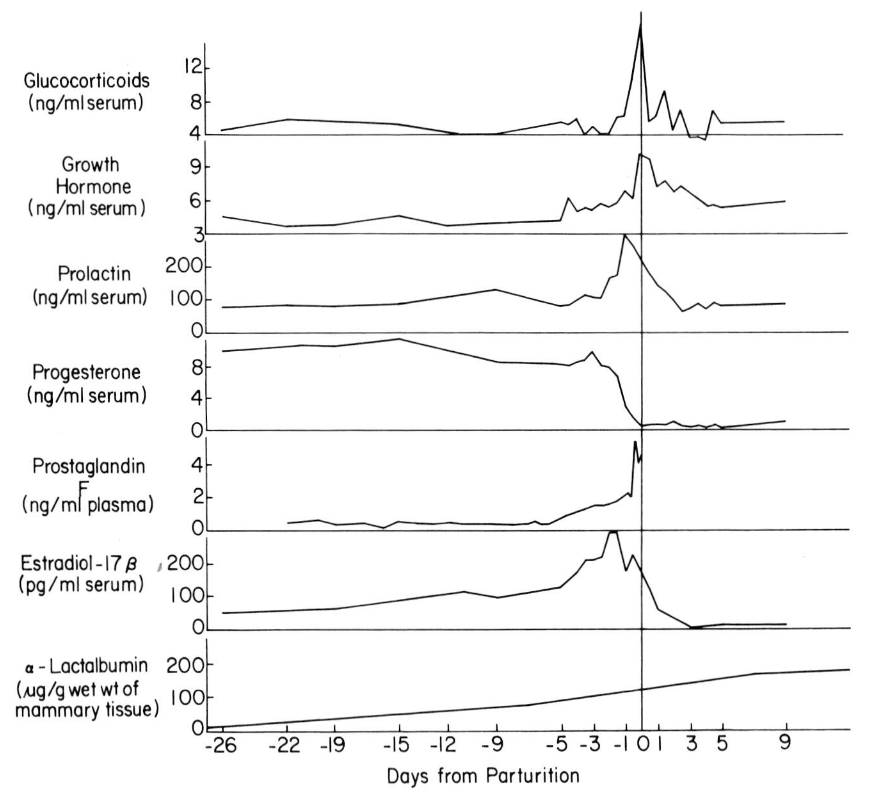

Fig. 2.8. Changes in concentrations of α-lactalbumin in mammary tissue and hormones in blood serum or plasma of cows during the periparturient period. (Modified from Tucker 1979)

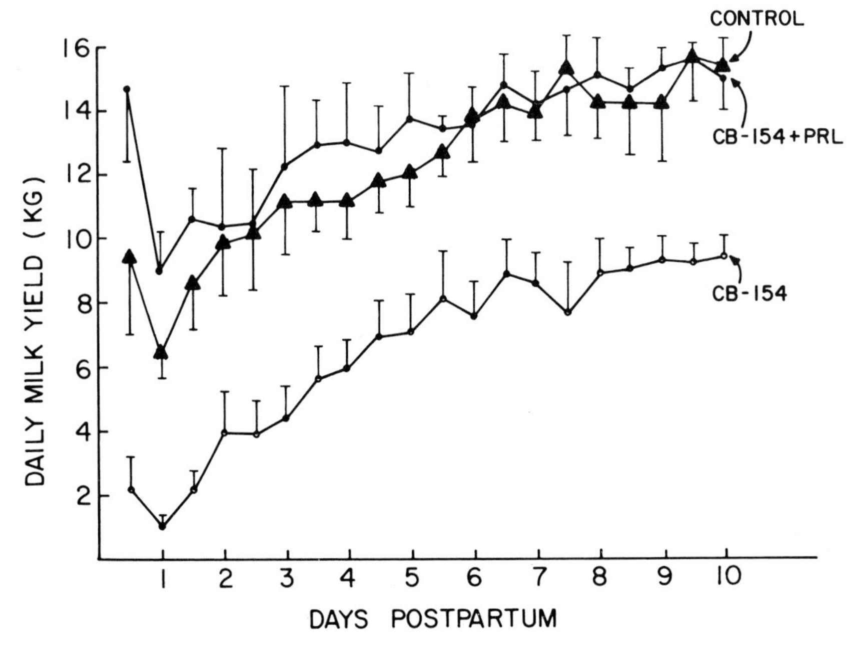

Fig. 2.9. Daily milk yields of untreated (*control*) cows, cows treated with 2-Br-α-ergokryptin (*CB-154*), or cows treated with CB-154 plus exogenous prolactin (*PRL*). CB-154 was administered from approximately 12 days before parturition through 10 days postpartum. Treatment with CB-154 reduced basal secretion of prolactin 80% and blocked the normal surge of prolactin at parturition. Exogenous prolactin was administered for 6 days beginning immediately before parturition. (From Akers et al. 1981)

ity of prolactin to induce milk protein synthesis. The receptors for the peptide hormones are located on the plasma membrane of the mammary epithelial cells (Fig. 2.2). In rabbits, numbers of prolactin receptors initially increase in mammary tissue coincident with initiation of the first phase of lactogenesis. Numbers of receptors remain constant until the second phase of lactogenesis in the immediate periparturient period, when they increase again. Such changes in receptor numbers are very likely involved in the mechanism of lactogenesis.

Prolactin is capable of regulating the concentration of its own receptor; this is a long-range control system and is termed "up-regulation." In this system, gradual increases in prolactin concentrations augment concentrations of the prolactin receptor. Progesterone antagonizes this effect of prolactin on the prolactin receptor. When the up-regulation system is blocked, receptor numbers for prolactin remain low and reduced milk production ensues. Up-regulation of prolactin receptors is associated with the appearance of cellular organelles during the first phase of lactogenesis.

Prolactin also has the ability to "down regulate" its receptor. This is a fast and reversible effect and is associated with sharp, acute releases of the hormone. Following an acute increase of prolactin, the number of prolactin receptors declines for about 6 hr, then gradually returns to normal within 24–30 hr. Thus, after binding to its receptor on the cell surface, the prolactin-receptor complex is internalized within the mammary cell. This process is believed to be concerned with degradation of existing prolactin-receptor complexes in the lysosomes and synthesis of new receptors. The receptor molecule for prolactin has a relatively short half-life, whereas the mRNA for the prolactin receptor is rather stable. Internalization and degradation of the prolactin-receptor complex is not related to induction of casein synthesis at lactogenesis, and its functional significance remains to be established.

Following binding of prolactin to the plasma membrane receptor, the prolactin-receptor complex evokes a series of reactions that depend on the microtubule network and the cell nucleus (Fig. 2.2). As previously noted, presence of the prolactin molecule is not required beyond initial binding to the prolactin receptor. Although many peptide hormones activate cAMP (Fig. 2.2), prolactin does not. Rather, the prolactin-receptor complex may activate the membrane-associated enzyme, phospholipase A, which leads to increased synthesis of prostaglandins. A few prostaglandins mimic some effects of prolactin on lactogenesis. For example, incubation of mammary tissue slices with certain prostaglandins stimulates synthesis of RNA in mammary tissue. Conversely, indomethacin, an inhibitor of prostaglandin synthesis, blocks the stimulatory effects of prolactin on synthesis of RNA.

The effects of prolactin and prostaglandin on RNA are abolished whenever intracellular cAMP concentrations are increased. On the other hand, addition of cyclic guanosine monophosphate (cGMP) mimics the effect of prolactin on synthesis of RNA. Thus, the stimulatory action of prolactin on RNA synthesis may be mediated by reduced intracellular cAMP and increased cGMP. Although prolactin does not activate adenyl cyclase, it induces synthesis of cAMP-dependent kinases (Fig. 2.2); some existing cAMP may still be essential to mediate the actions of prolactin.

In spite of the fact that some prostaglandins increase synthesis of RNA in the mammary cell, they do not stimulate casein synthesis, as does prolactin. A combination of polyamines (spermidine) plus prostaglandin mimics the effects of prolactin on RNA and casein synthesis. Hence, polyamines probably also are involved in the mechanism whereby prolactin affects milk protein synthesis in the mammary cell.

These reactions in response to the initial binding of prolactin to its receptor culminate in an increase in ribosomal RNA and in the accumulation of casein mRNA, due to severalfold increases in the rate of casein mRNA transcription and translation and an increase in the half-life of casein mRNA. Thus, prolactin controls expression of the casein gene and probably other genes as well. Many of these effects of prolactin on the casein gene are amplified by glucocorticoids and insulin and are inhibited by progesterone. There are several caseins secreted by the mammary gland (see Chap. 4), and each is controlled by its own mRNA. It appears that prolactin does not control expression of these genes coordinately; that is, the mRNAs increase independently of each other. In addition, cortisol is primarily responsible for the induction of at least one of the abundant mammary gland mRNAs, whose identity is still unknown. All of these intracellular events described above are consistent with a major role for prolactin in lactogenesis.

2.5-2: Placental lactogen. Pregnant rats and mice were first shown to secrete a polypeptide, lactogenic hormone, of placental origin. Subsequently, placental lactogens were found in many, but not all species. For example, rabbits do not secrete placental lactogen. In cattle, placental cotyledons are lactogenic when cocultured with mouse mammary explants. But, as described in 2.3-3, the role of bovine placental lactogen in mammary function is not established.

Placental lactogen will initiate milk secretion when injected intraductally into rabbits and will substitute for prolactin in inducing cultured mammary cells to secrete casein. As previously noted, placental lactogen binds to the prolactin receptor. There is an increased turnover of placental lactogen in serum coincident with the first phase of lactogenesis; thus, placental lactogen probably is of importance in the lactogenic process of some species.

2.5-3: Adrenal steroids. Adrenalectomy of pregnant animals markedly inhibits subsequent lactogenesis and lactation. Moreover, adrenalectomy blocks induction of synthesis of caseinlike proteins and RNA that normally occurs after ovariectomy of pregnant rats. Thus, adrenal gland secretions play a major role in lactogenesis.

2.5-3a: Administration of hormones. Injections of extracts of adrenal cortex plus prolactin synergize to induce secretion in mammary tissue of pseudopregnant rats. In hypophysectomized animals, minimal replacement therapy for lactogenesis is a combination of ACTH (or glucocorticoids) plus prolactin. Although administration of glucocorticoids will initiate lactation during pregnancy in dairy cows (Fig. 2.10), in most species a combination of prolactin and glucocorticoids is more effective. Such combinations have not been tested in cattle. Cortisol induces differentiation of rough endoplasmic reticulum and the Golgi apparatus of mammary epithe-

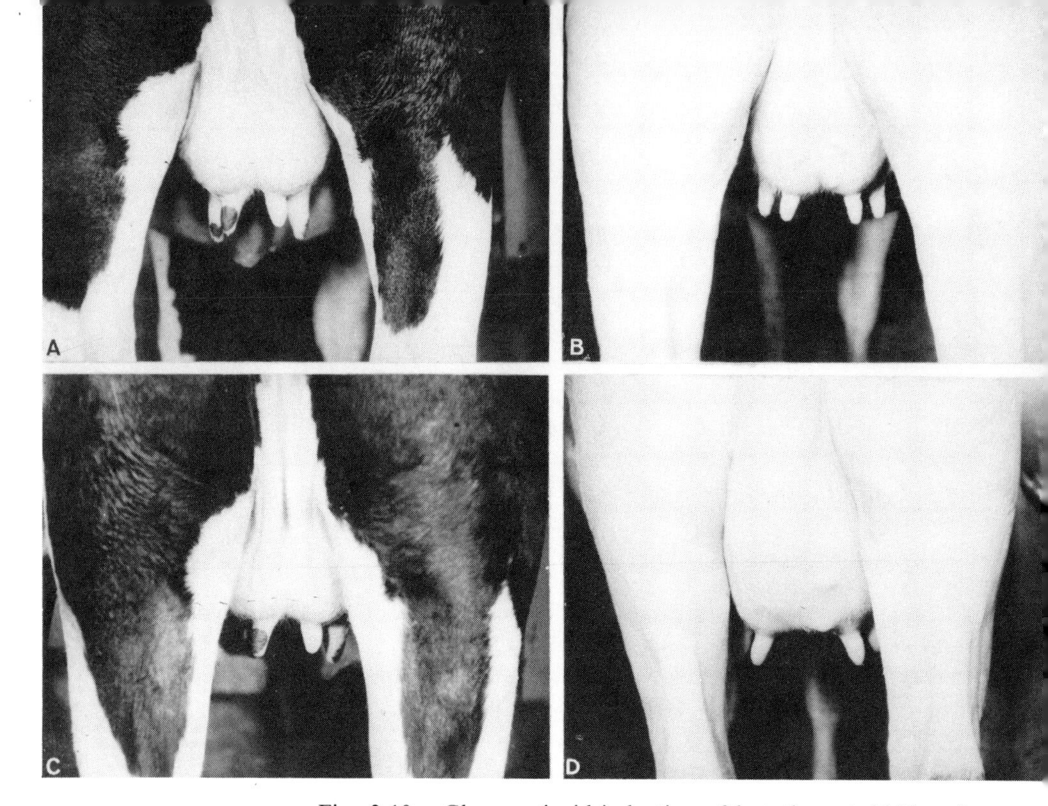

Fig. 2.10. Glucocorticoid induction of lactation. *A*. Udder of control heifer 7.5 mo pregnant at beginning of treatment. *B*. Udder of control heifer after 6 days of no treatment. *C*. Udder of experimental heifer 7.5 mo pregnant at beginning of treatment. *D*. Udder of experimental heifer after 6 days of injections of a synthetic glucocorticoid (9-α-fluoroprednisolone acetate). At first milking on day 7, controls produced no milk, whereas glucocorticoid-treated heifers produced 4.5 kg milk. (From Tucker and Meites 1965)

lial cells derived from midpregnant mice; this differentiation is essential to permit prolactin to induce synthesis of milk proteins. The glucocorticoids serve to amplify the effects of prolactin on lactogenesis.

2.5-3b: Hormone concentrations in serum. Studies of changes in concentrations of glucocorticoids in blood have provided additional insight into their potential role in lactogenesis. Secretion of glucocorticoids remains low for the greater part of gestation. Shortly before parturition, however, concentrations of glucocorticoids increase substantially in several species, including cattle, with peak concentrations coinciding with parturition (Fig. 2.8). As parturition approaches, secretion of fetal glucocorticoids occurs. This increased secretion of fetal glucocorticoids contributes to parturition in several species. Although the fetus may contribute small amounts of glucocorticoids to the maternal circulation, most evidence suggests that labor per se increases concentrations of glucocorticoids from the maternal adrenal during the periparturient period. Whether the periparturient surge of glucocorticoids is essential for lactogenesis or merely associated with stress of parturition is not established.

2.5-3c: Corticoid-binding globulin. Corticoid-binding globulin (CBG) is a protein that binds and inactivates glucocorticoids. Concentrations of this protein in blood are increased for the greater part of gestation. During pregnancy, CBG, also found in mammary tissue, is largely unsaturated and, therefore, is available to bind free glucocorticoids. These findings are consistent with the hypothesis that free, biologically active concentrations of glucocorticoids are reduced during pregnancy. Early reports on rats suggested that CBG capacity declined in the periparturient period, thereby increasing the availability of free glucocorticoids postulated to be involved in lactogenesis. However, recent research has failed to substantiate that CBG concentrations change in the periparturient period.

2.5-3d: Mechanism of action. Free glucocorticoids from blood bind receptor molecules within the cytosol of the mammary alveolar epithelial cell (Fig. 2.2). The cytosolic receptor-hormone complex migrates to the nucleus, where it induces synthesis of particular genes. Binding of glucocorticoids to mammary epithelial tissue increases dramatically during pregnancy and is maximal at parturition; thus, change in glucocorticoid receptor-site numbers is another factor circumstantially related to initiation of lactation.

The lactogenic effects of prolactin and cortisol probably are mediated by a decrease in concentrations of intracellular cAMP (Fig. 2.2). These hormones markedly reduce mammary tissue concentrations of cAMP, and if cAMP is added to mammary tissue explants cultured in vitro, the lactogenic effects of prolactin and cortisol are blocked. It is now established that cortisol is essential for prolactin to induce casein gene expression in mammary tissue. This constitutes additional evidence for the essential synergism between prolactin and the glucocorticoids to induce lactation.

2.5-4: Ovarian steroids. Secretions of the corpus luteum inhibit lactogenesis. Removal of the corpus luteum or other means of reducing progesterone secretion leads to initiation of lactation and abortion. However, reducing progesterone secretion in adrenalectomized or hypophysectomized animals does not result in lactogenesis. Thus, the major concept is that positive, as well as negative, factors work in concert to control initiation of lactation.

2.5-4a: Administration of hormones. The primary role of progesterone in lactogenesis is the inhibition of the process. Injection of progesterone during pregnancy prevents the normal induction of lactose, α-lactalbumin, and casein synthesis, as well as histological appearance of milk secretion. Progesterone also blocks prolactin-induced increases in these milk constituents and accumulation of casein mRNA. Progesterone acts directly on the mammary tissue to decrease the ability of prolactin to induce secretion of α-lactalbumin. Moreover, progesterone dramatically reduces the synergism between estrogen and prolactin, but the mechanism involved is not known.

Progesterone binds to the progesterone receptor in the mammary tissue and also competes with glucocorticoids for binding on the glucocorticoid receptor in the soluble cytoplasm (Fig. 2.2). It has been suggested that the large amounts of progesterone normally secreted during gestation saturate the glucocorticoid-binding sites, thereby preventing glucocorticoids from inducing lactation during the greater portion of gestation. Progesterone also inhibits the ability of prolactin to induce synthesis of prolactin receptors. These are antilactogenic effects.

In contrast to the inhibitory effects of progesterone on lactogenesis, administration of estrogens to animals with well-developed mammary glands induces milk secretion in a variety of species. Research shows that estrogens stimulate secretion of prolactin and possibly other hormones from the anterior pituitary. Thus, it is believed that pituitary hormones mediate a portion of the lactogenic responses associated with estrogen administration. In addition, there is now good evidence suggesting that estrogens also may directly stimulate mouse and bovine mammary tissue cultured in vitro to synthesize casein and α-lactalbumin. Combinations of prolactin and estrogens or of prolactin and glucocorticoids are synergistically lactogenic. Since estrogens and glucocorticoids increase numbers of prolactin receptors on the mammary membranes, this perhaps explains the synergistic effects among prolactin, glucocorticoids, and estrogens on lactogenesis at the mammary cell level.

Due to infertility problems, 15–20% of dairy cattle are culled from herds each year. Thus, there is interest in reinitiating secretion of large amounts of milk with exogenous hormones. To accomplish this goal, large numbers of mammary epithelial cells must be grown and lactation must be initiated. In most experiments, estrogens have been used alone or in combination with progesterone, but great variability in mammary development and subsequent milk yield precludes routine application of this research to barren cattle. Milk yields often were substantially lower than yields obtained following a normal pregnancy and parturition. The most consistent and greatest yields have been obtained by injecting barren cows subcutaneously at 12-hr intervals for 7 days with a combination of estradiol (0.05 mg/kg body weight) and progesterone (0.125 mg/kg body weight). Sufficient lactation requiring milking occurs in about 70% of the cows between days 14 and 21. Milk yield in cows that respond to the exogenous hormones usually averages about 70% of normal. Greater percentages of cows secrete significant quantities of milk if prolactin secretion is also stimulated between days 8 and 14, as has been accomplished by administration of the tranquilizing drug, reserpine. It should be understood, however, that none of these procedures have been legally approved in the United States for use in cattle.

2.5-4b: Hormone concentrations in serum. Of all the hormones measured in blood of periparturient cattle, the estrogens (estrone and estradiol) are the first to increase (Fig. 2.8). Concentations of these estrogens in serum of cattle begin to increase markedly about 1 mo before expected parturition, reach a maximum 2 days before parturition, then rapidly decline. Thus, changes in concentrations of these steroids generally overlap both phases of lactogenesis.

Changes in progesterone secretion in the periparturient period agree well with the inhibitory effects of this hormone on lactogenesis. In cattle, for example, there is a marked decrease in secretion of progesterone 1–2 days before parturition (Fig. 2.8). This reduction in serum progesterone in cattle coincides with the last phase of lactogenesis.

2.5-5: Prostaglandins. Prostaglandins (PGs) are fatty acids produced locally in a variety of tissues. They are not considered hormones in the usual sense, but they have profound effects on many physiological processes, including lactogenesis. In addition to the intracellular effects on lactogenesis described previously in 2.5-1c, prostaglandins also induce systemic effects, which may play a role in lactogenesis. For example, prostaglandin $F_{2\alpha}$($PGF_{2\alpha}$) is a well-established luteolytic agent, and administration of $PGF_{2\alpha}$ lyses the corpus luteum, which reduces secretion of progesterone. Accordingly, when $PGF_{2\alpha}$ is administered during pregnancy, abortion and lactogenesis subsequently occur. PG secretion into blood increases coincidently with the decrease in progesterone as the time of parturition approaches (Fig. 2.8). Increased estrogen secretion prepartum is the most likely cause of this increased PG secretion just prior to parturition. However, maximal concentrations of PG do not occur until parturition. In view of the late appearance of this surge, the precise role of systemic effects of $PGF_{2\alpha}$ on lactogenesis has not been established.

2.6: NEURAL CONTROL OF LACTOGENESIS

Afferent innervation of the mammary gland plays no role in the control of secretory activity of the mammary gland. However, afferent neural stimuli from the reproductive tract via the hypothalamus may be associated with periparturient releases of some of the hormones previously described (Fig. 2.3). In addition, prepartum milking generally initiates lactation in pregnant animals. This mechanism involves transmission of neural impulses from the teat to the hypothalamus, where secretion of the prolactin-inhibiting factor is suppressed, and the corticotrophin-releasing factor is stimulated. This stimulates secretion of prolactin and ACTH, and these two hormones, in turn, induce the mammary cell to secrete. However, neural components of the milking stimulus are not required to stimulate lactogenesis because the alveoli will be distended with milk, even if milking is not permitted before or immediately after parturition.

2.7: HORMONAL CONTROL OF LACTATION

There is a striking increase in milk yield in cattle, which reaches a peak 2–8 wk after parturition and then gradually declines. Maintenance of intense lactation requires maintenance of alveolar cell numbers, synthetic activity per mammary cell, and efficacy of the milk ejection reflex. A hormonal complex controls lactation, but unless milk is removed frequently from the udder, synthesis of milk will not persist despite an adequate hormonal status. Conversely, lactation will not be maintained indefinitely despite frequent milk removal. Thus, secretion and removal of milk are closely associated. The hormones required for maintenance of milk synthesis include prolactin, growth hormone, ACTH (or glucocorticoids), TSH (or thyroid hormones), insulin, and parathyroid hormone. Oxytocin is essential for milk removal and will be discussed in 2.9.

2.7-1: Anterior pituitary peptides. Hypophysectomy causes an immediate cessation of lactation (Fig. 2.7). Restoration of lactation in rabbits requires administration of only prolactin, whereas other species require prolactin, growth hormone, ACTH (or an adrenal glucocorticoid), and triiodothyronine. To date, complete restoration of lactation has been achieved with exogenous hormones only in the hypophysectomized goat (Fig. 2.7). Nonetheless, it is apparent that several anterior pituitary peptides are essential for maintenance of lactation.

2.7-1a: Administration of hormones. During early lactation, high doses of exogenous prolactin stimulate milk secretion in rats, primarily by increasing metabolism of the mammary epithelial tissue. Prolactin also reduces the time required for the mammary gland to refill with milk following nursing. During the declining phase of lactation, administration of prolactin in several laboratory species seems to be without effect on lactation. In rabbits, however, prolactin supplementation alone prevents the normal decline in milk yields.

Definitive studies of the response of ruminants to exogenous prolactin have not been performed because of very limited supplies of the peptide. Nevertheless, studies have been conducted suggesting that exogenous prolactin is not galactopoietic. Other approaches used to test the ability of prolactin to stimulate lactation involved the use of various drugs such as TRH and tranquilizers, which stimulate secretion of prolactin. Administration of TRH stimulates small increases in milk yields in cattle and women, but since TRH also causes release of growth hormone and thyroxine, one cannot ascribe the milk yield response solely to prolactin. Perphenazine increases secretion of prolactin but has no effect on milk yields in dairy ewes. Increasing daily light from 8 to 16 hr/day also increases secretion of prolactin and increases milk yields, but a direct cause-effect relationship has yet to be established.

In laboratory species, administration of growth hormone does not affect production of milk, but in ruminants, exogenous growth hormone is clearly galactopoietic. Purified growth hormone from bovine anterior pituitary glands administered three times per week stimulated milk production 18% and reduced feed requirements 29%. Recently, bovine growth hormone has been synthesized in the laboratory by recombinant DNA procedures. Growth hormone synthesized in this manner stimulated milk production in high-producing cows. It has been postulated that secretion of growth hormone increases diversion of nutrients from body stores to the mammary gland. Indeed, growth hormone stimulates milk yield at the expense of body tissue, probably adipose. Thus, whether or not growth hormone will have long-term beneficial effects on milk production and efficiency is yet to be determined.

The effects of TSH and ACTH on lactation are mediated through the thyroid and adrenal hormones, respectively. These aspects will be described in 2.7-2 and 2.7-5.

2.7-1b: Hormone concentrations in serum. In cattle, prolactin concentrations in blood are positively correlated with milk yield, but the coefficients are low. Increased clearance and secretion rates of prolactin are greater in early rather than late lactation, and these are associated with increased milk yields. In early lactation, milking or suckling will cause an acute increase in concentrations of serum prolactin in a variety of species (Fig. 2.11). However, as lactation progresses, quantities of prolactin released at each milking gradually diminish (Fig. 2.12). Increased secretion of prolactin is maintained as long as the milking stimulus is applied to the teat. Release of prolactin at milking is associated with a decrease in activity of PIF (and dopamine) in the hypothalamus. Furthermore, increasing the concentration of dopamine inhibits milking-induced release (as well as basal secretion) of prolactin. Changes in prolactin and dopamine with milking can be induced by stimulating the mammary nerve; thus, the mammary nerve, not exteroceptive stimuli from the offspring or milkers, mediates milking-induced release of prolactin. Moreover, washing the udder without removing milk from the mammary gland also causes prolactin release. In addition to reduced dopamine secretion at suckling, there is some evidence in rats that suckling stimulates release of TRH from the hypothalamus, which in turn induces release of prolactin and TSH.

Suppression of prolactin secretion in monogastric species markedly inhibits lactational performance. Surprisingly, in ruminants, suppression of

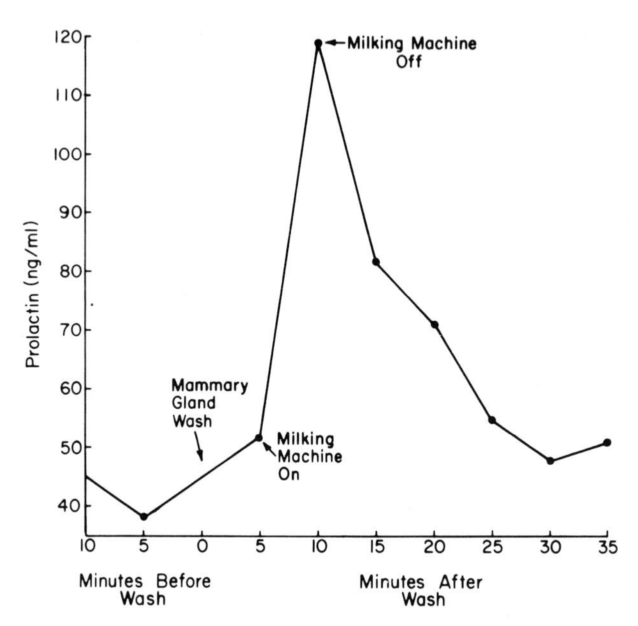

Fig. 2.11. Concentrations of serum prolactin during milking of cows in early stages of lactation. (Drawn from Tucker 1971)

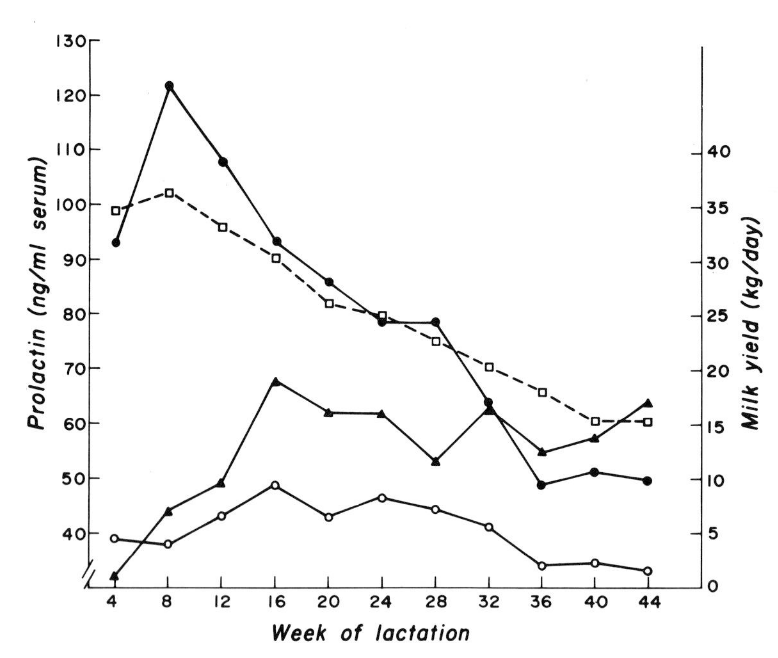

Fig. 2.12. Concentrations of serum prolactin during lactation of cows. Samples of blood were collected 1 hr before milking (○), 5 min after milking (●), and 1 hr after milking (▲). Average daily milk yield = □. (From Koprowski and Tucker 1973a)

prolactin secretion does not affect milk production during an established lactation.

Mammary uptake of prolactin from blood is greatest during acute release phases, such as during milking or after injection of TRH. Binding of prolactin to its receptor is obligatory for maximal milk secretion in rabbits. Similar information in dairy cattle has yet to be produced. Prolactin is bound to membranes of the rough endoplasmic reticulum, Golgi, and secretory vesicles. Prolactin is secreted into the alveolar lumen and therefore is present in milk; its function in milk remains unknown.

Acute nursing releases growth hormone in rats and goats, but concentrations of growth hormone in cows do not change during milking. Basal concentrations (Fig. 2.13) and TRH-induced releases of growth hormone are greatest in early and lowest in late stages of lactation in cattle. These changes parallel changes in intensity of milk secretion and nutrient demands on the animal. Mammary uptake of growth hormone occurs when growth hormone is acutely released, and there are reports that growth hormone is present in milk.

2.7-2: Thyroid hormones. Surgical removal of the thyroid gland reduces milk secretion. However, this response is difficult to interpret because the parathyroid glands, located on the thyroid, are also removed (Fig. 2.1), and the parathyroid glands also affect secretion of milk. Destroying only the thyroid cells with radiation (^{131}I) or suppression of endogenous secretion of thyroxine with a goitrogen has led to reduced yields of milk.

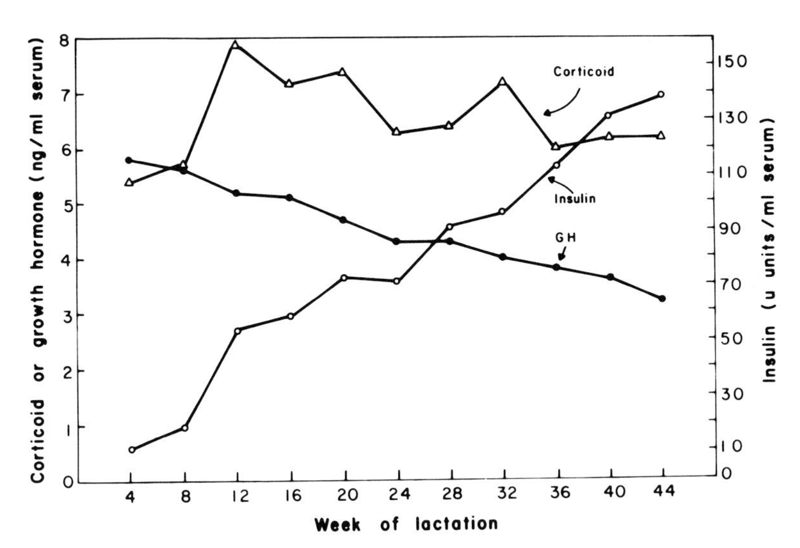

Fig. 2.13. Basal concentrations of growth hormone (*GH*), corticoids, and insulin in serum during lactation of cows. Data were adjusted for differences in stage of pregnancy and season of year. (From Koprowski and Tucker 1973b)

The conclusion is that thyroid secretions strongly influence milk synthesis, even though some milk secretion will continue in the absence of thyroid hormones.

2.7-2a: Administration of hormones. There is little doubt that exogenous thyroxine or triiodothyronine, given to normal animals, initially stimulates lactational performance. Thyroid-active compounds have been used commercially for many years to stimulate lactation in dairy cattle; the most common is iodinated casein (thyroprotein). Chemical iodination of casein leads to the formation of thyroxine and the product is orally active. Thus, feeding thyroprotein increases concentrations of thyroxine in blood. Feeding thyroprotein during early lactation raises milk production about 10%, and during late lactation, yield may be increased as much as 20%. Usually, the greatest milk producers have the greatest response. The galactopoietic effects of thyroprotein usually last only 2–4 mo, and subsequent yields are often below those normally expected. The net result shows there is no clear benefit over the entire lactation. Extra feed must be provided during the feeding of thyroprotein, and it should be fed only when cows are gaining in body weight, otherwise cows lose excessive amounts of weight. Milk yields usually decline when thyroprotein is removed from the diet.

2.7-2b: Hormone concentrations in serum. Thyroid secretion rates and concentrations of thyroxine and triiodothyronine in serum are reduced during lactation. Moreover, as milk yields increase, concentrations of serum thyroxine decrease (Fig. 2.14). In cattle, milking does not cause an acute release of thyroxine. There is no change in thyroxine-binding globulin, the major thyroxine-carrying blood protein, during lactation. Coupled with the decrease in concentrations of the thyroid hormones, the facts suggest the lactating animal is in a hypothyroid state. Providing extra thyroxine during lactation probably explains the galactopoietic effects of thyroprotein in dairy cattle. There is evidence that degradation of thyroxine in blood is heritable and correlated with a bull's transmitting ability for milk yield. Clearly, secretion of the thyroid hormones affects milk yield.

2.7-2c: Calcitonin. Calcitonin is a hormone released from the thyroid gland in response to high concentrations of calcium in blood. Calcitonin normally prevents increases in serum calcium and phosphorus, especially during lactation. Calcitonin concentrations in blood of lactating animals is greater than concentrations in nonlactating animals. Suppression of serum calcium and phosphorus is achieved more easily in lactating than in nonlactating rats. Calcitonin is undoubtedly of importance in the secretion of milk, especially in view of the high loss of calcium into milk (see Chap. 5).

2.7-3: Parathyroid hormone. Parathyroidectomy reduces milk production and calcium in blood during lactation. Conversely, administration of parathyroid hormone stimulates milk yields and increases concen-

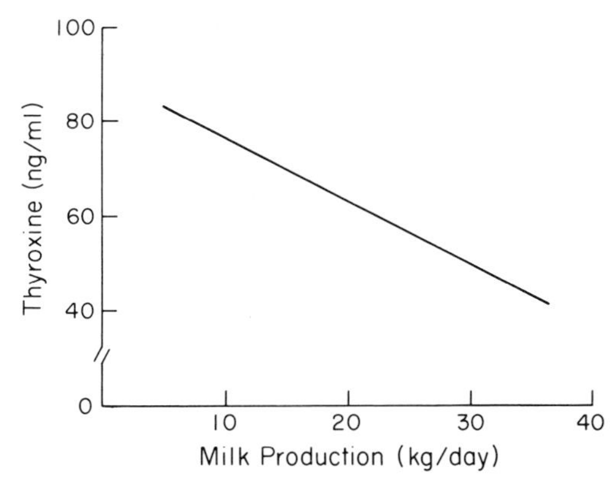

Fig. 2.14. Relationship between concentrations of serum thyroxine and milk yield in cows. (Modified from Vanjonack and Johnson 1975)

trations of serum calcium. Vitamin D is metabolized to 25-hydroxyvitamin D, which, under the influence of the parathyroid hormone, is converted to 1,25-dihydroxyvitamin D (1,25-OHD). The 1,25-OHD then acts on the intestine to stimulate calcium absorption and, in concert with parathyroid hormone, increases calcium mobilization from bone. Hypocalcemia induces secretion of parathyroid hormone, which in turn stimulates production of 1,25-OHD. Parathyroidectomy of lactating rats inhibits the normally observed increase in 1,25-OHD, indicating parathyroidectomy is a primary modulator of 1,25-OHD. In view of the large calcium drain of lactation (see Chap. 5), interaction of the parathyroid hormone and vitamin D metabolites are important for maintaining lactation. Indeed, the concentrations of 1,25-OHD in serum are markedly elevated during lactation.

2.7-4: Endocrine pancreas. Exogenous administration of insulin suppresses lactation and, paradoxically, insufficiency of insulin decreases milk yield. When extra glucose is supplied, exogenous insulin stimulates lactation. Concentrations of insulin are negatively correlated with milk yield, being low in early and high in late stages of lactation (Fig. 2.13). Mammary uptake of insulin, associated with uptake of glucose, is maintained throughout and is essential for maintenance of lactation.

2.7-5: Adrenal steroids. Removal of adrenal glands impairs milk secretion, enzymatic function, and casein mRNA synthesis. Administration of individual mineralo- or glucocorticoids partially restores milk yield in adrenalectomized animals, but a combination of mineralo- and glucocorticoids is more effective. This suggests the reduced lactation following adrenalectomy is due to defects in electrolyte, protein, and carbohydrate metabolism. Administration of glucocorticoids to intact laboratory species retards the normal decline in milk yield, as measured by litter weight gain (Fig. 2.15). Many of these effects of glucocorticoids are exerted by maintenance of mammary cell numbers and metabolic activity.

In contrast to results in laboratory species, the role of adrenal steroids in lactation in ruminants is less clear. For example, administration of therapeutic doses of ACTH or adrenal glucocorticoids almost invariably leads to reduced milk secretion. In one study, when smaller doses of glucocorticoids were given, milk yields were increased, whereas in another study, low doses of supplemental glucocorticoids were without effect. Basal secretion of glucocorticoids does not change during lactation (Fig. 2.13). In cattle, glucocorticoids are released acutely in response to milking stimuli and the response does not change as lactation progresses. However, in rats, basal and suckling-induced increases in glucocorticoids decrease with advancing lactation and declining milk yields. Moreover, CBG is reduced during early lactation and increased during late stages of lactation, which may indicate

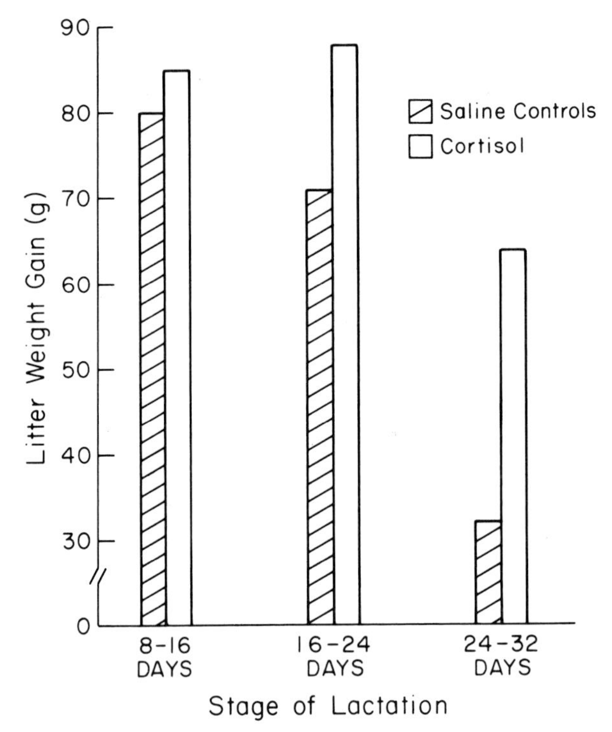

Fig. 2.15. Litter weight of rats injected with saline or cortisol between days 16 and 32 of lactation. To maintain an intense nursing stimulus, when litters attained 16 days of age, they were replaced with 8-day-old foster litters (at days 16 and 24 of lactation). (Drawn from Thatcher and Tucker 1970)

that decreased milk synthesis is coupled with reduced availability of glucocorticoids. At relatively low ambient temperatures (15°C), high-producing cows have greater concentrations of glucocorticoids than low-producing cows. In contrast, at 30°C high producers secrete much lower quantities of glucocorticoids than low producers. This may explain, in part, why high producers are less persistent than low producers during hot weather. The conclusion is that glucocorticoids are essential for lactation, but either increased secretion rates above normal or decreased secretion rates (as may occur during hot weather) decrease milk production.

Glucocorticoids are taken up from blood at milking and are bound to specific receptors in the cytosol of the mammary cell (Fig. 2.2). Mammary tissue from lactating cows possesses about four times as many mammary receptors for glucocorticoids as tissue from nonlactating cows. Glucocorticoid-binding activity is correlated positively with glucose uptake into mammary tissue. Concentrations of corticosterone in milk are about equal to those found in blood serum, but the primary glucocorticoid in cattle, cortisol, is found in much lower concentrations in milk than in blood. The functional significance of the glucocorticoids in milk remains to be elucidated.

2.7-6: Ovarian steroids. Ovariectomy during lactation has little effect on milk secretion. However, exogenous estrogens have been used clinically to inhibit lactation. There is evidence that estrogen receptors are present in mammary tissue and are undoubtedly involved in the inhibitory response. Indeed, estrogens have been reported to interfere with milk ejection by causing the disappearance of myofilaments of the myoepithelial cells. Thus, the inhibitory effects of estrogens are exerted directly on the mammary tissue.

There is some evidence that low doses of estrogens stimulate milk secretion, and these effects are probably mediated by alteration of secretion of other galactopoietic hormones from the anterior pituitary gland.

Although progesterone inhibits lactogenesis, it does not affect milk yields when given during the postpartum period. This lack of effect may be associated with a marked decrease in the number of progesterone-binding sites in lactating mammary tissue. Therefore, with fewer receptors, the biological action of progesterone would not occur. Another possible explanation for the lack of effect of progesterone during lactation may be that progesterone has a greater affinity for milk fat than for receptors; thus, milk fat may sequester progesterone, thereby nullifying its biological activity.

Progesterone is sequestered in the milk fat droplets and is released into the alveolar lumen as fat is secreted. Progesterone concentrations in milk parallel very closely the concentrations in blood. Milk progesterone concentrations have been used in cattle to diagnose pregnancy by collecting a milk sample 20–22 days after insemination. If progesterone concentration in milk is elevated, the cow may be pregnant (about 70% would be expected) or in the luteal phase of the estrous cycle. However, if progesterone is reduced in milk, one may be approximately 90% certain the animal is not pregnant.

2.8: NEURAL CONTROL OF LACTATION

There is no convincing evidence that secretory nerves directly affect secretory activity of the mammary alveolar epithelium. In fact, completely denervated glands will secrete milk. There is no doubt, however, that stimulation of the mammary afferent nerves transmits impulses via the spinal cord to the hypothalamus, causing a variety of hormonal responses, which have been described in previous sections. These hormones affect cell numbers and metabolic processes of the mammary alveolar cells.

Feed intake and water consumption markedly affect rates of milk secretion, and both of these processes are regulated by the hypothalamus. Feed intake is increased postpartum, even when milk is not removed from the udder for prolonged periods. Feed and water intake are believed to be regulated by the central nervous system. The most dramatic evidence for the role of the nervous system in lactation is associated with the milk ejection reflex, a process described in 2.9.

2.9: MILK EJECTION

To remove milk, resistance of the streak canals in the teats must be overcome, and contraction of the myoepithelial cells must occur to force milk from the alveoli through the ducts. Contraction of myoepithelial cells involves activation of a neurohormonal reflex (milk ejection) and is associated with release of the octapeptide, oxytocin. Milk ejection can occur under water or on land and usually, although not always, occurs at the time of milking or nursing. Nursing may be continuous, as in the kangaroo; or may occur at intervals as short as 30 min, as in dolphins; every 4–6 hr in cattle; once a day in rabbits; or once a week, as in northern fur seals.

2.9-1: Neural components. The milk ejection reflex involves activation of nerve receptors in the skin of the teat that are sensitive to pressure. Mechanical stimulation of the teats activates these receptors, which leads to increased impulse transmission in the afferent mammary nerves (Fig. 2.16). Nerve impulses destined to evoke release of oxytocin enter the spinal cord bilaterally via the dorsal roots. The nerve fibers ascend the spinal cord in the dorsal funiculus to the midbrain, where the bilateral pathway projects into dorsal and ventral paths into the posterior hypothalamus. There are two hypothalamic sites, the paraventricular and supraoptic nuclei, that synthesize oxytocin and its carrier protein, neurophysin. It is likely that the afferent neural pathway innervates the paraventricular nuclei and/or the pituitary stalk. The afferent neural pathway to the supraoptic nucleus has not been clearly defined; it is part of the spinothalamic system, which is usually activated by abrupt stimuli. Hence, milk ejection occurs from stimuli of high intensity and relatively long duration, such as milking or suckling stimuli.

On the other hand, there is little doubt that cues arising from the external environment, cerebral cortex, or conditioned responses can cause release of oxytocin. For example, milk frequently leaks from teats of ani-

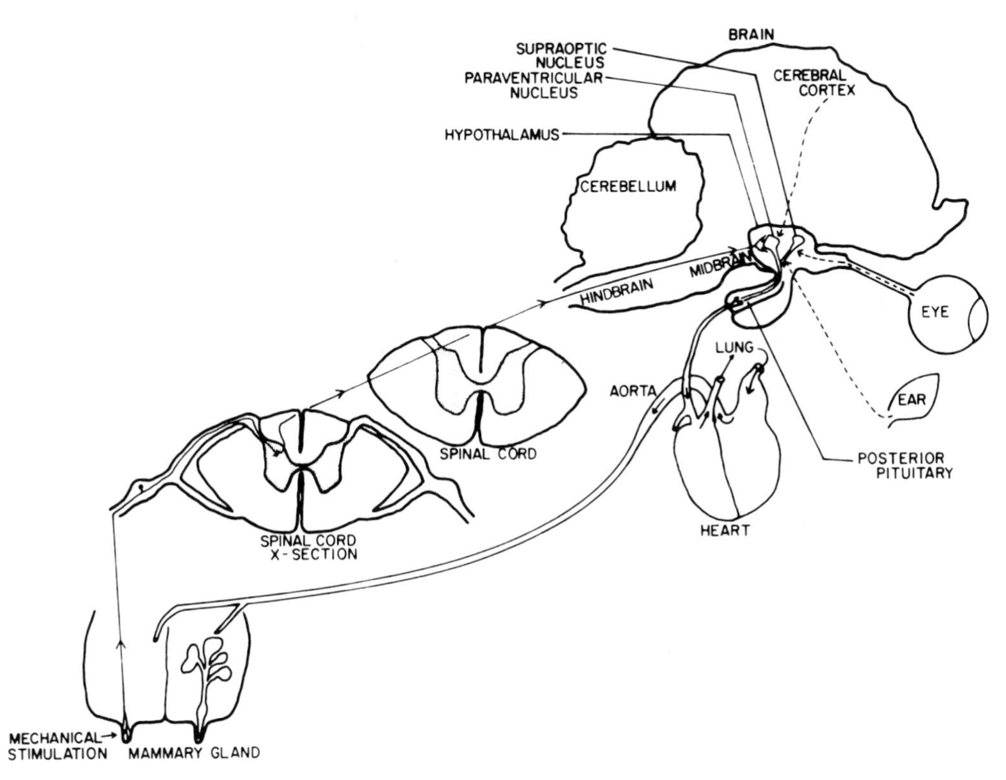

Fig. 2.16. Neural pathway for the milk ejection reflex. Mechanical (sensory) stimulation of the teats initiates a neural reflex that travels from the teats to the spinal cord, to the paraventricular and supraoptic nuclei of the hypothalamus, and then to the posterior pituitary gland, where oxytocin is discharged into the blood. Oxytocin binds to and causes contraction of the myoepithelial cells, thereby completing the circuit and evoking ejection of milk. Signals via the cerebral cortex, eyes, and ears also may elicit release of oxytocin. (From Tucker 1978)

mals immediately before milking or nursing. Moreover, direct stimulation of higher brain centers also causes release of oxytocin.

The final common pathway from the paraventricular and supraoptic nuclei consists of neurosecretory axons of the hypothalamo-neurohypophysial tract that pass through the pituitary stalk and terminate in the posterior pituitary (Fig. 2.3); the cell bodies of these nerves are in the paraventricular and supraoptic nuclei. These nuclei receive excitatory (cholinergic), as well as inhibitory (noradrenergic), neurons from other parts of the brain (Fig. 2.17). These stimulatory and inhibitory neurons represent part of the mechanism whereby oxytocin secretion is controlled. There is substantial evidence that neurons of the hypothalamo-neurohypophysial tract are capable of transmitting nerve impulses in response to milking, and these impulses are involved in release of oxytocin into blood.

2.9-2: Hormonal component. Following synthesis in the paraventricular and supraoptic nuclei, oxytocin becomes weakly bound to neurophysin and forms secretory granules (Fig. 2.17). Granules move down the axons to the posterior pituitary at a rate of 2–3 mm/hr. Within the posterior pituitary, there are numerous swellings along the neurosecretory axons termed Herring bodies, which are storage depots for the neurosecretory granules of oxytocin-neurophysin. At the time of milking, oxytocin is released from the granules by exocytosis in response to electrical activity associated with nerve impulse propagation. Potential factors controlling exocytosis include cholinergic and adrenergic neurons in the hypothalamus, nerve impulse propagation down the hypothalamo-neurohypophysial tract, influx of calcium from the neuron into the vesicle that activates ATPase, and prostaglandins. Neurophysin is released coincidently with oxytocin but is probably not bound to oxytocin in blood. In cattle, oxytocin increases rapidly in blood following mechanical stimulation of teats and reaches a peak within 2 min (Fig. 2.18). Concentrations then rapidly decline, reaching basal conditions within 10 min. Therefore, to achieve maximal removal of milk in cattle, it is important to attach the milking machine to teats within 30–60 sec of stimulating the teats, before efficacy of oxytocin disappears. Secondary discharges of oxytocin may occur late in the milking process of cattle. In rats, oxytocin release may occur repeatedly, provided the stimulus to the teats is periodic rather than sustained.

An essential component of the milk ejection reflex is the binding of oxytocin, specifically and with high affinity, to protein receptor sites on the myoepithelial cells. This results in contraction of the myoepithelial cell and expulsion of milk from the mammary gland. The number of oxytocin receptors increases to maximal amounts during the first lactation, then probably persists for the lifetime of the myoepithelial cell.

2.9-3: Stimulation of milk ejection. Suckling and milking are the most potent natural stimuli that cause milk ejection. Other stimuli ranked

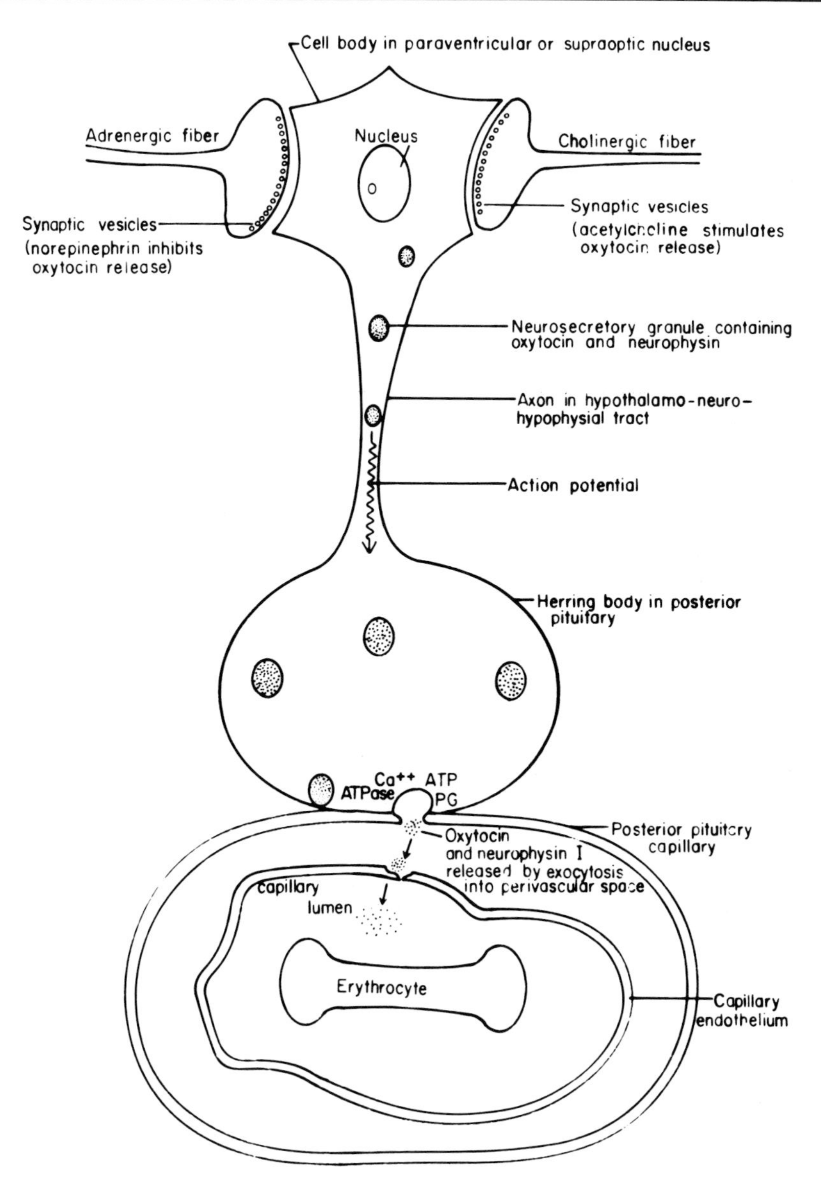

Fig. 2.17. Anatomical relationship between neurons in the paraventricular, or supraoptic nucleus, where oxytocin and neurophysin are synthesized, and the Herring body of the posterior pituitary gland, where oxytocin and neurophysin are discharged into capillaries in response to an action potential of nerve impulse. The action potential stimulates synthesis as well as release of oxytocin. *ATP* = adenosine triphosphate; *PG* = prostaglandins. (From Tucker 1978)

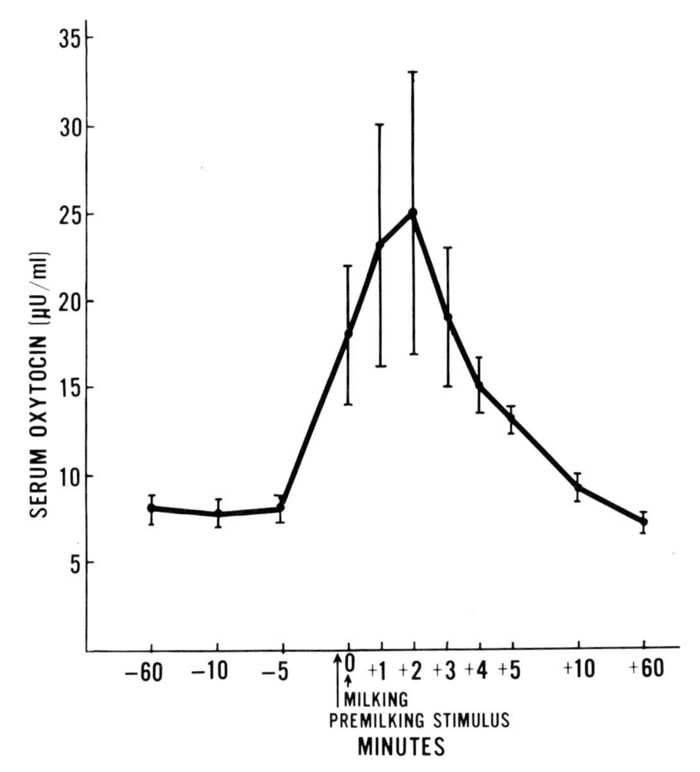

Fig. 2.18. Concentrations of serum oxytocin during milking of cows. (From Gorewit 1979)

in decreasing order of effectiveness are washing the udder plus presentation of calf to mother, washing the udder, and, finally, presentation of the calf. Visual and auditory cues associated with milkers and milking routines may also cause milk ejection.

2.9-4: Inhibition of milk ejection. Various stressful stimuli that inhibit milk ejection are associated with increased activity of the sympathetic nervous system. In fact, sympathectomy increases the rate of milk flow. Increased secretion of catecholamines during stressful activities increases discharge of epinephrine and norepinephrine. These catecholamines increase the tone of the smooth muscles of the mammary ducts and blood vessels, resulting in the reduction of oxytocin reaching the myoepithelial cells and partial occlusion of the mammary ducts. Moreover, epinephrine directly blocks oxytocin from binding to myoepithelial cells; this is termed peripheral inhibition of milk ejection. Thus, exogenous oxytocin will not cause milk ejection in animals exhibiting peripheral inhibition.

The most common cause of failure of milk ejection is associated with stress of milking in the early postpartum period, which sometimes inhibits release of oxytocin from the posterior pituitary gland. Primiparous cows frequently exhibit this central inhibition of milk ejection. In these circumstances, exogenous oxytocin is administered, causing milk ejection, and this practice is warranted because failure to remove milk, especially in early lactation, may reduce milk yields for the duration of that lactation. Recent evidence in mice suggests that acute thermal stress inhibiting suckling-induced release of oxytocin can be overcome with exogenous oxytocin. This example of central inhibition of milk ejection is mediated by endogenous opioid peptides in the hypothalamus. Other evidence suggests that catecholamines are involved in the central, as well as peripheral, inhibition of milk ejection. In any event, it seems most probable that milk ejection occurs as a result of oxytocin release, which is normally coupled with inhibition of the central and peripheral inhibitory controls.

REFERENCES

Akers, R. M., D. E. Bauman, A. V. Capuco, G. T. Goodman, and H. A. Tucker. 1981. Prolactin regulation of milk secretion and biochemical differentiation of mammary epithelial cells in periparturient cows. Endocrinology 109:23.

Anderson, R. R. 1974. Endocrinological control. In Lactation, 1:97. See Larson and Smith 1974.

Bath, D. L., F. N. Dickinson, H. A. Tucker, and R. D. Appleman. 1978. General endocrinology in dairy cattle. In Dairy Cattle: Principles, Practices, Problems, Profits. 2d ed., 267. Philadelphia: Lea & Febiger.

Bauman, D. E., M. J. de Geeter, C. J. Peel, G. M. Lanza, R. C. Gorewit, and R. W. Hammond. 1982. Effect of recombinantly derived growth hormone (bGH) on lactational performance of high yielding dairy cows. J. Dairy Sci. Suppl. 1, 65:121. Abstract.

Bolander, F. F., K. R. Nicholas, J. J. Van Wyk, and Y. J. Topper. 1981. Insulin is essential for accumulation of casein mRNA in mouse mammary epithelial cells. Proc. Natl. Acad. Sci. 78:5682.

Bradley, T. R., and P. M. Clarke. 1956. The response of rabbit mammary glands to locally administered prolactin. J. Endocrinol. 14:28.

Cowie, A. T. 1969. General hormonal factors involved in lactogenesis. In Lactogenesis: The Initiation of Milk Secretion at Parturition, ed. M. Reynolds and S. J. Folley, 157. Philadelphia: Univ. Penn. Press.

de Greef, W. J., and T. J. Visser. 1981. Evidence for the involvement of hypothalamic dopamine and thyrotrophin-releasing hormone in suckling-induced release of prolactin. J. Endocrinol. 91:213.

Delouis, C., J. Djiane, L. M. Houdebine, and M. Terqui. 1980. Relation between hormones and mammary gland function. J. Dairy Sci. 63:1492.

Djiane, J., C. Delouis, and P. A. Kelly. 1982. Prolactin receptor turnover in explants of pseudopregnant rabbit mammary gland. Mol. Cell. Endocrinol. 25:163.

Eakle, K. A., Y. Arima, P. Swanson, H. Grimek, and R. D. Bremel. 1982. A 32,000 molecular weight protein from bovine placenta with placental lactogen-like activity in radioreceptor assays. Endocrinology 110:1758.

Falconer, I. R. 1980. Aspects of the biochemistry, physiology, and endocrinology of lactation. Aust. J. Biol. Sci. 33:71.

Ganguly, R., P. K. Majumder, N. Ganguly, and M. R. Banerjee. 1982. The mechanism of progesterone-glucocorticoid interaction in regulation of casein gene expression. J. Biol. Chem. 257:2182.

Gorewit, R. C. 1979. Method for determining oxytocin concentrations in unextracted sera; characterization in lactating cattle. Proc. Soc. Exp. Biol. Med. 160:80.

Grosvenor, C. E., and F. Mena. 1974. Neural and hormonal control of milk secretion and milk ejection. In Lactation, 1:227. See Larson and Smith 1974.

Haldar, J., and V. Bade. 1981. Involvement of opioid peptides in the inhibition of oxytocin by heat stress in lactating mice. Proc. Soc. Exp. Biol. Med. 168:10.

Hobbs, A. A., D. A. Richards, D. J. Kessler, and J. M. Rosen. 1982. Complex hormonal regulation of rat casein gene expression. J. Biol. Chem. 257:3598.

Houdebine, L. M. 1980. Role of prolactin, glucocorticoids and progesterone in the control of casein gene expression. In Hormone and Cell Regulation, vol. 4, ed. J. Dumont and J. Nunez, 175. Amsterdam: Elsevier/North-Holland.

Koprowski, J. A., and H. A. Tucker. 1973a. Serum prolactin during various physiological states and its relationship to milk production in the bovine. Endocrinology 92:1480.

______. 1973b. Bovine serum growth hormone, corticoids, and insulin during lactation. Endocrinology 93:645.

Larson, B. L., ed. 1978. Lactation: A Comprehensive Treatise, vol. 4. New York: Academic.

Larson, B. L., and V. R. Smith, eds. 1974. Lactation: A Comprehensive Treatise, vol. 1. New York: Academic.

Mena, F., P. Pacheco, N. S. Whitworth, and C. E. Grosvenor. 1980. Recent data concerning the secretion and function of oxytocin and prolactin during lactation in the rat and rabbit. Front. Horm. Res. 6:217.

Plotsky, P. M., and J. D. Neill. 1982. The decrease in hypothalamic dopamine secretion induced by suckling: Comparison of voltametric and radioisotopic methods of measurement. Endocrinology 110:691.

Shiu, R. P. C., and H. G. Friesen. 1980. Mechanism of action of prolactin in the control of mammary gland function. Annu. Rev. Physiol. 42:83.

Soloff, M. S. 1982. Oxytocin receptors and mammary myoepithelial cells. J. Dairy Sci. 65:326.

Thatcher, W. W., and H. A. Tucker. 1970. Lactational performance of rats injected with oxytocin, cortisol-21-acetate, prolactin, and growth hormone during prolonged lactation. Endocrinology 86:237.

Tindal, J. S. 1978. Neuroendocrine control of lactation. In Lactation, 4:67. See Larson 1978.

Topper, Y. J., and C. S. Freeman. 1980. Multiple hormone interactions in the developmental biology of the mammary gland. Physiol. Rev. 60:1049.

Tucker, H. A. 1969. Factors affecting mammary gland cell numbers. J. Dairy Sci. 52:721.

______. 1971. Hormonal response to milking. J. Anim. Sci. Suppl. 1, 32:137.

______. 1974. General endocrinological control of lactation. In Lactation, 1:277. See Larson and Smith 1974.

______. 1978. The role of physiological factors in stimulating the milk ejection reflex. In Proceedings of International Symposium on Machine Milking, 21. 17th Annual Meeting National Mastitis Council, Inc. Washington, D.C.: National Mastitis Council.

______. 1979. Endocrinology of lactation. Semin. Perinatol. 3:199.

______. 1981. Physiological control of mammary growth, lactogenesis, and lactation. J. Dairy Sci. 64:1403.

Tucker, H. A., and J. Meites. 1965. Induction of lactation in pregnant heifers with 9-fluoroprednisolone acetate. J. Dairy Sci. 48:403.

Vanjonack, W. J., and H. D. Johnson. 1975. Effects of moderate heat and milk yield on plasma thyroxine in cattle. J. Dairy Sci. 58:507.

CHAPTER 3

NUTRITIONAL, METABOLIC, AND ENVIRONMENTAL ASPECTS OF LACTATION

ROBERT J. COLLIER

3.1: INTRODUCTION

Lactation is much more energy expensive than pregnancy. At parturition, transfer of nutrients from the maternal unit to the neonate shifts from the uterus to the mammary gland. The rapidly increasing body mass and growth rate of the offspring is reflected in increasing nutrient drain from the mother.

Just prior to parturition, the fetal calf requires approximately 10% of the dam's net energy intake. However, at peak lactation, the energy requirement for milk synthesis can approach 80% of net energy intake, far exceeding maintenance requirements of the mature animal. Homeorhesis, a shift in nutrient partitioning, requires a number of adaptations within the animal; it is defined as orchestrated changes for the priorities of a physiological state. This type of control is different from homeostasis, in which the classic feedback systems maintain a steady state of a given physiological function.

Both homeostatic and homeorhetic mechanisms are required for the lactating animal to maintain metabolic and physiological equilibrium while sustaining a large net energy turnover. The net energy demand of lactation often exceeds the animal's ability to eat, resulting in a negative energy balance. The fate of nutrients taken up for various productive processes in mammals is illustrated in Figure 3.1. How these nutrients are partitioned to various tissues is to a large extent determined by the endocrine system. Endocrine control of lactation is discussed in Chapter 2.

As lactation commences, feed intake, which is controlled by the hypothalamus, increases, thereby increasing the intake nutrient pool. In addition, during lactation mammals develop cravings for specific types of nutrients, such as salt or water. These cravings are also controlled by the hypothalamus. As feed intake increases, flow rate of digesta through the alimentary canal increases, and the small and large intestine increase in size to accommodate the increased nutrient intake pool.

Nutrients absorbed from the digestive tract enter a metabolizable nutrient pool. Plasma volume increases with onset of lactation, and the circulating pool size of many nutrients also increases.

Nutrients in the metabolizable pool are deposited in reserve or utilized in a productive process. To meet lactation requirements, many nutrient reserve sites, such as adipose and bone, change from nutrient deposition of calcium in bone and fatty acids in adipose tissue to mobilization of these nutrients. This change from deposition to mobilization is under endocrine control.

The metabolizable nutrient pool is stored in the depot nutrient pool or utilized to meet maintenance, growth, reproduction, or lactation requirements. Partitioning of the metabolizable nutrient pool occurs on several levels of mammalian organization: distribution of cardiac output and nu-

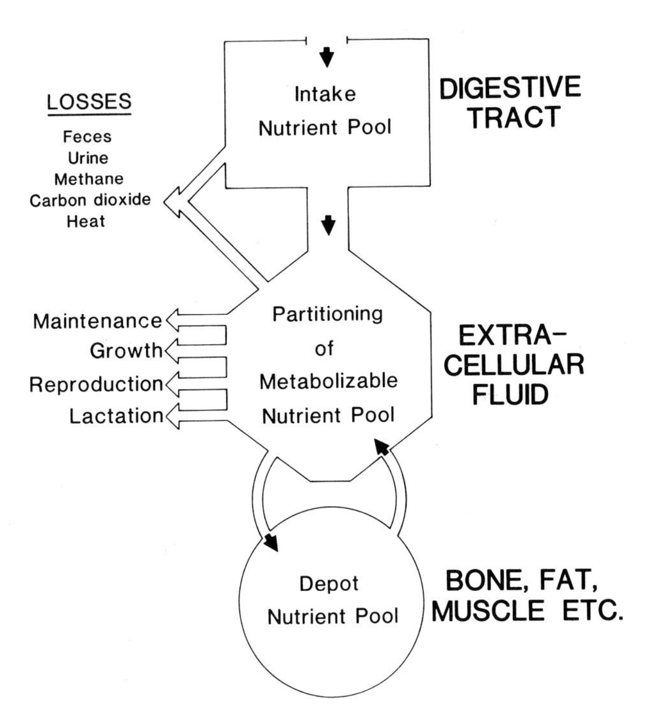

Fig. 3.1. Routes of nutrient flow.

trients to given organs, metabolic activity of the cell types and their ability to transport nutrients from blood, and the activity of the endocrine system, which regulates the entire process.

The objective of this chapter is to delineate the formation of milk product precursors and describe their partitioning with onset of lactation.

3.2: DIGESTION

3.2-1: Digestive tract anatomy. The digestive system takes in raw food materials and converts them to readily usable substrates. The variety of plant and animal food sources available has resulted in variations in the pattern of digestion in a given species. However, basic similarities exist among all mammals. These include the process of mastication and salivation, gastric digestion, proteolysis and lipolysis in the small intestine, bacterial fermentation in the large intestine, and absorption of various substrates and by-products at key points along the digestive tract. The residue of this process is removed from the tract by the process of defecation.

The class Mammalia has been divided by feeding habits and alimentary development into four major groups.

1. Carnivorous and insectivorous mammals. Foregut fermentation is not present and the large intestine is short. The caecum is either not present or very simple.
2. Omnivorous mammals. Foregut fermentation is not present. However, digestion of plant fiber can take place in the large intestine, which is well developed.
3. Herbivorous mammals with a foregut fermentation chamber. All ruminants belong to this group. The foregut may have three or four chambers. The large intestine is well developed and may or may not include a caecum.
4. Herbivorous mammals without a foregut fermentation chamber. The stomach is simple, and the large intestine displays its greatest development in this group. The caecum may be larger than the remainder of the large intestine.

Regardless of the food source and type of digestive tract, the process of digestion requires not only physical breakdown by mastication and mixing but also chemical cleavage of the bonds that hold substrates together. Gastric acids and enzymes are responsible for the majority of the chemical changes occurring in food as it moves along the digestive tract. Table 3.1 summarizes the enzymes and acids involved in the digestive process and substrates utilized.

Table 3.1. Location of digestive processes in the mammalian digestive system

Location	Enzyme	Substrate	End Product
Mouth	Amylase	Starch and carbohydrates	Maltose, dextrose
Rumen	β-1,4 glucosidase	Cellulose	Cellobiose, glucose
	Maltase	Maltose	Glucose
	β-1,4 glucosidase	Hemicellulose	Pentose
	Microbial enzymes	Simple sugars	Volatile fatty acids
Stomach (abomasum)	Pepsin	Proteins	Proteoses, peptones
	Lipase	Fats	Glycerol, long-chain fatty acids
Duodenum	Trypsin	Proteins, peptides	Amino acids
	Chymotrypsin	Peptones, proteoses	Peptides
	Amylase	Starch	Maltose
	Lipase	Fats	Long-chain fatty acids, glycerol
	Carboxypeptidase	Peptides	Amino acids, peptides
	Bile	Fats	Emulsified fats
Small intestine	Peptidase	Peptides	Amino acids, dipeptides
	Sucrase	Sucrose	Glucose, fructose
	Maltase	Maltose	Glucose
	Polynucleotidase	Nucleic acid	Mononucleotides
Large intestine	β-1,4 glucosidase	Cellulose	Cellobiose
Caecum	Microbial enzymes		Glucose, volatile fatty acids

Source: Adapted from Campbell and Lasley 1975.

Digestion begins in the mouth with mastication and initial stages of starch breakdown via amylase. Mastication is repeated in ruminants as fibrous material is brought back up from the rumen during the process of rumination. This allows consumption of large quantities of food in a short period without having to complete the mastication process. The primary digestive process in the rumen completes the breakdown of carbohydrates via salivary amylase, microbial cellulases, and uptake of sugars by bacteria and protozoa. In ruminants, very little carbohydrate escapes digestion in the rumen. In nonruminants, carbohydrates are further digested in the small intestine. Initial steps in breakdown of protein and fat begin in the stomach of nonruminants or abomasum of ruminants. Completion of fat and protein breakdown and uptake occurs in the small intestine. In some animals, such as rabbits and horses (group 4), appreciable fermentation occurs in the large intestine and/or caecum.

Metabolic pathways involved in the major aspects of digestion and absorption sites of the end products are discussed in 3.3.

3.2-2: Control of digesta flow. The four major factors that influence the rate at which nutrients flow from the digestive tract into the circulating substrate pool are feed quality, quantity of feed intake, passage rate of digesta in the alimentary canal, and efficiency of digestion. Feed quality will be discussed in 3.4. Food intake is a voluntary motor activity primarily under control of the hypothalamic feed intake centers. The major nuclei in the hypothalamus controlling feed intake are the ventromedial nucleus (satiety center) and the lateral hypothalamus (feeding center). Factors known to influence the hypothalamic feed intake centers are the physiological state of the animal, feedback from digestive tract sensory receptors, environmental temperature, and concentration of circulating substrates. Receptors identified in the richly innervated gut wall include stretch receptors, pH receptors, chemoreceptors, and osmoreceptors. Thus, degree of feed intake is influenced by several factors. Feed requirements can easily be calculated if age, level of milk production, and quality of feed are known (see 3.4).

Passage rate of digesta is primarily controlled by motility of the digestive tract. Food is subjected to several processes involving muscle contraction during digestion. These include mastication, insalivation, deglutition, rumination (in ruminants), gastric contraction, and movement through the small and large intestines. These movements can be broken down into three major groups: fragmentation, mixing, and propulsion. Fragmentation occurs primarily during mastication and/or rumination. Mixing occurs throughout the digestive tract but is most prominent in the rumen and stomach. Propulsive movements are required all along the tract to move the digesta.

Additional factors that influence the rate of passage are the quantity, quality, and size of fiber ingested; environmental temperature; osmolality; and pathological conditions. Fiber digestibility and size influence the time required in the rumen for digestion. Environmental heat stress directly influences digestive tract motility, slowing passage rate and thereby increasing digestive efficiency. Increasing the osmolality of the rumen also has been shown to affect the rate of rumen turnover.

3.2-3: Nonruminant digestion. Since all mammals without foregut fermentation (see 3.2-1: groups 1, 2, and 4) have no bacterial fermentation of food before entering the stomach, glucose is absorbed from the digestive tract. However, some herbivores (e.g., rabbit, horse) carry out fermentation in the large intestine, and the organic acids generated are produced after the main site of absorption in the small intestine. Any bacterial protein and vitamins produced in the large intestine are poorly absorbed. Thus, the advantage of nonruminant digestion is a better utilization of carbohydrates of dietary origin. The disadvantage is the relatively poor utilization of plant structural polysaccharides (e.g., cellulose). Some herbivores partially alleviate the poor utilization of organic acids, microbial protein, and vitamins produced in the large intestine by ingesting fecal material (coprophagy).

3.2-4: Ruminant digestion. Ruminants are particularly suited to take advantage of plant cellulose digestion to provide energy and carbon skeletons for product formation. Most animals domesticated for milk production (except the horse) are ruminants. One of the primary reasons for this is that humans can harvest a crop (milk) from land unsuitable for cereal grain production.

The ruminant stomach has four compartments. The first of these is the reticulum, which has three openings. The first opens into the rumen, the second communicates with the esophagus, and the third is the reticuloomasal orifice. The primary functions of the reticulum are to control the direction of food mass flow and to form the bolus for passage back up the esophagus during the process of rumination.

The second and largest compartment is the rumen, where fermentation occurs. The rumen wall is muscular and contractions serve to mix rumen contents. The lining is covered with papillae and subdivided by projections termed pillars. The papillae greatly increase surface area of the rumen and are the site of volatile fatty acid absorption.

The third compartment is the omasum, which opens anteriorly into the reticulum and posteriorly into the abomasum. The omasum also is termed the manyplies, which refers to the large number of folds within the organ. The omasum is believed to be involved in absorption of water and some fatty acids by papillae on the folds. Digesta is pumped from the omasum directly into the abomasum.

The abomasum, or fourth compartment, resembles the simple stomach of the nonruminant. Anteriorly, it communicates with the omasum and posteriorly with the small intestine. This is the site of gastric acid production and initiation of proteolysis.

The remainder of the digestive tract of ruminants is similar to that of nonruminants; digesta flow through the small and large intestines to complete the process of digestion.

3.2-5: Microbiology of the rumen. One of the main features of the rumen is its relatively constant anaerobic environment. This permits a continuous growth of bacteria and protozoans, both anaerobic populations. It also results in a continual flow of products, such as organic acids, directly from the rumen into the bloodstream or further down the digestive tract, as is the case for protein of bacterial or protozoan origin.

Table 3.2 lists representative examples of rumen bacteria. As can be noted, some are cellulose degrading, others use the products of cellulose breakdown or act on starches or sugars, which may be present in feed. The bacterial populations break down plant polysaccharides to volatile fatty acids. Their second function is to participate in protein production either by utilizing nonprotein nitrogen to produce ammonia, which is then used to synthesize bacterial protein, or by the protozoan population consuming the bacteria and utilizing them as a nitrogen source for protein production. This is further discussed in 3.4-3.

Protozoa, which populate the rumen, are primarily ciliates of two families, Isotrichadae (holotrichs) and Ophryoscolecidae (oligotrichs). As mentioned earlier, all rumen protozoa are anaerobes, which obtain energy for growth and function by fermenting carbohydrates. Bacteria of the rumen provide a nitrogen source, as well as some lipids, for rumen protozoa. Although protozoa are not essential for rumen fermentation, they appear to increase the efficiency of rumen fermentation and, thus, are believed to be beneficial to the host animal.

3.2-6: Pathways of volatile fatty acid synthesis. Several species of bacteria, the majority of which are coccoid forms, have been isolated from rumen fluid. Substrates required by these bacteria are primarily sugars of plant origin or by-products of fermentation. The rumen microbial

Table 3.2. Representative microbes of the rumen

Species	Type	Gram Stain	Energy Source	Fermentation Products
Bacteroides succinogenes	Cellulose fermenting	−	Cellulose, glucose, starch	Acetate, succinate
Ruminococcus flavefaciens	Cellulose fermenting	−	Cellulose, xylan, glucose	Succinate, acetate, formate
Butyrivibrio fibrosolvens	Cellulose fermenting	−	Glucose, xylan, starch, cellulose	Butyrate, formate, lactate
Bacteroides ruminocola	Deaminating	−	Glucose, xylan, starch	Formate, succinate, acetate, isobutyrate, isovalerate
Methanobacterium ruminantium	Methanogenic	+	Hydrogen, formate	Methane
Veillonella alcalescens	Lactic acid fermenting	−	Lactate	Acetate, propionate
Peptostreptococcus elsdenii	Lactic acid fermenting	−	Glucose, lactate	Acetate, propionate, butyrate, valerate
Succinivibrio dextrinosolvens	Starch and sugar fermenting	±	Glucose	Formate, succinate, acetate
Selenomonas ruminantium	Starch and sugar fermenting	−	Glucose, starch, lactate	Acetate, propionate
Streptococcus bovis	Starch and sugar fermenting	+	Glucose, starch	Lactate

Source: Adapted from Bryant 1970 and McDonald et al. 1973.

community is specialized to break down cellulose and hemicellulose from plant fiber. Cellulose is constructed of long chains of glucose bonded by β-1,4 linkages (Fig. 3.2). Hemicelluloses are not related to cellulose but are polymers of pentose. Cellulase, the enzyme that breaks the β-1,4 linkage, is not produced by mammalian tissue; only bacteria found in the rumen and large intestine produce this enzyme. Thus, anaerobic bacteria of the rumen or large intestine have a symbiotic relationship with the host animal. Fiber digestion in the large intestine is most important to those herbivores lacking foregut fermentation (see 3.2-3).

The stages of carbohydrate breakdown are shown in Figure 3.3. The process of plant polysaccharide digestion to yield volatile fatty acids occurs in three main stages. The first stage involves breaking down the complex sugars to simple sugars, which can enter the glycolytic cycle, or second stage of metabolism. The end product of the glycolytic pathway is pyruvate, which serves as a substrate for the third and final stage of fermentation. Different bacteria are involved in the various stages of fermentation and provide precursor substrates for each other (Table 3.2). The major sugars entering the rumen are cellulose, hemicellulose, starch, and water-soluble carbohydrates, such as fructans. Cellulose is first broken into smaller cellobiose units by action of bacterial β-1,4 glucosidase. Cellobiose is then converted to glucose, which is readily taken up by bacteria and metabolized to pyruvate via the Embden-Meyerhoff glycolytic pathway. Hemicellulose is converted by action of β-1,4 glucosidase into pentose sugars that can be converted to fructose-6-phosphate or fructose-1-6-diphosphate, which enter the glycolytic pathway. Starches are acted upon by salivary amylase and converted to maltose or isomaltose, which in turn are converted to glucose or glucose-1-phosphate and then enter the glycolytic pathway. Fructans are converted to fructose by hydrolytic enzymes and sucrose is broken into fructose and glucose, which then readily enter the glycolytic pathway.

Once the initial phase of polysaccharide digestion is complete, the simple sugars are metabolized in the glycolytic pathway, which is anaerobic and, thus, of great importance to energy utilization in rumen microbes and protozoa.

The end product of the glycolytic pathway is pyruvate, which is an important intermediate in the production of the end products of rumen fermentation: acetate, butyrate, and propionate. Other important intermediates are succinate and lactate.

3.3: DIGESTION AND ABSORPTION

3.3-1: Background. Metabolism of nutrients in the digestive tract and their absorption into the vascular system and extracellular fluid or

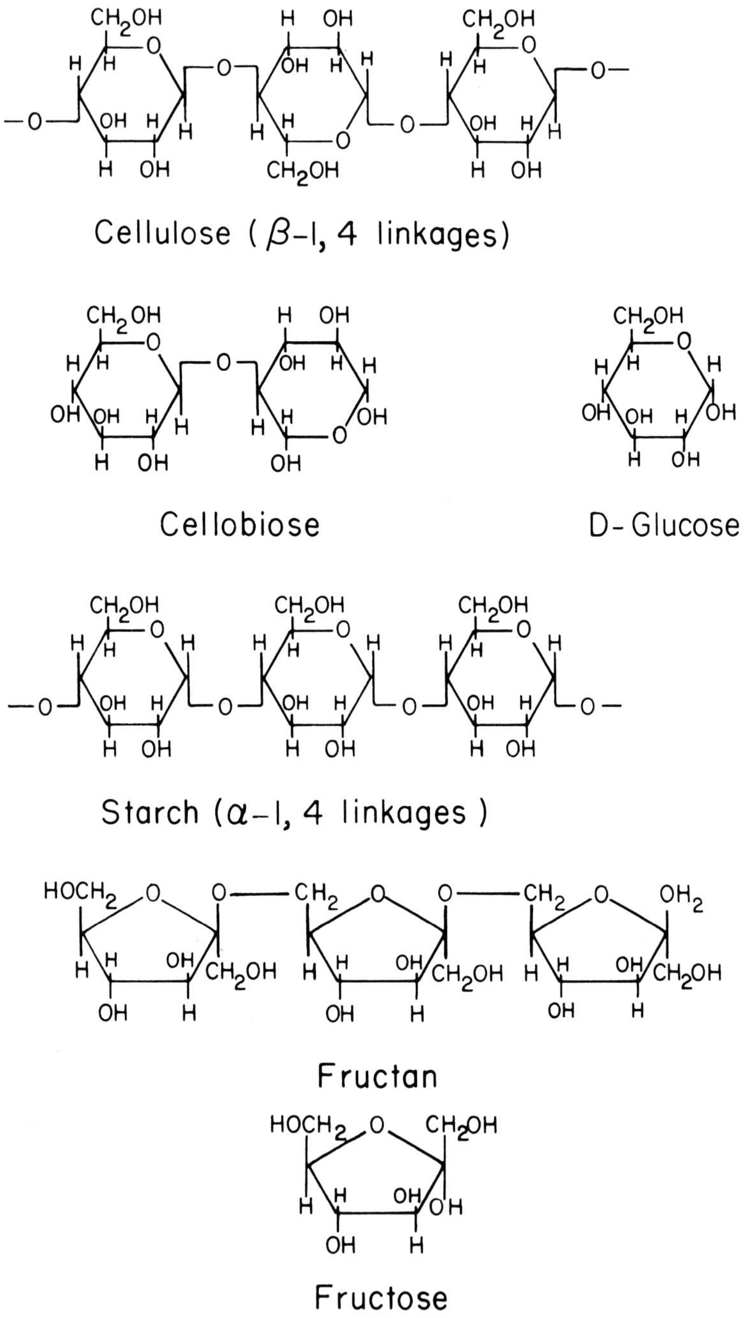

Cellulose (β-1, 4 linkages)

Cellobiose

D-Glucose

Starch (α-1, 4 linkages)

Fructan

Fructose

Fig. 3.2. Structures of common carbohydrates found in ruminant diets.

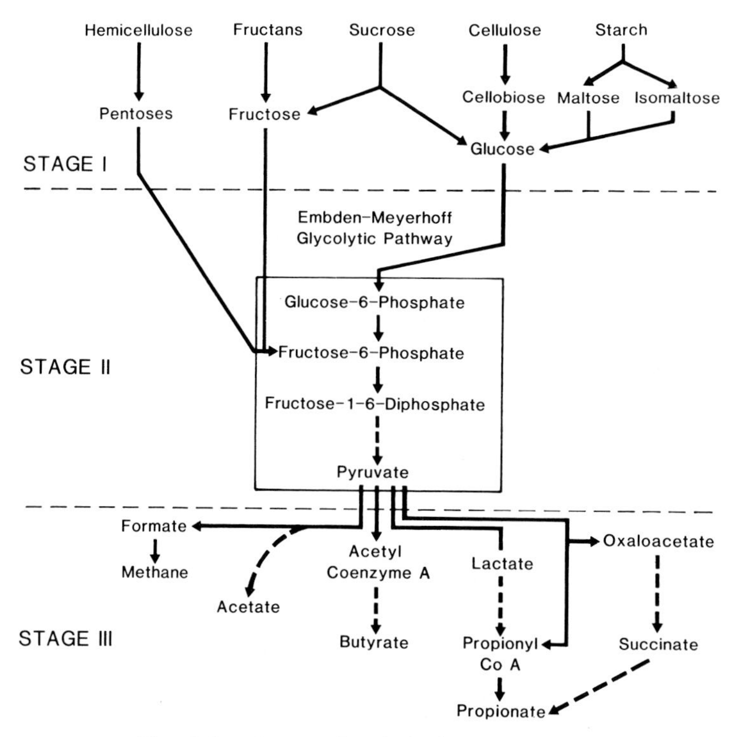

Fig. 3.3. Stages of carbohydrate metabolism in ruminants.

metabolizable nutrient pool are outlined in Figure 3.1. Digestion is not complete because some nutrients are lost in feces, in heat production, in the rumen, and/or in the large intestine to CO_2 and methane. The loss of carbon in CO_2 and methane is most pronounced in ruminants. Nutrients not lost in the digestive process are termed digestible nutrients, and they are available for absorption or diffusion into the vascular system.

3.3-2: Volatile fatty acids. The end products of rumen fermentation are predominantly volatile fatty acids, such as acetate, propionate, and butyrate (Fig. 3.3). Absorption of these volatile fatty acids (VFAs) occurs primarily in the rumen and omasum. There is appreciable metabolism of butyrate, but not acetate or propionate, by the rumen epithelium. Acetate is the predominant acid produced in the rumen, accounting for about 65% of total VFAs present. The molar proportion of propionate is approximately 20% and butyrate 10%, and the remaining 5% consists of fatty acids produced in small quantities, such as isovaleric, valeric, and isobutyric acids.

Diet greatly influences the type and quantity of VFAs produced. Animals on an all-forage diet have higher production of acetate; grain diets favor production of propionate. If animals are placed on all-concentrate diets, the proportion of propionate may even exceed that of acetate.

Acid production is greatest following feeding. Since the rumen is buffered primarily by salivary bicarbonate, a large amount of CO_2 is produced during this period. Methane and CO_2 also are produced by the fermentation process, leading to appreciable gas production (up to 30 l/hr), which is lost by eructation. Conditions that prevent loss of CO_2 result in bloat.

The absorption of VFAs across the rumen epithelium is associated with sodium transport. Following feeding, VFA production increases but the concentration of sodium in rumen fluid declines as VFAs are absorbed across the rumen epithelium. Acetate and propionate are not metabolized as they pass across the rumen wall. On the other hand, butyric acid is converted to β-hydroxybutyric acid (BHBA). The VFAs are absorbed into the portal circulation and carried to the liver, where all the propionate is extracted from the blood for glucose production (Fig. 3.4). Acetate and BHBA pass through the liver and are distributed to various tissues for energy production and fatty acid synthesis.

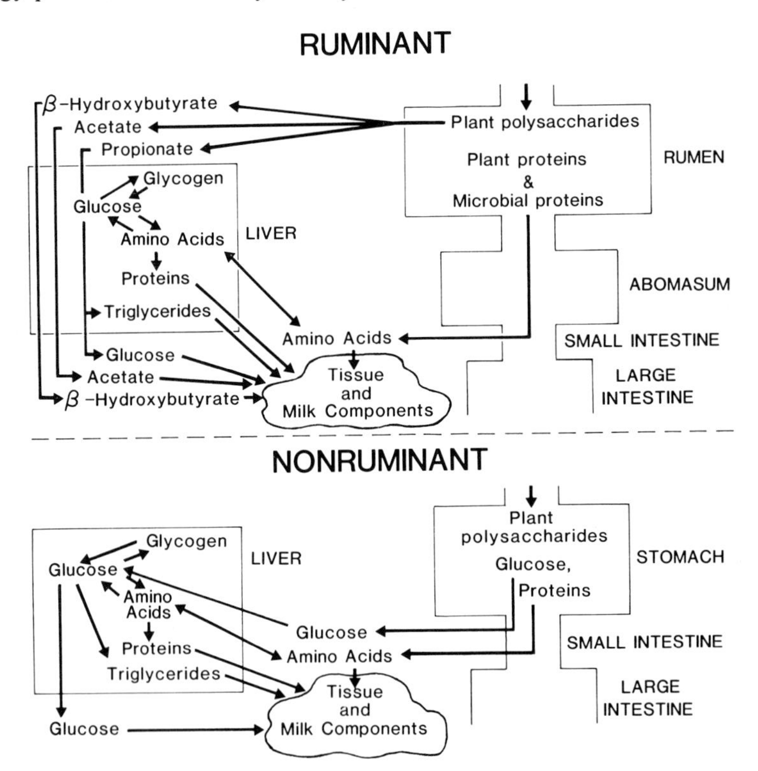

Fig. 3.4. Routes of carbohydrate utilization in ruminants and nonruminants.

3.3-3: Carbohydrate metabolism. In nonruminants, polysaccharides and disaccharides are reduced to simple sugars prior to absorption. The monosaccharide unit formed is primarily D-glucose. Enzymes involved in these conversions are salivary and pancreatic amylases and α-dextrinases, disaccharidases, and maltases in the brush border of the small intestine. The majority of the absorption of D-glucose occurs in the upper half of the small intestine (duodenum and jejunum).

Lactose (milk sugar) is a disaccharide composed of a glucose and galactose molecule. The enzyme lactase, in the brush border of the small intestine, hydrolyzes the lactose molecule, yielding the two monosaccharides. Glucose absorption from the small intestine against a concentration gradient is energy dependent and also involves transport of sodium (Na^+) and potassium (K^+). Currently, it is believed that the transport of glucose per se is not energy dependent but that the energy expenditure is related to the Na^+/K^+ ATPase pump.

Once glucose leaves the intestinal epithelial cells, it is transported primarily into the portal circulation and then to the liver, where a portion is extracted for glycogen synthesis and storage of triacylglycerol (triglyceride) (Fig. 3.4). The remainder enters the circulating nutrient pool and is partitioned to tissues according to their metabolic requirements for glucose.

In adult ruminants, little if any carbohydrate escapes rumen fermentation. Prior to onset of rumen fermentation, the young ruminant utilizes carbohydrates in a manner similar to that of nonruminants. However, once rumen fermentation begins, gluconeogenesis from propionate in the liver is the primary source of circulating glucose.

Blood glucose concentrations tend to be lower in ruminants, approximating 40–80 mg%, while nonruminants normally have blood glucose concentrations from 100–120 mg%. Due to the low blood concentration of glucose and availability of acetate for energy production, ruminants have developed glucose-sparing strategies in several tissues, most noticeably in the mammary glands to prevent hypoglycemia under conditions of great metabolic demand, such as lactation (see 3.6).

3.3-4: Protein and amino acid metabolism. In ruminants and nonruminants, protein metabolism in the foregut differs in the production of microbial protein and hydrolysis of plant protein by microbes in the rumen. Protein metabolism in the lower digestive tract is similar.

Proteins are made of amino acids linked together by peptide bonds. The peptide bond is composed of the nitrogen of the amino group of one amino acid linked to a carbonyl group of a neighboring amino acid. This linkage requires the loss of water. Proteases, which are hydrolytic enzymes, attack these bonds, releasing the individual amino acids. This process begins in the stomach or abomasum with production of hydrochloric acid and the enzyme pepsin. Further hydrolysis occurs in the small intestine via the enzymes trypsin, chymotrypsin, aminopeptidase, and carboxypeptidase, in addition to pepsin. These enzymes are produced in the pancreas and secreted into the small intestine. Each proteolytic enzyme attacks a different point along the peptide chain to free the individual amino acids.

Amino acids are actively absorbed by epithelial cells lining the proximal jejunum. Several transport systems are involved in this uptake, with individual transport systems specific for certain amino acids.

Amino acids in the metabolizable nutrient pool may be utilized for protein synthesis or gluconeogenesis. A detailed description of milk protein synthesis is given in 4.7.

3.3-5: Lipid metabolism. Lipid digestion is carried out almost exclusively in the small intestine. Bile from the gall bladder and pancreatic juice flow into the duodenum, where the bile salts act on lipids to form spherical emulsion particles. These emulsion particles contain primarily triacylglycerols. Pancreatic lipase attacks the triacylglycerols to form mono- and diacylglycerols, as well as free fatty acids. The free fatty acids, monoacylglycerols, and diacylglycerols enter the epithelial cells of the brush border of the small intestine, where the long-chain free fatty acids are converted to fatty acyl compounds, which are then attached to mono- and diacylglycerols to form triacylglycerols. The fatty acids in these triacylglycerols all have long chain lengths (more than 12 carbons). A protein coat is added to the surface of the lipid droplet and the droplet (chylomicron) is extruded into the lymph circulation by reverse pinocytosis. The chylomicron averages 500 Å in diameter and primarily is composed of triacylglycerols with small amounts of phospholipid, protein, and free fatty acids. The chylomicra are transported via lymphatic circulation to the portal venous drainage.

Blood lipids arise from three main sources: lipids of dietary origin, lipids mobilized from adipose tissue depots, and lipids synthesized in the liver (Fig. 3.5). Plasma chylomicra may be taken up by liver, adipose tissue, or peripheral tissues, such as the mammary gland; liver cells take up chylomicra directly from the plasma. Other tissues rely on lipoprotein lipase to break down triacylglycerols in chylomicra before uptake of the fatty acids, mono- or diacylglycerols, and glycerol. Lipoprotein lipase is located on capillary endothelial cells and, therefore, can act on the chylomicra as they leave the circulation.

The triacylglycerols of chylomicra taken up by liver also are hydrolyzed, producing glycerol and free fatty acids. Glycerol returns to circulation, while the free fatty acids are utilized to form new triacylglycerols or are released into plasma, bound to albumin or high-density lipoprotein. Albumin is synthesized in the liver as well. The albumin–fatty acid complex dissociates in the target tissue, and the free fatty acid crosses the capillary wall to be taken up by the target tissue.

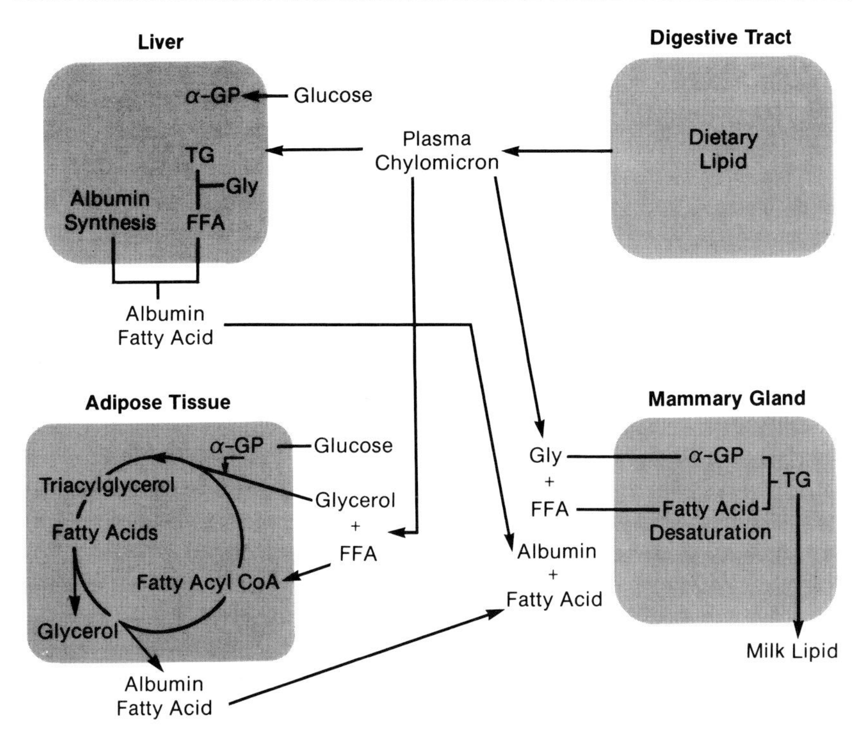

Fig. 3.5. Sources, mobilization, and metabolism of lipids. *GP* = glycerol phosphate; *TG* = triglycerides; *FFA* = free fatty acids; *Gly* = glycerol.

The primary objective of adipose tissue is to lay down adipose stores during periods of positive energy balance and mobilize these stores during periods of negative energy balance. Both processes occur continuously. However, the energy status of the animal will dictate which process is favored. Thus, both triacylglycerol synthesis and mobilization occur in the adipocyte.

In contrast to liver and adipose tissue, the mammary gland is a one-way avenue of lipid uptake and formation of milk triacylglycerols. This involves hydrolysis and uptake of triacylglycerols at the capillary wall and desaturation and formation of milk triacylglycerols. Milk fat synthesis is further discussed in 3.6-4.

3.4: NUTRIENT REQUIREMENTS

3.4-1: Background. Optimum growth and lactation require adequate supplies of nutrients, which can be divided into five major classes: energy, water, protein, vitamins, and minerals. Energy incorporates under one term both fat and carbohydrate requirements and any protein utilized in energy production. Aside from water, energy is considered the most limiting nutrient, since it is required for proper utilization of all remaining nutrients. Nutrient requirements for various productive processes in domestic animals have been studied for several years and are published by the National Research Council (NRC). These tables of nutrient requirements are referred to as NRC recommendations. An adapted version of the NRC recommendations for growth, pregnancy, and lactation in cattle, sheep, and swine are listed in Tables 3.3–3.6. These can be used to calculate feed requirements of animals at a given point in their life cycle. Primary productive processes in animals are growth, reproduction, and lactation. In addition to these processes, each animal has a maintenance requirement to meet the nutrient needs required to maintain basal metabolism and activity at a given body weight.

3.4-2: Energy. Approaches used to express energy requirements of animals include the terms total digestible nutrients (TDN), digestible energy (DE), metabolizable energy (ME), and net energy (NE). The values for TDN and DE are approximately similar but are derived differently. The value for TDN is derived by the formula

$$\% \text{ TDN} = \frac{\text{crude protein} + (\text{digestible ether extract} \times 2.25) + \text{nitrogen-free extract}}{\text{feed consumed}} \times 100$$

The value for DE is calculated by the formula

$$\text{DE} = \text{energy consumed} - \text{energy lost in feces}$$

Neither TDN nor DE take into account energy lost in gas production, urine, or heat production (Fig. 3.6).

NE is considered the most accurate measure of energy requirements and has been adopted by the NRC as the official standard. NE is derived by determining the energy content of feed, energy lost in digestion via feces and gas production, energy lost in urine, and energy lost as heat. The NE value is then calculated by subtracting energy lost in feces, gas, urine, and heat from the gross energy. The remaining NE can be utilized for maintenance, growth, lactation, or reproduction. The approximate percentages of energy in each of these categories for a lactating cow are shown in Figure 3.7. Considerable energy is lost in feces, urine, and gas, leaving only 20% of total energy consumed available for maintenance and production.

Since NE is derived by subtracting energy lost as heat from ME, efficiency of utilization of ME influences availability of NE. Table 3.7 demonstrates differences in efficiency of utilization of ME from different nutrients and foods. Fat is utilized with greater efficiency than protein because of the

Table 3.3. Nutrient requirements of beef cattle

			Energy								Total Protein in Diet		Calcium in Diet		Phosphorus in Diet		Vitamin A[d]
			Daily				In diet DM										
Weight[a] (kg)	Gain[b] (kg)	Daily DM[c] (lb)	ME (Mcal)	TDN (kg)	NE_m (Mcal)	NE_g (Mcal)	ME (Mcal/kg)	TDN (%)	NE_m (Mcal/kg)	NE_g (Mcal/kg)	Daily (kg)	DM (%)	Daily (G)	DM (%)	Daily (G)	DM (%)	Daily (1,000 IU)
Pregnant yearling heifers–last third of pregnancy																	
318	0.4	7.0	13.9	3.9	7.95	NA[e]	0.41	55.4	0.24	NA[e]	0.59	8.4	19	0.27	14	0.20	19
318	0.6	7.2	15.7	4.4	7.95	0.87	0.45	60.3	0.27	0.15	0.64	9.0	24	0.33	15	0.21	20
318	0.9	7.2	17.4	4.8	7.95	1.89	0.50	67.0	0.32	0.20	0.68	9.8	27	0.33	16	0.21	20
341	0.4	7.3	14.6	4.0	8.25	NA	0.41	55.1	0.24	NA	0.59	8.3	20	0.27	14	0.19	20
341	0.6	7.5	16.4	4.5	8.25	0.92	0.45	59.9	0.27	0.15	0.68	8.9	24	0.32	16	0.21	21
341	0.9	7.5	18.2	5.0	8.25	1.99	0.50	66.5	0.31	0.19	0.72	9.5	28	0.37	17	0.23	21
364	0.4	7.6	15.2	4.2	8.56	NA	0.41	54.8	0.23	NA	0.64	8.2	21	0.28	15	0.20	21
364	0.6	7.9	17.1	4.7	8.56	0.96	0.45	59.6	0.27	0.15	0.68	8.8	25	0.33	16	0.21	22
364	0.9	8.0	19.0	5.3	8.56	2.09	0.49	66.1	0.31	0.19	0.72	9.3	28	0.35	17	0.21	22
386	0.4	8.0	15.7	4.4	8.85	NA	0.40	54.5	0.23	NA	0.64	8.2	21	0.26	16	0.20	22
386	0.6	8.3	17.8	4.9	8.85	1.01	0.44	59.3	0.27	0.15	0.72	8.6	25	0.30	17	0.21	23
386	0.9	8.3	19.8	5.5	8.85	2.19	0.49	65.7	0.31	0.19	0.77	9.1	28	0.34	18	0.22	23
409	0.4	8.3	16.3	4.5	9.15	NA	0.40	54.3	0.23	NA	0.68	8.1	22	0.26	17	0.20	23
409	0.6	8.6	18.5	5.1	9.15	1.05	0.44	59.1	0.26	0.15	0.72	8.5	26	0.30	18	0.21	24
409	0.9	8.7	20.6	5.7	9.15	2.28	0.49	65.4	0.31	0.19	0.77	9.0	28	0.32	19	0.21	24
432	0.4	8.6	16.9	4.7	9.44	NA	0.40	54.1	0.23	NA	0.68	8.0	23	0.27	17	0.20	24
432	0.6	9.0	19.1	5.3	9.44	1.09	0.44	58.9	0.26	0.15	0.77	8.4	26	0.29	19	0.21	25
432	0.9	9.1	21.3	5.9	9.44	2.38	0.49	65.1	0.30	0.18	0.82	8.8	29	0.32	19	0.21	25
Dry pregnant mature cows–last third pregnancy																	
364	0.4	7.6	15.0	4.2	8.56	NA	0.40	54.5	0.23	NA	0.64	8.2	20	0.26	15	0.20	21
409	0.4	8.3	16.2	4.5	9.15	NA	0.40	54.0	0.23	NA	0.68	8.0	22	0.27	17	0.21	23
454	0.4	8.9	17.3	4.8	9.72	NA	0.40	53.6	0.23	NA	0.72	7.9	23	0.26	18	0.20	25
500	0.4	9.5	18.3	5.1	10.28	NA	0.40	53.2	0.22	NA	0.72	7.8	25	0.26	20	0.21	26
545	0.4	10.1	19.4	5.4	10.83	NA	0.40	52.9	0.22	NA	0.77	7.8	26	0.26	21	0.21	28
591	0.4	10.7	20.4	5.7	11.37	NA	0.40	52.7	0.22	NA	0.82	7.7	28	0.26	23	0.21	30
636	0.4	11.3	21.5	6.0	11.90	NA	0.39	52.5	0.22	NA	0.86	7.6	29	0.26	24	0.21	32

Source: From National Research Council 1984.

[a] Average weight for a feeding period.

[b] Approximately 0.4 ±0.09 kg weight gain/dry matter (kg DM) over the last third of pregnancy is accounted for by the products of conception. Daily 2.15 Mcal of Ne_m and 0.01 kg of protein are provided for this requirement for a calf with a birth weight of 36.4 kg.

[c] Dry matter consumption should vary depending on the energy concentration of the diet and environmental conditions. These intakes are based on the energy concentration shown in the table and assuming a thermoneutral environment without snow or mud conditions. If the energy concentrations of the diet to be fed exceed the tabular value, limit-feeding may be required.

[d] Vitamin A requirements per kg of diet are 2800 IU for pregnant heifers and cows and 3900 IU for lactating cows and breeding bulls.

[e] Not applicable.

Table 3.3. (*Continued*)

			Energy								Total Protein in Diet		Calcium in Diet		Phosphorus in Diet		Vitamin A[d]
			Daily				In diet DM										
Weight[a] (kg)	Gain[b] (kg)	Daily DM[c] (lb)	ME (Mcal)	TDN (kg)	NE_m (Mcal)	NE_g (Mcal)	ME (Mcal/kg)	TDN (%)	NE_m (Mcal/kg)	NE_g (Mcal/kg)	Daily (kg)	DM (%)	Daily (G)	DM (%)	Daily (G)	DM (%)	Daily (1,000 IU)
Two-year-old heifers nursing calves–first 3–4 mo postpartum–4.5 kg milk/day																	
318	0.2	7.2	17.0	4.7	9.20[f]	0.87	0.49	65.1	0.30	0.18	0.82[g]	11.3	26	0.36	17	0.24	28
341	0.7	7.6	17.7	4.9	9.51[f]	0.92	0.48	64.4	0.30	0.18	0.82[g]	11.0	26	0.34	18	0.24	30
364	0.2	8.0	18.4	5.1	9.81[f]	0.96	0.48	63.8	0.30	0.18	0.86[g]	10.8	27	0.34	19	0.24	31
386	0.2	8.4	19.1	5.3	10.11[f]	1.01	0.47	63.2	0.30	0.17	0.86[g]	10.6	27	0.33	19	0.23	33
409	0.2	8.7	19.8	5.5	10.40[f]	1.05	0.47	62.7	0.29	0.17	0.91[g]	10.4	28	0.32	20	0.23	34
432	0.2	9.1	20.5	5.7	10.69[f]	1.09	0.46	62.3	0.29	0.17	0.91[g]	10.2	28	0.31	21	0.23	35
454	0.2	9.5	21.1	5.9	10.98[f]	1.14	0.46	61.9	0.28	0.16	0.95[g]	10.0	29	0.31	22	0.23	37
Cows nursing calves–average milking ability–first 3–4 mo postpartum–4.5 kg milk/day																	
364	0.0	7.9	16.6	4.6	9.81[f]	NA	0.44	58.2	0.26	NA	0.82[g]	10.2	23	0.30	17	0.22	31
409	0.0	8.5	17.7	4.9	10.40[f]	NA	0.43	57.3	0.25	NA	0.86[g]	9.9	24	0.28	19	0.22	33
454	0.0	9.2	18.8	5.2	10.98[f]	NA	0.42	56.6	0.25	NA	0.91[g]	9.6	25	0.28	20	0.22	36
500	0.0	9.8	19.9	5.5	11.54[f]	NA	0.42	56.0	0.25	NA	0.91[g]	9.4	27	0.27	22	0.22	38
545	0.0	10.5	21.0	5.7	12.09[f]	NA	0.41	55.5	0.24	NA	0.95[g]	9.3	28	0.27	23	0.22	41
591	0.0	11.0	22.0	6.1	12.63[f]	NA	0.41	55.1	0.24	NA	1.00[g]	9.1	30	0.27	25	0.22	43
636	0.0	11.6	23.0	6.4	13.15[f]	NA	0.41	54.7	0.23	NA	1.05[g]	9.0	31	0.27	26	0.22	46
Cows nursing calves–superior milking ability–first 3–4 mo postpartum–9.0 kg milk/day																	
364	0.0	7.1	19.9	5.5	13.22[f]	NA	0.58	77.3	0.39	NA	1.00[g]	14.2	34	0.48	22	0.31	28
409	0.0	8.5	21.5	6.0	13.81[f]	NA	0.52	69.8	0.34	NA	1.09[g]	12.9	35	0.41	24	0.28	33
454	0.0	9.4	22.7	6.3	14.38[f]	NA	0.50	67.0	0.32	NA	1.14[g]	12.3	36	0.39	25	0.27	37
500	0.0	10.1	23.8	6.6	14.94[f]	NA	0.49	65.2	0.30	NA	1.18[g]	11.9	38	0.38	27	0.27	40
545	0.0	10.8	24.9	6.9	15.49[f]	NA	0.48	63.7	0.30	NA	1.23[g]	11.5	39	0.36	28	0.26	42
591	0.0	11.5	26.0	7.2	16.03[f]	NA	0.47	62.6	0.29	NA	1.27[g]	11.2	41	0.36	30	0.26	45
636	0.0	12.1	27.1	7.5	16.56[f]	NA	0.46	61.7	0.28	NA	1.32[g]	11.0	42	0.35	31	0.26	47

[f]Includes 0.15 Mcal NE_m/kg milk produced.
[g]Includes 0.01 kg protein/kg milk produced.

energy cost of urea production. Glucose is also utilized with high efficiency. Reduction in efficiency of glucose administered via the rumen is due to heat losses in fermentation. Stored energy is utilized with high efficiency. In the mature ruminant, energy is stored primarily as fat. Thus, mobilization of fat reserves during periods of peak energy demand is a highly efficient method of meeting extra energy requirements.

A negative energy balance occurs when animals cannot meet energy requirements because of low energy content of feed or if the energy requirements exceed the animals' ability to physically take in enough energy in feed to meet their requirements. Animals in a negative energy balance will utilize

Table 3.4. Daily nutrient requirements of lactating and pregnant dairy cattle

	Feed Energy				Total Crude Protein (g)	Calcium (g)	Phosphorus (g)	Vitamin A (1,000 IU)
	NE_l (Mcal)	ME (Mcal)	DE (Mcal)	TDN (kg)				
Maintenance of mature lactating cows[a] (kg body wt)								
350	6.47	10.76	12.54	2.85	341	14	11	27
400	7.16	11.90	13.86	3.15	373	15	13	30
450	7.82	12.99	15.14	3.44	403	17	14	34
500	8.46	14.06	16.39	3.72	432	18	15	38
550	9.09	15.11	17.60	4.00	461	20	16	42
600	9.70	16.12	18.79	4.27	489	21	17	46
650	10.30	17.12	19.95	4.53	515	22	18	50
700	10.89	18.10	21.09	4.79	542	24	19	53
750	11.47	19.06	22.21	5.04	567	25	20	57
800	12.03	20.01	23.32	5.29	592	27	21	61
Maintenance plus last 2 mo of gestation of mature dry cows (kg body wt)								
350	8.42	14.00	16.26	3.71	642	23	16	27
400	9.30	15.47	17.98	4.10	702	26	18	30
450	10.16	16.90	19.64	4.47	763	29	20	34
500	11.00	18.29	21.25	4.84	821	31	22	38
550	11.81	19.65	22.83	5.20	877	34	24	42
600	12.61	20.97	24.37	5.55	931	37	26	46
650	13.39	22.27	25.87	5.90	984	39	28	50
700	14.15	23.54	27.35	6.23	1035	42	30	53
750	14.90	24.79	28.81	6.56	1086	45	32	57
800	15.64	26.02	30.24	6.89	1136	47	34	61
Milk production–nutrients/kg milk of different fat percentages (% fat)								
2.5	0.59	0.99	1.15	0.260	72	2.40	1.65	
3.0	0.64	1.07	1.24	0.282	77	2.50	1.70	
3.5	0.69	1.16	1.34	0.304	82	2.60	1.75	
4.0	0.74	1.24	1.44	0.326	87	2.70	1.80	
4.5	0.78	1.31	1.52	0.344	92	2.80	1.85	
5.0	0.83	1.39	1.61	0.365	98	2.90	1.90	
5.5	0.88	1.48	1.71	0.387	103	3.00	2.00	
6.0	0.93	1.56	1.81	0.410	108	3.10	2.05	
Body weight change during lactation–nutrients/kg weight change								
Weight loss	−4.92	−8.25	−9.55	−2.17	−320			
Weight gain	5.12	8.55	9.96	2.26	500			

Source: From National Research Council 1978.

[a]To allow for growth of young lactating cows, increase the maintenance allowances for all nutrients except vitamin A by 20% during the first lactation and 10% during the second lactation.

Table 3.5. **Nutrient concentration in diet dry matter for ewes**

Body Wt (kg)	Daily Gain/ Loss (g)	Daily DM/ Animal[a] (kg)	Live Wt (%)	Energy TDN (%)	DE[b] (Mcal/ kg)	ME (Mcal/ kg)	TP[c] (%)	DP[d] (%)	Ca (%)	P (%)	Carotene (mg/ kg)	Vitamin A (IU/ kg)	Vitamin D (IU/ kg)
Maintenance													
50	10	1.0	2.0	55	2.4	2.0	8.9	4.8	0.30	0.28	1.9	1275	278
60	10	1.1	1.8	55	2.4	2.0	8.9	4.8	0.28	0.26	2.0	1391	303
70	10	1.2	1.7	55	2.4	2.0	8.9	4.8	0.27	0.25	2.2	1488	323
80	10	1.3	1.6	55	2.4	2.0	8.9	4.8	0.25	0.24	2.3	1569	342
Nonlactating and first 15 wk of gestation													
50	30	1.1	2.2	55	2.4	2.0	9.0	4.9	0.27	0.25	1.7	1159	253
60	30	1.3	2.1	55	2.4	2.0	9.0	4.9	0.24	0.22	1.7	1177	256
70	30	1.4	2.0	55	2.4	2.0	9.0	4.9	0.23	0.21	1.9	1275	277
80	30	1.5	1.9	55	2.4	2.0	9.0	4.9	0.22	0.21	2.0	1360	296
Last 6 wk of gestation or last 8 wk of lactation suckling singles[e]													
50	175(+45)	1.7	3.3	58	2.6	2.1	9.3	5.2	0.24	0.23	3.6	2500	164
60	180(+45)	1.9	3.2	58	2.6	2.1	9.3	5.2	0.23	0.22	3.9	2684	175
70	185(+45)	2.1	3.0	58	2.6	2.1	9.3	5.2	0.21	0.20	4.2	2833	185
80	190(+45)	2.2	2.8	58	2.6	2.1	9.3	5.2	0.21	0.20	4.5	3091	202
First 8 wk of lactation suckling singles or last 8 wk of lactation suckling twins[f]													
50	−25(+80)	2.1	4.2	65	2.9	2.4	10.4	6.2	0.52	0.37	3.0	2024	132
60	−25(+80)	2.3	3.9	65	2.9	2.4	10.4	6.2	0.50	0.36	3.3	2217	145
70	−25(+80)	2.5	3.6	65	2.9	2.4	10.4	6.2	0.48	0.34	3.5	2380	155
80	−25(+80)	2.6	3.2	65	2.9	2.4	10.4	6.2	0.48	0.34	3.8	2615	171
First 8 wk of lactation suckling twins													
50	−60	2.4	4.8	65	2.9	2.4	11.5	7.2	0.52	0.37	2.6	1771	116
60	−60	2.6	4.3	65	2.9	2.4	11.5	7.2	0.48	0.36	2.9	1962	128
70	−60	2.8	4.0	65	2.9	2.4	11.5	7.2	0.48	0.34	3.1	2125	139
80	−60	3.0	3.7	65	2.9	2.4	11.5	7.2	0.48	0.34	3.3	2267	148

Source: From National Research Council 1975.

Note: Values are for ewes in moderate condition, not excessively fat or thin. Fat ewes should be fed at the next lower weight, thin ewes at the next higher weight. Once maintenance weight is established, such weight would follow through all production phases.

[a]To convert dry matter to an as-fed basis, divide dry matter by percentage of dry matter.

[b]1 kg TDN = 4.4 Mcal DE (digestible energy). DE may be converted to ME (metabolizable energy) by multiplying by 82%.

[c]TP = total protein.

[d]DP = digestible protein.

[e]Values in parentheses are for ewes suckling singles last 8 wk of lactation.

[f]Values in parentheses are for ewes suckling twins last 8 wk of lactation.

Table 3.6. Nutrient requirements of breeding swine

Air-Dry Feed Components	Bred Gilts, Sows: Young and Adult Boars	Lactating Gilts and Sows		
	1,800g[a]	4,000g	4,750g	5,500g
		(*amounts/animal/day*)		
Digestible energy (kcal)	6,120[b]	13,580	16,130	18,670
Metabolizable energy (kcal)	5,760[b]	12,780	15,180	17,750
Crude protein (g)	216	520	618	715
Indispensable amino acids				
arginine (g)	0	16.0	19.0	22.0
histidine (g)	2.7	10.0	11.9	13.8
isoleucine (g)	6.7	15.6	18.5	21.4
leucine (g)	7.6	28.0	33.2	38.5
lysine (g)	7.7	23.2	27.6	31.9
methionine+cystine (g)[c]	4.1	14.4	17.1	19.8
phenylalanine+tyrosine (g)[d]	9.4	34.0	40.4	46.8
threonine (g)	6.1	17.2	20.4	23.6
tryptophan (g)[e]	1.6	4.8	5.7	6.6
valine (g)	8.3	22.0	26.1	30.2
Mineral elements				
calcium (g)	13.5	30.0	35.6	41.2
phosphorus (g)[f]	10.8	20.0	23.8	27.5
sodium (g)	2.7	8.0	9.5	11.0
chlorine (g)	4.5	12.0	14.2	16.5
potassium (g)	3.6	8.0	9.5	11.0
magnesium (g)	0.7	1.6	1.9	2.2
iron (mg)	144	320	380	440
zinc (mg)	90	200	238	275
manganese (mg)	18	40	48	55
copper (mg)	9	20	24	28
iodine (mg)	0.25	0.56	0.66	0.77
selenium (mg)	0.27	0.40	0.48	0.55
Vitamins				
vitamin A (IU)	7,200	8,000	9,500	11,000
β-carotene (mg)	28.8	32.0	38.0	44.0
vitamin D (IU)	380	800	950	1,100
vitamin E (IU)	18.0	40.0	47.5	55.0
vitamin K (IU)	3.6	8.0	9.5	11.0
riboflavin (mg)	5.4	12.0	14.2	16.5
niacin (mg)[g]	18.0	40.0	47.5	55.0
pantothenic acid (mg)	21.6	48.0	57.0	66.0
vitamin B_{12} (μg)	27.0	60.0	71.2	82.5
choline (mg)	2,250.0	5,000.0	5,940.0	6,875.0
thiamin (mg)	1.8	4.0	4.8	5.5
vitamin B_6 (mg)	1.8	4.0	4.8	5.5
biotin (mg)[h]	0.18	0.4	0.48	0.55
folacin (mg)[h]	1.08	2.4	2.8	3.3

Source: From National Research Council 1979.

Note: Requirements reflect the estimated levels of each nutrient needed for optimal performance when a fortified grain–soybean meal diet is fed. Concentrations are based upon amounts per unit of air-dry diet (i.e., 90% dry matter).

[a]An additional 25% should be fed to working boars.

[b]Individual feeding and moderate climatic conditions are assumed. An energy reduction of about 10% is possible when gilts and sows are tethered or individually penned in a stall in environmentally controlled housing. An energy increase of about 25% is suggested for cold climatic (winter) conditions.

[c]Methionine can fulfill the total requirement; cystine can meet at least 50% of the total requirement.

[d]Phenylalanine can fulfill the total requirement; tyrosine can meet at least 50% of the total requirement.

[e]It is assumed that usable tryptophan content of corn does not exceed 0.05%.

[f]At least 30% of the phosphorus requirement should be provided by inorganic and/or animal product sources.

[g]It is assumed that most of the niacin present in cereal grains and their by-products is in bound form and thus unavailable to swine. The niacin contributed by these sources is not included in the requirement listed. In excess of its requirement for protein synthesis, tryptophan can be converted to niacin (50 mg tryptophan yields 1 mg niacin).

[h]These levels are suggested; no requirements have been established.

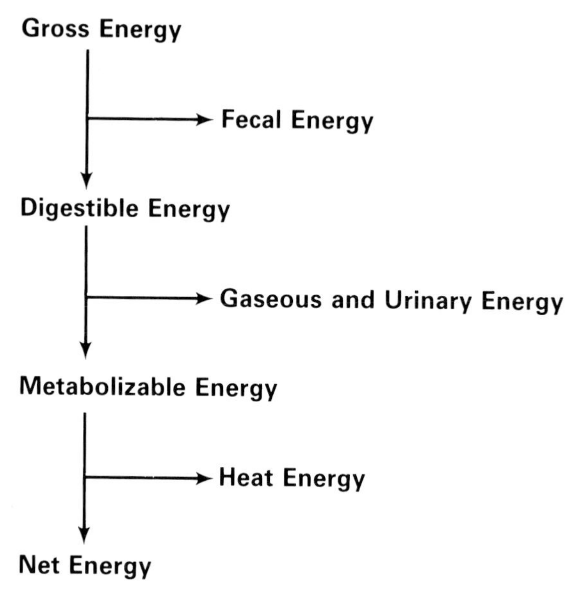

Fig. 3.6. Partition of feed energy.

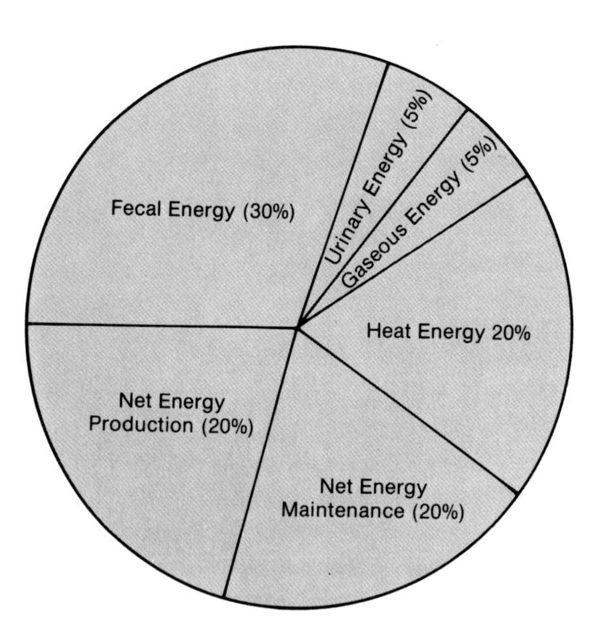

Fig. 3.7. Approximate percentages of gross energy in a lactating cow. (Modified from Foley et al. 1972)

body fat reserves to meet energy requirements. When body fat reserves are exhausted, available energy will be used for maintenance and pregnancy requirements at the expense of lactation and growth requirements.

3.4-3: Protein requirements. Protein is utilized following breakdown into individual amino acids and absorption across the digestive tract. Some protein is lost in feces. Thus, crude protein is the term used to define the protein content of feed, while digestible protein refers to the crude protein of feed minus protein lost in feces. Proteins on average contain 16% nitrogen. Multiplication of the nitrogen content by 6.25 gives the approximate value for crude protein.

Nonruminants require dietary protein containing sufficient amounts of essential amino acids since these cannot be synthesized. Ruminants have the advantage of microbial synthesis of protein to aid in meeting requirements of essential amino acids. In fact, if a source of nitrogen, such as urea, is supplied in the diet, the microbes in the rumen utilize available carbon from

Table 3.7. Efficiency of utilization for maintenance of metabolizable energy in various nutrients and foods

Food or Nutrient	Animal	Efficiency (%)
Carbohydrates		
glucose	Dog	95
glucose (per rumen)	Sheep	94
glucose (per abomasum)	Sheep	100
glucose	Fowl	89
starch	Fowl	97
starch	Rat	88
Fats		
olive oil	Dog	95
olive oil	Rat	99
Proteins		
casein	Rat	76
casein (per abomasum)	Sheep	82
Volatile Fatty Acids		
acetic	Sheep	59
propionic	Sheep	86
butyric	Sheep	76
Roughages		
dried ryegrass (young)	Sheep	78
dried ryegrass (mature)	Sheep	74
meadow hay	Sheep	70
lucerne hay	Steer	66
sudan grass hay	Cow	75
Concentrates		
maize	Sheep	78
maize	Steer	82

Source: From McDonald et al. 1973.

plant carbohydrates to synthesize enough amino acids to meet requirements of nonlactating animals.

Protein requirements of animals depend on age and stage of lactation. The three major routes of protein utilization are growth, maintenance, and lactation. As in energy requirements for lactation, each increase in milk production requires an additional increase in crude protein content of the diet. Requirements for growth, lactation, and maintenance are given in Tables 3.3–3.6.

3.4-4: Mineral requirements. Mineral requirements of animals are influenced by stage of life cycle. Lactation imposes large mineral demands on animals due to the mineral content of milk and minerals required in nutrient transport and metabolism. Milk contains large amounts of calcium, phosphorus, and potassium, resulting in increased metabolism of these minerals during lactation. Sodium, chloride, magnesium, and sulfur requirements of animals also increase during lactation, due to increased energy metabolism. Collectively, these minerals are grouped into the category of major mineral requirements.

Balance studies indicate that cattle are in negative calcium and phosphorus balance in early lactation but replace these stores in late lactation and during the dry period. Inability of cattle to mobilize sufficient calcium from bone during early lactation is the basis of one of the major metabolic diseases of cattle, milk fever. Milk fever is further discussed in 3.9-3. In addition to milk fever, calcium- and phosphorus-deficient animals undergo weakening of bone and teeth. Because phosphorus is heavily involved in energy metabolism via ATP production, deficiency of this mineral also results in impaired energy metabolism.

Overfeeding of calcium and phosphorus during late pregnancy was once practiced to prevent calcium and phosphorus deficiency in early lactation. However, this practice is harmful to animals because it inhibits endogenous mobilization of calcium and phosphorus during early lactation and thus results in animals being more prone to develop milk fever. Calcium and phosphorus requirements for cattle, sheep, and swine are presented in Table 3.3–3.6.

Magnesium deficiency is ordinarily not a problem since sufficient quantities are available in most diets. However, cattle grazing on fresh-growth pastures may develop a deficiency, which can be overcome by supplementation with 0.06% magnesium.

Sodium and potassium also are required in large quantities in lactating animals. Sodium concentrations are low in milk; however, increased sodium requirements during lactation are due to increased nutrient transport. Sodium may be added directly to the diet or made available in salt blocks. In both cases, sodium supplied as sodium chloride provides any chloride needed in the diet.

Potassium concentrations in milk are high, and lactation imposes increased potassium requirements. Forages, which normally supply all potassium needed for ruminants, contain large amounts of potassium. However, certain feeding practices, such as feeding of by-products, may provide only minimal potassium. This may be further exacerbated in hot humid areas, which cause cattle to sweat. Sweat of ruminants contains large quantities of potassium, increasing potassium requirements of heat-stressed cattle as much as 15%. Presently, NRC recommendations for potassium content in diets of cattle is 0.8%. Research has shown that heat-stressed cattle require as much as 1% potassium in the diet to avoid decreases in milk yield. Potassium deficiency is characterized by loss of appetite, weight loss, rough hair coat, and decreased milk yield. The NRC recommended levels of sodium are 0.18% and potassium 0.8% for a ratio of 0.22. Until better information becomes available, this ratio is the only one recommended.

Trace minerals, which include iron, manganese, copper, molybdenum, zinc, cobalt, selenium, and iodine, are usually supplied in sufficient quantities in the diet. However, certain areas have soil deficiencies of one or more of these elements, resulting in potential deficiencies in animals fed forages or grain grown on these soils. Trace elements can be added to diets to avoid deficiency-related disease.

3.5: PARTITIONING OF NUTRIENTS

3.5-1: Background. At various stages of an animal's life cycle, certain tissues achieve metabolic priority over other tissues of the body. Well-known examples are the metabolic requirements of the fetus and placenta during pregnancy, the mammary gland during lactation, and bone and muscle during growth. To accommodate the increased requirements of high-priority tissues, the animal must alter the pattern with which nutrients are partitioned among the tissues. This shift in nutrient partitioning was identified in 3.1 as homeorhesis and is associated with altered physiological states requiring a shift in the division of the circulating nutrient pool. The shift in nutrient partitioning occurs at several levels and is largely controlled by the central nervous system. Along with changes in body metabolism, changes may occur in animal behavior, such as "salt drive," which occurs with onset of lactation, and the dipsogenic response to suckling in many mammals. On the other hand, homeostasis is a process that is constantly at work at all points of an animal's life cycle.

The most dramatic examples of homeorhesis are the changes that occur with onset of lactation. The metabolic requirements of lactation far exceed maintenance requirements of the adult animal. Lactogenesis signals the commencement of a massive nutrient drain from the dam to support growth and development of the neonate. This requires a tremendous alteration in maternal metabolism and underscores the high priority placed on lactation to ensure survival of the species. Many behavioral and metabolic adaptations have evolved in various species to assist the dam in meeting this metabolic challenge. These adaptations are well defined in only a few species. The endocrine regulation of metabolism during lactation is even less understood.

Two excellent examples of homeorhesis occur in certain pinniped species and in ruminants. Most species double or triple food intake during lactation. In contrast, the Weddell seal and northern and southern elephant seals neither eat nor drink during the entire lactation of approximately 28 days. To accomplish this feat, milks of these species contain no detectable lactose, which spares glucose for maternal maintenance requirements. Instead, the milk is extremely high in fat content, ranging from 15% in early lactation to 55% in late lactation in the northern elephant seal. Water for milk synthesis is derived from maternal fat catabolism, and water conservation is further enhanced as lactation progresses, due to the steadily rising fat content of milk. Likewise, in the offspring energy and water conservation mechanisms develop as they reduce heat loss via increased insulation of developing blubber and reduce water loss via apneustic breathing and low urine output.

Ruminants also have evolved mechanisms to spare glucose. However, the glucose-sparing mechanisms are oriented toward sparing glucose for lactose production and utilization. These mechanisms are well defined and include utilization of propionate for glucose production, utilization of acetate for fat and energy production, and absence of the citrate cleavage pathway in adipose and mammary tissue, which prevents utilization of glucose in fat synthesis. The ruminant neonate is able to utilize the glucose in lactose because onset of rumen fermentation is delayed for several weeks. If rumen fermentation were not delayed, no lactose would escape rumen degradation.

Homeorhesis involves changes at several levels of mammalian organization. Major alterations, which will be discussed in this section, deal with redistribution of cardiac output toward mammary circulation and uptake of nutrients, alteration in turnover of key metabolites via alteration in cellular metabolism of key tissues, and change in endocrine status of the dam.

3.5-2: Metabolic adaptations associated with onset of lactation. To some degree, virtually every mammalian tissue participates in the redirection of nutrient flow toward neonatal nourishment. In addition, metabolic adaptations that have evolved in a given species achieve their fullest expression in meeting the nutrient demand of lactation.

It is not possible in this section to deal with all the metabolic changes in various tissues associated with homeorhetic adaptation to lactation. Attention will be given to metabolism of substrates for key milk constituents. Table 3.8 is a partial list of metabolic adaptations associated with onset of lactation.

Intake of feed and water is usually increased in mammals with onset of lactation; exceptions are pinnipeds previously mentioned in 3.5-1. Increased feed intake necessarily involves the feeding intake centers of the hypothalamus. Neuropeptides and neurotransmitters involved in increasing feed intake are not well identified. Digestive tract hypertrophy occurs during pregnancy and into lactation to accommodate increased gut fill, resulting in an increased capacity for nutrient absorption and increased nutrient flow into the metabolizable nutrient pool (Fig. 3.1).

Water, the greatest contributor to milk volume, contributes from 34–89% of the total volume in milk, depending on the species; however, as a constitutent it has been studied the least. Increased uptake of water by the mammary gland triggers the thirst drive in mammals, leading to increased water intake and flow of water across the digestive tract. If water intake is in excess or is inadequate, kidney outflow of water is regulated by antidiuretic hormone (ADH) to conserve or excrete water. Normally, water availability is not limiting. However, suckling has been shown to cause release of ADH, which is associated with the thirst drive and water conservation.

Table 3.8. Partial list of metabolic adaptations associated with onset of lactation

Physiological Function	Metabolic Change	Tissues Involved
Milk synthesis	Increased use of nutrients	Mammary gland
Intake and digestion	Increased food and water consumption	Central nervous system
	Hypertrophy of digestive tract Increased capacity for nutrient absorption	All segments of digestive tract
Lipid metabolism	Increased lipolysis Decreased lipogenesis	Adipose tissue
Glucose metabolism	Increased gluconeogenesis, increased glycogenolysis	Liver
	Utilization of acetate for energy[a]	Mammary gland
Protein metabolism	Mobilization of protein reserves	Muscle and other body tissues
Mineral metabolism	Increased absorption and mobilization of reserves	Gut, bone, kidney, liver
Water metabolism	Increased absorption and expansion of plasma volume	Gut, kidney, central nervous system

Source: Adapted from Bauman and Currie 1980.
[a]Ruminants.

Fat represents a major component of milk, especially from an energy standpoint, since it supplies the greatest percentage of calories in milk. The two major sources of fat in milk are de novo synthesis from acetate (BHBA and/or glucose) and the uptake of preformed fatty acids. Lipids may be of dietary origin or from adipose tissue stores. Extensive mobilization of lipid reserves often is necessary to meet energy demand of lactation. This requires increased lipolysis and decreased lipogenesis in adipose tissue during early and peak lactation (Fig. 3.5). These stores of fat are then replaced during late lactation and the dry period.

Glucose utilization for energy and lactose synthesis represents another major energy demand on the dam. Increased hepatic gluconeogenesis and decreased peripheral glucose utilization are essential to meet this demand, especially in ruminants, since dietary glucose does not escape rumen fermentation. Nonruminants can normally meet glucose requirements by increasing food consumption and reducing peripheral glucose utilization. However, gluconeogenesis from amino acids is an additional glucose source in early lactation, when the dam may be in a negative energy balance. In addition to increased glucose production during lactation, there is a concomitant reduction in glycogen deposition in liver and muscle. Ruminants utilize all the above-mentioned alterations in glucose metabolism during lactation. They also have evolved a glucose-sparing mechanism to shunt glucose toward lactose production and away from energy production (see 3.6).

Increased protein synthesis in the mammary gland requires an increase in amino acid flow across the digestive tract. If amino acid flow across the digestive tract is insufficient to meet protein synthesis requirements, mobilization of protein reserves from muscle and other tissues will occur.

Major minerals in milk are calcium, phosphorus, and potassium. Normally milk has a low sodium concentration because lactose serves as the major osmotic determinant of milk; however, sodium is required to move nutrients across the digestive tract. Thus, the salt drive known to occur in mammals during lactation is due to increased sodium requirement to assist in increased nutrient flow through the various nutrient pools. Roughages and muscle contain high concentrations of potassium. Therefore, herbivores and carnivores normally can find sufficient dietary potassium to meet requirements. Exceptions are by-product and high-concentrate rations, which may be low in potassium, necessitating the addition of potassium. This may be further exacerbated if ruminants are heat stressed, since their sweat contains large quantities of potassium (see 3.8). Calcium and phosphorus are obtained from dietary sources and mobilization of bone reserves. Failure to absorb and mobilize sufficient calcium results in milk fever, a major problem in high-yielding dairy cattle (see 3.9).

Numerous tissues are involved in absorbing and mobilizing nutrients to meet the metabolic requirements of lactation. In many cases, reduced utilization by peripheral tissues also is required to ensure that adequate nutrients are available for milk synthesis. This requires a delicate balancing of tissue needs and available nutrients, largely controlled by the central nervous system operating through hormones, neuropeptides, and neurotransmitters. Hormonal control of lactation is discussed in Chapter 2. Involvement of the endocrine system in nutrient partitioning during lactation is further discussed in 3.5-5.

3.5-3: Mammary blood flow. Rate of milk synthesis and secretion depends on availability of milk precursors, which in turn depends on rate of mammary blood flow and uptake by the mammary gland. Thus, control of mammary blood flow is a possible mechanism to control nutrient partitioning. Increasing blood flow through the mammary vascular bed, relative to other tissues, has the net effect of diverting nutrients away from peripheral tissues toward the process of milk synthesis and secretion in the mammary gland. Three considerations necessary to understand the relationship of mammary blood flow to nutrient partitioning are total mammary blood flow, mammary blood flow as a percentage of total cardiac output, and extraction efficiency of the tissue. Increasing blood flow to the mammary gland has no effect on diverting nutrients if cardiac output is also increased, which increases blood flow to other tissues. Likewise, if extraction efficiency of mammary tissue declines as blood flow increases, there is little or no net gain in substrate uptake.

Mammary blood flow in several species has been investigated in various physiological states using a variety of methods. The most prominent methods include radioactive microspheres, electromagnetic flowmeter, thermal dilution, antipyrine, and Evans blue dye techniques. Generally these methods are in agreement, with the exception that the indicator dye techniques tend to overestimate flow rates.

Because there is wide variation among mammals in location and number of mammary glands, there is also a wide diversity in location of arterial supply. The anatomy of mammary circulation is discussed in 1.5. The cow, sheep, and goat have been utilized most often to study mammary blood flow since the arterial supply is simple and readily accessible. The additional advantage of using domestic animals is that the venous system is readily cannulated. The study of mammary uptake of milk precursors can be obtained by multiplying mammary blood flow by arterial-venous difference of the substrate or hormone of choice. Accurate measurement of mammary uptake requires steady-state conditions in which mammary blood flow and substrate or hormone concentrations are not rapidly changing.

arterial concentration − venous concentration = arterial-venous difference

mammary uptake = arterial-venous difference × blood flow

Alterations in the physiological state of the mammary gland are associated with changes in mammary blood flow. Growth of the mammary gland during pregnancy is synchronized with growth of the mammary vascular system and increased blood flow. However, it is with onset of lactation that mammary blood flow increases most dramatically.

Resting blood flow through the mammary gland in nonlactating animals is related primarily to mass of tissue present. Older, nonlactating animals with large mammary glands have a higher resting blood flow than younger animals (Table 3.9).

3.5-4: Mammary uptake of milk precursors. The uptake of milk precursors by the mammary gland is limited more by rate of blood flow than by large changes in extraction. Work done mainly with goats and cows indicates little change in arterial-venous difference with low or high flow rates or low or elevated substrate concentrations; therefore, total uptake of various nutrients by the mammary gland is primarily flow limited. Elevation of a key substrate concentration, such as glucose, lowers blood flow rate but has no effect on extraction efficiency. Thus, there is considerable autoregulation of blood flow directly at the mammary gland. Factors that control dilation and constriction of the mammary vascular bed are not well understood. Several compounds have been shown to cause vasodilation, including acetylcholine, histamine, adenosine, and bradykinen, but whether or not these compounds actually control rate of mammary blood flow is not documented.

Since all milk precursors are derived from blood, it is not surprising that blood flow rate is highly correlated with milk yield. The average ratio of blood flow to milk yield is approximately 500:1. This means that a cow producing 45 kg milk per day requires 22,727 l blood to pass through the mammary vascular tree in 24 hr, or a blood flow rate of 15.78 l/min. The figure of 500:1 is an average of reported values. It should be noted that this relationship changes with stage of lactation and considerable animal varia-

Table 3.9. Comparative resting blood flow in nonlactating dairy cows

Cow	Previous Production[a] (kg)	Body Wt (kg)	Arterial Size[b] (mm)	Blood Flow (ml/min)
A	975	496	6.0	380
B	3367	509	6.0	510
C	7493	506	6.5	640
D	11410	571	9.0	1107

Source: Adapted from Heeken et al. 1983.
[a]Actual milk yield at time of experiment.
[b]External pudendal artery supplying one udder half.

Table 3.10. Arterial-venous differences across the mammary gland of cows, goats, and pigs

	% Substrate Extracted		
Substrate	Cow	Goat	Pig
Glucose	25	33	30
Acetate	56	63	45
β-Hydroxybutyrate	40	57	15
Lactate	10	28	15
Triglycerides	58	40	22
Free fatty acids	4	3	
Methionine	57	72	37
Phenylalanine	43	63	33
Leucine	44	63	33
Threonine	34	60	23
Lysine	59	49	26
Arginine	47	48	27
Isoleucine	45	47	31
Histidine	27	42	25
Valine	27	37	26
Glutamate	56	58	39
Tyrosine	45	39	25
Asparagine		37	1
Proline		36	31
Ornithine	42	36	16
Aspartate	50	33	13
Alanine	19	25	9
Glutamine		23	9

Source: Adapted from Linzell 1974.

tion exists. Ratios in early lactation of 1000:1 are not uncommon and late lactation estimates have been reported as low as 400:1.

Uptake of a specific nutrient by mammary tissue is directly related to the requirement of that nutrient for milk synthesis. Table 3.10 lists various substrates and the percentage of substrate extracted from blood or plasma across the mammary gland of cows, goats, and pigs. Species differences exist and are related to milk composition and intermediary metabolism of the mammary tissue of that species. For example, acetate and BHBA extraction is greater in ruminants (cows and goats) than in pigs. The percentage extraction of a given amino acid is representative of the proportion of that amino acid appearing in milk protein and varies considerably among and within species. Because of the high requirement of methionine and lysine for milk protein synthesis in cattle, these amino acids are considered limiting.

Substrates leave the capillary bed by various routes. Chylomicra are taken up by capillary endothelial cells, where the triacylglycerols are hydrolyzed by lipoprotein lipase. Subsequently, the free fatty acids and some glycerol are then taken up by the mammary epithelial cells. Glycerol and fatty acids not taken up by the epithelial cells appear in lymph and venous circulation. Amino acids diffuse out of the capillary beds passively but require an active transport system, gamma glutamyl transpeptidase, on the epithelial cell membrane for transport into the mammary epithelial cell. The affinity of the transpeptidase system for a given amino acid agrees with the percentage extraction of that amino acid for blood. In cattle, gamma glutamyl transpeptidase has a greater affinity for taking up methionine than alanine, which agrees with the extraction rate (Table 3.10). Uptake of milk precursors is further discussed in 4.4-1.

3.5-5: Endocrine involvement in nutrient partitioning. Control of homeostasis and homeorhesis on several levels of mammalian organization demands a high degree of cellular and organismal communication that is carried out by the central nervous system through a variety of organic compounds, broadly classified as hormones.

Hormones are intimately involved in regulation of metabolism and the process of lactation is hormone dependent. Previously, research on the endocrinology of lactation centered on the hormonal control of the mammary gland (see Chap 2). Recently, interest in endocrinology of lactation has been widened to include the involvement of the endocrine system in nutrient partitioning.

Table 3.11 lists some of the known adaptations that occur in hormone release or sensitivity of tissues to a hormone with onset of lactation. Knowledge of the endocrine adaptations occurring with onset of lactation is limited and reflects the relatively recent interest in this area.

Glucose is a limiting nutrient required for lactose synthesis; in turn, lactose controls milk volume. Several adaptations are known to occur that establish priority of the mammary gland in glucose metabolism. In goats and cattle, insulin is not required for glucose uptake or milk synthesis. This

Table 3.11. Partial list of endocrine adaptations associated with onset of lactation

Physiological Function	Tissues Involved	Adaptation
Glucose metabolism	Adipose[a]	Reduced insulin binding
	Mammary[a]	Lack of insulin requirement for lactose synthesis
	Pancreas[b]	Reduced insulin response to glucose load
Glucose metabolism	Liver[a]	Reduced insulin receptor numbers
	Peripheral[b]	Reduced insulin concentrations during early lactation
Lipid metabolism	Adipose[b]	Increased lipolytic response to epinephrine and norepinephrine
		Increased numbers of β-adrenergic receptors
	Mammary[a]	Increased prolactin binding
		Prolactin stimulated increase in lipoprotein lipase
Protein metabolism	Mammary[a]	Prolactin induced increase in activity of gamma glutamyl transpeptidase

[a]Measured in the rat.
[b]Measured in cattle.

removes a possible antagonism between peripheral tissues and the mammary gland in competing for available glucose. In addition, insulin concentrations are low during early lactation and rise as milk yield declines, reducing peripheral glucose uptake during early lactation when lactose synthesis rates are highest. The lower insulin concentrations during early lactation are not due to lower glucose flux. Glucose intake and gluconeogenesis are highest during this period. Instead, the pancreas releases less insulin in response to a glucose load. In rats, adipose tissue has been shown to have lower insulin receptor numbers with onset of lactation, which contributes to a lower glucose utilization for lipid synthesis in adipose tissue.

Lipid metabolism is markedly altered with onset of lactation (see 3.5-2). Mobilizing body fat reserves is an important adaptation to meet the energy requirements of lactation, especially when the animal is in a negative energy balance. Thus, adipose tissue switches from lipid synthesis to mobilization of lipid. Concomitantly, there is a decline in lipoprotein lipase activity in adipose tissue and an increase in lipoprotein lipase activity in mammary tissue. In rats, these changes can be induced by prolactin. In nonruminants, which utilize glucose for lipid synthesis, adipose tissue insulin receptor numbers and the responsiveness of adipose to insulin both decline with onset of lactation, reducing glucose uptake for lipid synthesis. In ruminants, the β-adrenergic receptor population increases with onset of lactation and is related to the increased lipolytic response of adipose tissue to epinephrine and norepinephrine during lactation (Table 3.11).

In summary, the endocrine environment during lactogenesis and lactation reduces peripheral utilization of nutrients and increases peripheral mobilization of fat, protein, and glucose. In concert with these changes is a shift in cardiac output distribution, which permits the mammary gland to take up these nutrients from the metabolizable nutrient pool.

3.6: MAMMARY GLAND METABOLISM

3.6-1: Background. The lactating mammary epithelial cell is one of the most metabolically active cells found in nature. Integration of mammary gland metabolism and peripheral metabolism is critical to prevent metabolic disorders. The redistribution of nutrient flow is the major physiological mechanism linking whole body metabolism to metabolism of the mammary gland. In addition to homeorhesis, within mammary epithelial cells, several adaptations occur that complement the organismal change in nutrient flux. The objective of this section is to describe energy metabolism in mammary epithelial cells and its relationship to milk fat synthesis. See Chapter 4 for further aspects of milk synthesis.

3.6-2: Structure and function. Lactating mammary epithelial cells are highly differentiated and easily discernible from nonlactating cells at the ultrastructural level. One of the general rules of biology is that form follows function, and this rule applies to the differentiated mammary epithelial cell. Individual structures in the lactating cell are associated with certain metabolic functions. This correlates with another general rule of biology; specialization requires compartmentalization. In other words, metabolic pathways are compartmentalized to increase efficiency and to avoid interfering with other metabolic pathways.

The major metabolic events associated with milk synthesis are illustrated in Figure 3.8. Transport of milk precursors occurs primarily at cell membranes. Synthesis of the nucleic acid code and messenger and ribosomal RNA occurs in the nucleus. The endoplasmic reticulum is the site of protein synthesis, esterification of fatty acids to glycerol to form triacylglycerols, phospholipid synthesis, and fatty acid desaturation. The mitochondrion is the site of production of ATP, nonessential amino acid precursors, and fatty acid precursors. The Golgi apparatus is where lactose synthesis, glycoprotein synthesis, casein phosphorylation, and packaging of water, K^+, lactose, and casein occurs. The cytosol is the site of the Embden-Meyerhoff glycolytic pathway, α-glycerol phosphate synthesis, reduced nicotinamide adenine dinucleotide phosphate (NADPH) generation, and amino acid activation for protein synthesis. Obviously, during the process

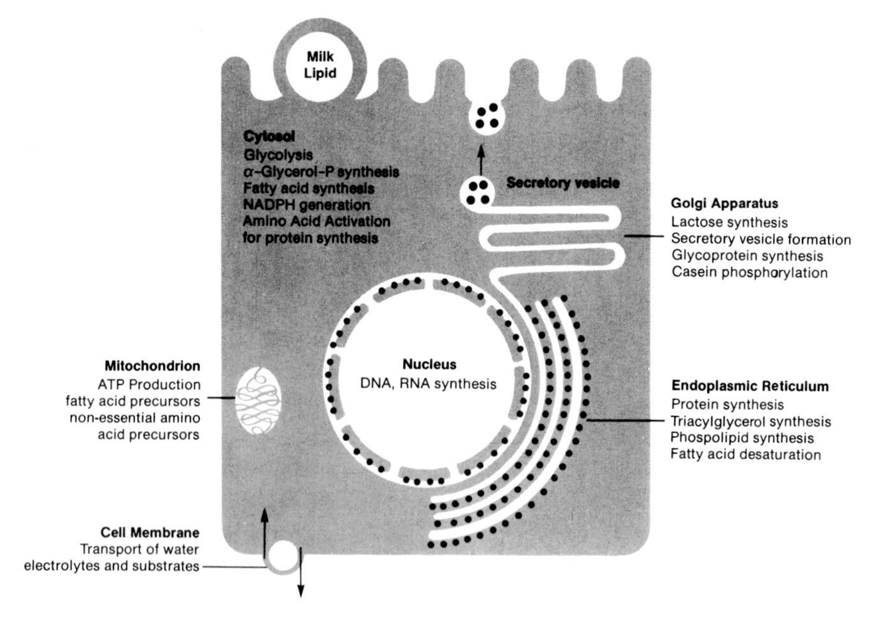

Fig. 3.8. Structure-function relationships in mammary epithelial cells. (Adapted from Davis and Bauman 1974)

of milk synthesis, there is interchange of substrates, intermediates, and nucleic acids between various compartments.

The process of regulating the flow of nutrients, synthetic products, and intermediates through the lactating cell and through the cell membrane is only partially understood (see Chap. 4). Membrane permeability influences movement of molecules in and out of various compartments. For instance, glucose can cross the membrane of the Golgi appratus but lactose cannot; citrate can exit the mitochondrion, but once in the cytoplasm, citrate does not readily reenter the mitochondrion. Microtubules and microfilaments are in some way involved because colchicine, which inhibits microtubule synthesis, halts milk secretion. The exact role of these cellular structures in cell organization and product flow in the cell is not yet fully understood.

3.6-3: Energy metabolism. The primary energy substrates for mammary cells are glucose and acetate. The major differences between ruminants and nonruminants with respect to the utilization of these compounds at the mammary epithelial cell are mirrored in the differences in concentrations in blood. Nonruminants have relatively high blood glucose and low blood acetate concentrations, while ruminants have much lower blood glucose and relatively high blood acetate concentrations. This difference in blood substrate concentration dictates a greater requirement for glucose utilization in fat synthesis in nonruminants and a requirement in ruminants to spare glucose as much as possible for lactose synthesis.

Glucose plays a central role in milk synthesis in both ruminants and nonruminants. Figure 3.9 illustrates the four major routes of glucose metabolism in lactating mammary epithelial cells. As glucose enters the cell,

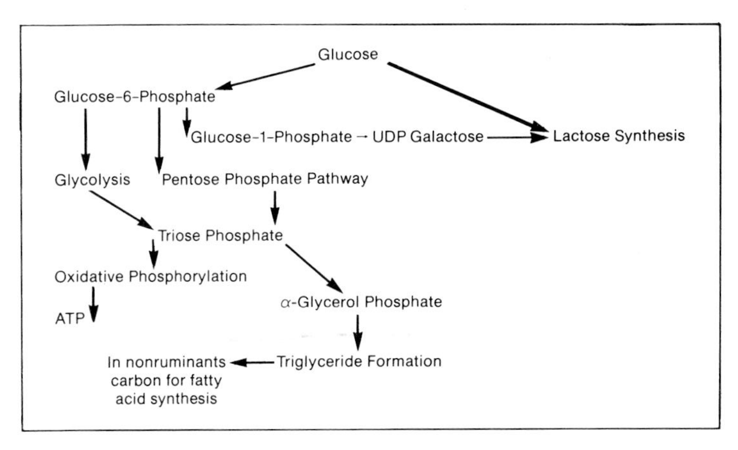

Fig. 3.9. Routes of glucose metabolism in mammary epithelial cells.

some is directly utilized in lactose synthesis in the Golgi apparatus. This reaction involves the terminal step in lactose synthesis whereby glucose acts as the galactosyl acceptor of UDP-galactose to form lactose and uridine diphosphate (UDP). The enzyme catalyzing this step is lactose synthase.

Glucose not immediately utilized in lactose synthesis is phosphorylated by the enzyme hexokinase to form glucose-6-phosphate. Glucose-6-phosphate may be utilized in one of three possible pathways that include formation of galactose, glycolysis, or formation of pentose phosphates. Galactose synthesis is further discussed in 4.6. Glycolysis and pentose phosphate formation utilize the remaining glucose phosphate. Glycolysis (Embden-Meyerhoff pathway) functions to provide energy to drive cellular metabolism, provide triose phosphates used in the formation of glycerol, and produce carbon for amino acid and fatty acid synthesis. The pentose phosphate cycle is interlocked with the pathways involving fatty acid synthesis via the production of the cofactor NADPH by the pentose phosphate cycle. This cofactor is utilized to provide hydrogen ions (reducing equivalents) needed for fatty acid synthesis. The fatty acid synthesis pathway, in turn, produces the oxidized form of the cofactor nicotinamide adenine dinucleotide phosphate (NADP) utilized by the pentose phosphate pathway. The pentose sugars produced by the pentose phosphate pathway can also be used to synthesize pyridine nucleotides and nucleic acids. These three pathways of glucose phosphate metabolism in lactating mammary epithelial cells are summarized in Figure 3.9.

Triose phosphate is an intermediate in the glycolytic pathway, an intermediate in the pentose phosphate pathway, and is the major precursor for production of α-glycerol phosphate. Triacylglycerol formation uses α-glycerol phosphate as the carbon backbone to which fatty acids are attached.

Alternatively, triose phosphate can be used to produce pyruvate for the tricarboxylic acid (TCA) cycle, which results in production of reduced nicotinamide adenine dinucleotide (NADH), shown in Figures 3.10 and 3.11. The NADH produced may provide reducing equivalents for production of α-glycerol phosphate from triose phosphate or may participate in the production of malate from oxaloacetate in the malate transhydrogenation cycle. There is a difference between ruminants and nonruminants with respect to utilization of the NADH generated by pyruvate production from triose phosphate (Figs. 3.10 and 3.11). This difference, which is due to a much greater activity of the malate transhydrogenation cycle in nonruminants, is further discussed in 3.6-4.

Pyruvate readily enters the mitochondrion, which is the site of ATP generation, via the TCA cycle. Acetate also readily enters the mitochondrion and participates in the formation of ATP via its oxidation. Thus, in ruminants acetate taken up by the mammary cell participates in energy production and fatty acid synthesis. This has a glucose-sparing effect since less glucose is required for energy production and glucose provides essentially no carbons for fatty acid synthesis. The major reason for little participation of acetate in energy production and fat synthesis in nonruminants is its low concentration in blood.

BHBA is another by-product of rumen fermentation found in blood of ruminants and taken up by mammary tissue. However, BHBA is used pri-

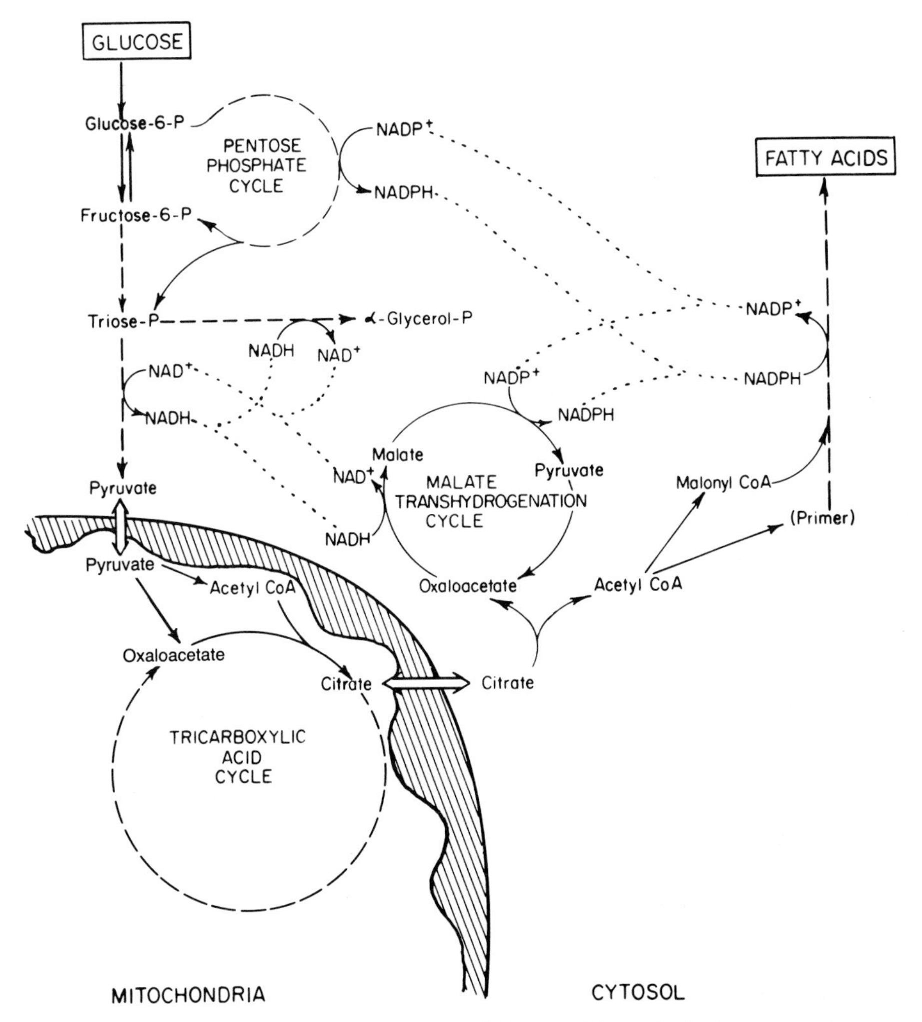

Fig. 3.10. Pathways of fatty acid synthesis in nonruminant mammary tissue. Triglycerides = triacylglycerols. (From Bauman and Davis 1974)

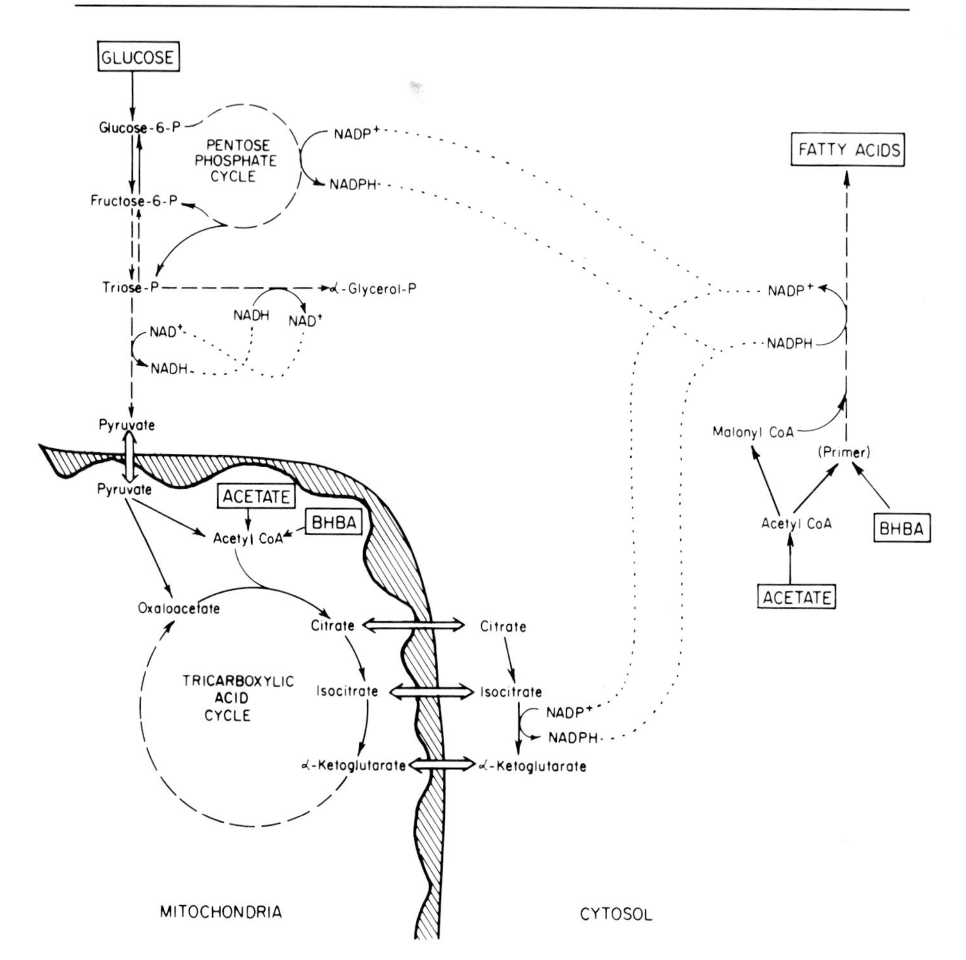

Fig. 3.11. Pathways of fatty acid synthesis in ruminant mammary tissue. (From Bauman and Davis 1974)

marily in fatty acid synthesis and does not appreciably participate in energy production.

3.6-4: Fatty acid synthesis. Fat is a major constituent and the greatest caloric component of milk. Fat in milk is composed primarily of triacylglycerols, either of dietary and blood origin or synthesized de novo in the mammary gland. Considerable species variation exists both in chain length and degree of saturation of milk lipids. Lipids of dietary origin are more highly saturated in ruminant animals, due to the hydrogenation of fatty acids in the rumen. Mammary epithelial cells of ruminants contain an active desaturase enzyme, which reduces the ratio of stearic and oleic acids in ruminant milk to that found in nonruminant species. Generally, lipids of dietary or blood origin are of longer chain length, $\geq C_{16}$, than those synthesized de novo, C_4-C_{16}. Data from several species indicate that at least 50 molar% of fatty acids in milk are synthesized de novo in the mammary gland.

Fatty acid synthesis occurs in the cytoplasm of the mammary epithelial cell and is essentially a two-step sequence (Fig. 3.12). The first reaction, catalyzed by acetyl CoA carboxylase, requires the substrate acetyl CoA. The second step is carried out by the fatty acid synthetase complex, which has been isolated from several mammalian tissues. In all mammalian tissues studied except the mammary gland, the predominant product of fatty acid synthesis is palmitic acid. However, fatty acid synthetase in mammary tissue has been modified to produce short- and medium-chain fatty acids. The reason for this difference in chain length is the presence of an additional enzyme, thioesterase II, which changes the products formed toward medium-chain fatty acids and away from palmitic acid.

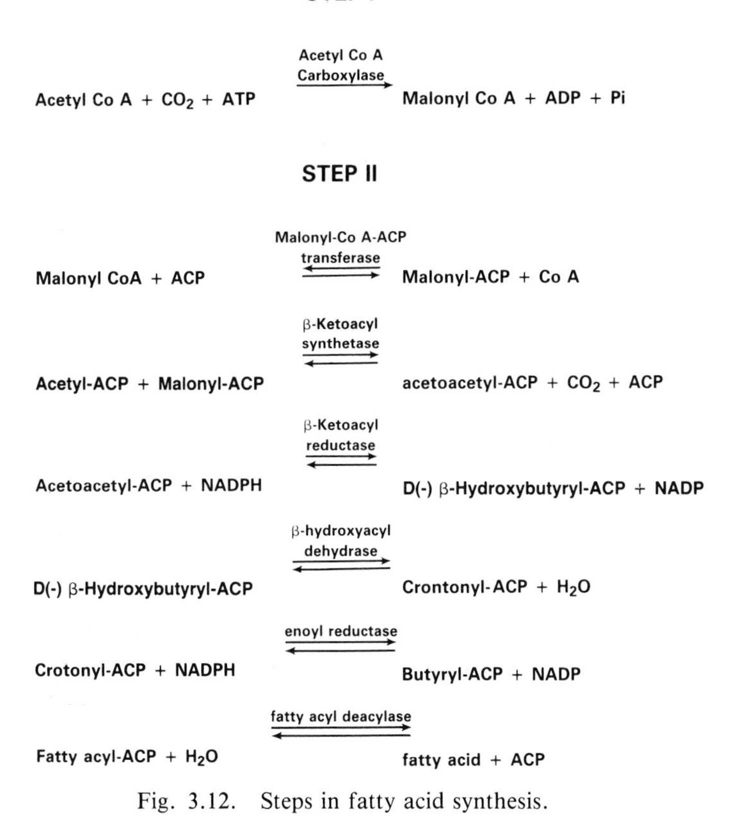

Fig. 3.12. Steps in fatty acid synthesis.

Major differences occur between ruminant and nonruminant species in two aspects of fatty acid synthesis; the generation of acetyl CoA is required for step 1, the generation of reducing equivalents in the form of NADPH for step 2 (Figs. 3.10 and 3.11).

In nonruminants (Fig. 3.10), acetyl CoA is generated in the mitochondrion by oxidative decarboxylation of pyruvate. However, acetyl CoA does not easily diffuse across the mitochondrial membrane. Citrate, which is formed by combining acetyl CoA and oxaloacetate, crosses the mitochondrial membrane and enters the cytoplasm. In the cytoplasm, citrate is cleaved by ATP-citrate lyase to form acetyl CoA and oxaloacetate. The acetyl CoA provides carbons for fatty acid synthesis; the oxaloacetate is used as a substrate for the malate transhydrogenation cycle, which generates pyruvate and NADPH for fatty acid synthesis. Pyruvate generated by the malate transhydrogenation cycle is then available to enter the mitochondrion. The pentose phosphate cycle is the other source of reducing equivalents in nonruminants.

In ruminants (Fig. 3.11), acetate and BHBA taken up from blood supply essentially all the carbons for fatty acid synthesis. Utilization of glucose for fatty acid synthesis is prevented by the absence of the citrate lyase enzyme in the cytosol of mammary tissue. Citrate, which leaves the mitochondrion, either is converted to isocitrate and subsequently to α-ketoglutarate, generating reducing equivalents, or may diffuse into the Golgi vesicle and subsequently into milk. Milk of ruminants has much higher citrate concentrations than that of nonruminants, which permits the use of citrate in secretions from mammary glands of ruminants as a marker for onset of lactogenesis during the periparturient period. Reducing equivalents for step 2 in fatty acid synthesis of ruminant animals, therefore, are generated by the pentose phosphate cycle and conversion of citrate to α-ketoglutarate (Fig. 3.11).

Acetyl CoA carboxylase activity increases dramatically with onset of lactation; this enzyme is considered regulatory in milk fat synthesis, since it is required for formation of malonyl CoA. The second step in fatty acid synthesis (Fig. 3.12) begins with the binding of malonyl or butyryl CoA to the fatty acid synthetase complex via a thioester linkage. This complex is composed of seven enzyme subunits and an acyl carrier protein (ACP) to which all the intermediates are bound. Once the malonyl or butyryl CoA binds to the ACP, the reaction sequence is condensation, ketoreduction, dehydration, and enoylreduction. This completes one cycle of chain-length addition. Subsequently, malonyl CoA is added to the carboxyl end of the newly synthesized fatty acid by repeating the cycle. The cycle is repeated until the chain is terminated by the fatty acyl deacylase (thioesterase II), with formation of fatty acids of short- or medium-chain length.

Milk fat is composed primarily of triacylglycerols, which are formed de novo in the mammary gland. Fatty acid and glycerol components of triacylglycerols may be of dietary or adipose store origin or synthesized within the mammary epithelial cell (see 4.5 and Fig. 4.10). Triacylglycerols in blood chylomicra and low-density lipoproteins are acted on by lipoprotein lipase, providing glycerol, free fatty acids, and 2-monoacylglycerol for uptake by mammary epithelial cells. In mammary epithelial cells, formation of triacylglycerols takes place by esterification of the fatty acids to the glycerol backbone; the primary pathway involves esterification of fatty acids to α-glycerol phosphate, which may arise from triose phosphate during glycolysis. It also may be derived by phosphorylating glycerol, which is taken up following lipolysis of blood-borne triacylglycerols. Formation of the triacylglycerol completes the process of milk fat synthesis. Secretion of milk fat is discussed in 4.8.

3.7: MILK QUALITY

3.7-1: Background. Milk composition is discussed thoroughly in Chapter 5. The objective of this section is to discuss nutritional and environmental effects on milk quality. The quality of milk is determined by its composition, bacterial content, and flavor. Milk composition and bacterial content are determined by standard laboratory tests. Milk flavor, which is determined by the consumer, is a combination of the taste, texture, and smell of milk.

3.7-2: Nutritional effects. Diet can influence composition and flavor of milk. High-grain and/or low-roughage diets alter rumen fermentation, favoring production of propionate and shifting of the acetate:propionate ratio, often resulting in a decline in milk fat content. Milk fat depression also can be caused by certain types of roughage, such as pearl millet or fresh lush pastures, or roughage that is ground too finely. To avoid depression in milk fat content, feed 15–17% crude fiber in the diet.

Various off-flavors can be secreted into milk from feed sources such as fresh pasture, garlic, onions, and strong silage. These are due to volatile oils present in the plant material that are taken up by the mammary gland and appear in the milk fat.

Contamination of feed with pesticides, herbicides, antibiotics, aflatoxins, or other chemical contaminants is always a potential problem. This area has been extensively researched, and milk is routinely examined for commonly detected residues of these compounds. In addition, many feed companies analyze rations for these compounds as well. Legal tolerance levels are established for most compounds. Examples are 5 parts per million (ppm) for polychlorinated biphenyls and 1.25 ppm for DDT. Constant vigilance by the producer, consumer, and regulatory agencies is a must as the use of chemicals in agriculture increases.

3.7-3: Seasonal effects. Environmental temperature extremes influence milk composition. Heat stress reduces roughage intake, which results in decline in milk yield as well as percentage of milk fat. Solids-not-fat also are lower during hot months. Cows calving during cooler months produce more fat and solids during their lactation than cows calving during warm months. The majority of seasonal effects on milk composition are attributed to temperature.

3.8: ENVIRONMENTAL EFFECTS

3.8-1: Background. Environment in its broadest sense refers to all factors other than genotype that influence an animal's productivity and health.

The environment of an animal directly affects production level by affecting basal metabolism, food intake, rate of digesta passage, maintenance requirements, reproduction, growth, and milk production. Indirect environmental effects are associated with quality and availability of feed.

The range of effective environmental temperature to which an animal can be exposed without changing its basal metabolism to maintain constant body temperature is referred to as the thermoneutral zone (Fig. 3.13). The upper and lower critical temperatures mark the upper and lower boundaries of this zone, within which thermoregulation is carried out without any additional metabolic cost to the animal. This range of temperatures, therefore, permits maximum milk production.

Both heat and cold stress increase maintenance requirements of cattle (Fig. 3.13). However, cold stress increases feed intake, which prevents a decline in milk yield until temperatures go below −5°C. In contrast, heat stress reduces feed intake and increases water intake, causing a rapid decline in milk yield as maintenance requirements increase and nutrient intake decreases.

3.8-2: Environmental factors. Figure 3.14 depicts the physical parameters of the environment that influence heat gain and loss in animals. Heat loss is influenced by wind speed, relative humidity, cloud cover, and surrounding ambient temperature. Heat gain is influenced by cloud cover, solar radiation, air temperature, vegetation, and geography. Latitude has a large effect on thermal environment because of its relationship to the angle of solar radiation and daylength. Latitudes between 30° north and 30° south are considered tropical or subtropical. Approximately 50% of the world's cattle are located in this region, where environmental heat stress greatly restricts milk production and growth. Latitudes between 30° and 60° north and south are generally considered temperate. However, in some locations and times of year, environmental stress may occur in these areas.

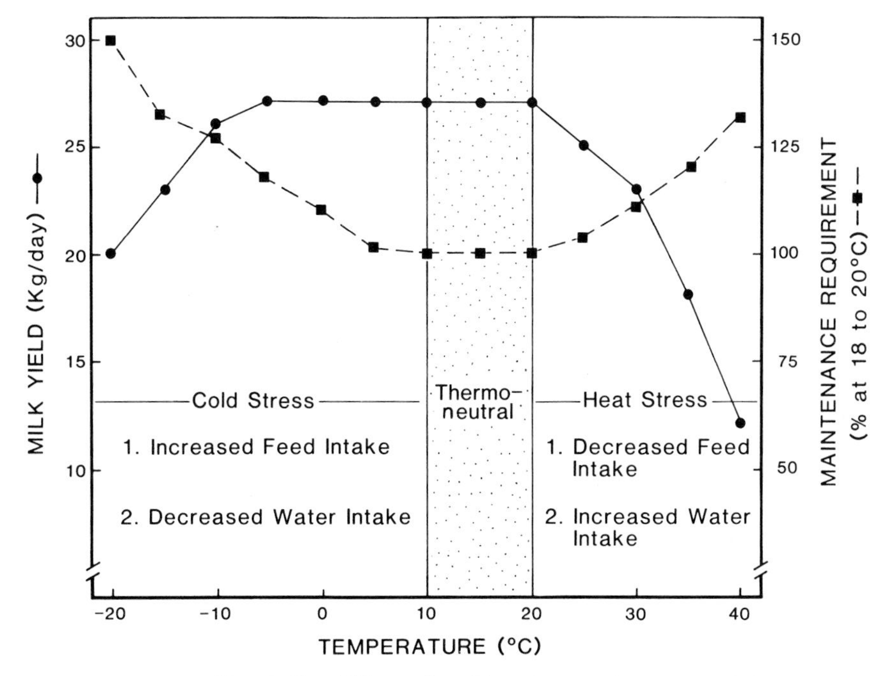

Fig. 3.13. Effect of ambient temperature on maintenance requirements and milk yields in 600-kg cattle. (Adapted from McDowell 1981)

Four routes of heat loss are available to animals: convection, conduction, radiation, and evaporation. The first three routes operate on a thermal gradient, while evaporation operates along a vapor pressure gradient. Air temperature and solar radiation affect the ability of animals to lose heat by convection, conduction, and radiation; relative humidity influences evaporative heat loss.

3.8-3: Animal factors. Factors influencing an animal's response to a given environment include age, degree of insulation, production level, and genotype. Young and neonates with less insulation and higher surface area:mass ratios gain and lose heat more rapidly than older animals. Lactating animals are more cold resistant and heat sensitive because milk production increases feed intake and metabolic heat production. Certain genetic strains or breeds of animals are adapted to hot or cold ambient conditions. The *Bos indicus* cattle, for example, which evolved in tropical regions, are more heat stress resistant than *Bos taurus* cattle. The primary reasons for the greater heat tolerance of *B. indicus* cattle are lower milk yield, feed intake, and basal metabolic rate.

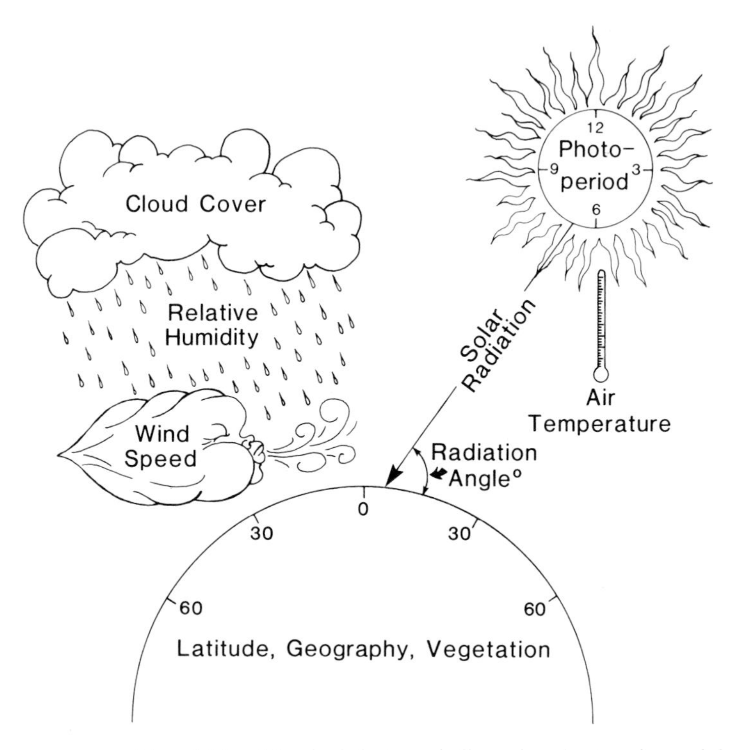

Fig. 3.14. Physical factors influencing heat gain and loss in domestic animals.

3.8-4: Feed and water consumption. Feed intake is increased by cold stress and decreased by heat stress. The increase in feed intake during cold stress is caused by increased maintenance requirements, primarily for metabolic heat production, and is not associated with increased milk yield (Fig. 3.13). In contrast, feed intake is reduced during heat stess despite the increase in maintenance requirements. This is related to the heat increment associated with feed intake. A number of physiological factors involved in heat stress effects on feed intake are direct effects of the heat stress on hypothalamic feed intake centers, the increased gut fill due to reduced rate of passage and increased water intake, and the increase in respiration rate. Increase in respiration rate is also associated with reduced rumination, since panting animals do not have time to eat or ruminate. Animals that do not pant, such as the horse and rat, also display a reduced feed consumption during hot weather. Animals exposed to daytime heat stress will shift their eating behavior to cooler night hours. Decreased food consumption during heat stress is the major reason for the decline of milk production.

Water intake slightly decreases during cold stress and rapidly increases during heat stress due to increased water requirement for evaporative heat loss. If ambient temperature is above the animal's body temperature, the only available route of heat loss is evaporation. Water may be evaporated at the skin surface by sweating or by increasing the respiratory water loss via panting, which is an extremely costly means of losing heat from a metabolic standpoint because it greatly reduces feed intake and, hence, milk yield. Furthermore, panting can result in excess CO_2 removal from blood, creating respiratory alkalosis.

3.8-5: Metabolic adaptation. Animals exposed to chronic environmental stress undergo metabolic adaptations to alleviate the effects of the stress. These include changes in endocrine function, basal metabolism, metabolism of water and electrolytes, acid-base balance, and (in ruminants) an alteration in rumen fermentation.

Ruminal VFA production is increased in cold stress, due to increased feed intake, and decreased in heat stress. The high heat increment associated with forage causes ruminants to selectively reduce forage consumption while maintaining concentrate intake. Reduction in forage intake may alter rumen fermentation, since acetate production may be decreased while propionate production may not. The alteration in acetate:propionate ratio is the probable cause of reduced milk fat yield during heat stress.

Heat stress also alters dietary protein utilization and protein metabolism. Reduced feed intake lowers dietary protein intake and also may reduce nitrogen balance. Several studies have shown a reduced nitrogen retention during heat stress.

Electrolyte metabolism, as well, is significantly affected by heat stress. Animals that utilize sweating as a means of increasing evaporative heat loss produce sweat that is either high in sodium, as in humans, or contains high potassium, as in cattle. Increased sweat loss of either potassium or sodium will increase dietary requirements of these electrolytes. Cattle normally are able to obtain potassium from forages, which contain large amounts of potassium. However, by-products such as sugar, bagasse, citrus pulp, and cotton seed hulls contain much lower quantities. Rations containing by-products or feeds low in potassium may not provide enough potassium in the diet to meet increased demands for potassium in cattle exposed to chronic thermal stress. Studies have shown that increasing the potassium concentration in rations low in potassium increased the milk yield in cattle exposed to chronic thermal stress.

3.8-6: Endocrine changes. Environmental stress has major effects on the endocrine system of animals due to the alteration in metabolism.

Cold stress increases secretion of hormones associated with increasing metabolic rate, elevating thyroxine and glucocorticoid concentrations in blood. In laboratory animals, growth hormone concentrations are elevated during cold stress, as well. However, no seasonal change in growth hormone concentrations has been detected in cattle. Prolactin concentrations are markedly decreased by cold stress in all species studied. The reason for this decrease is not clear but may be associated with reduced water and electrolyte metabolism during cold exposure. Prolactin is associated with osmoregulation in lower vertebrates. Epinephrine concentrations increase during cold exposure, and this is related to effects of epinephrine on lipolysis as energy requirements increase.

Chronic heat stress decreases circulating concentrations of thyroxine, growth hormone, and glucocorticoids. Reduction in concentrations of these hormones is related to reduced metabolic rate during heat stress.

Prolactin concentrations increase during heat stress, possibly due to increased water and electrolyte metabolism. Another hormone associated with electrolyte metabolism is aldosterone. Aldosterone acts at the distal convoluted tube of the kidney nephron to conserve sodium at the expense of potassium. In animals that secrete sweat high in sodium, aldosterone concentrations are elevated by heat stress. In contrast, animals that secrete sweat high in potassium display reduced aldosterone concentrations during thermal stress. The increase in sodium loss via the kidney resulting from lower aldosterone concentrations is related to the need to conserve potassium.

3.8-7: Milk yield. Milk yield is decreased by cold and heat stress. Decrease in milk yield during cold stress is due primarily to increased maintenance requirements to maintain body core temperature. Decrease during heat stress is due to direct effects of heat stress during lactation and indirect or carry-over effects of heat stress during pregnancy.

Direct effects of heat stress on milk yield are due to increased maintenance requirements to dissipate excess heat load, decreased metabolic rate, and decreased feed intake. Heat stress results in a much faster decrease in milk yield than cold stress (Fig. 3.13), due to the fact that during cold stress, animals increase feed intake to meet their increased maintenance requirement. However, heat stress reduces feed intake, despite the increased maintenance requirement, which results in a more rapid decline in milk yield.

In addition to direct effects of heat stress on lactation, there is a carry-over effect if animals are heat stressed during pregnancy. This is in part responsible for the seasonal trend in milk yield in cattle. Cows calving in cool winter months produce more milk in subsequent lactations than cows calving during hot summer months. Studies of sheep, cattle, and laboratory animals have shown that heat stress during pregnancy reduces fetal and placental growth and, in cattle, placental production of estrone sulphate. This alteration in endocrine status of the dam may reduce mammary growth. Alternatively, heat stress during pregnancy may alter the metabolic status of the dam, reducing her subsequent capability to respond to the metabolic challenge of lactation.

3.8-8: Milk composition. This section discusses environmental effects on milk composition. See Chapter 5 for a more thorough discussion of milk composition.

Milk yield and, therefore, composition yield is adversely affected by environmental stress. There are pronounced seasonal variations in milk composition of cattle. Fat percent, total solids, and solids-not-fat (SNF) are highest during winter. Seasonal variation in SNF is due primarily to variation in protein content of milk. Fat and protein are generally lowest during hot months and highest during cooler months. These changes are in part compounded by seasonal changes in forage type and availability.

Studies examining temperature effects on milk composition report a negative effect of high temperature on milk fat, protein, and lactose content. Decrease in milk fat concentration during heat stress has been related to alteration in rumen fermentation. Decreased forage consumption leads to an altered acetate:propionate ratio in rumen fluid, which is associated with reduced milk fat.

Changes in milk composition due to environment are related to altered feed intake and metabolism. Presently, there is no evidence that thermal environment directly affects the milk synthetic pathways of mammary epithelial cells.

3.9: METABOLIC DISEASES

3.9-1: Background. Lactating animals are susceptible to a variety of metabolic diseases, due to the occurrence of negative nutrient balance in early lactation. Metabolic disease also can be caused by poor management practices, such as overfeeding during the dry period.

Major diseases examined in this section are ketosis, milk fever, and hypomagnesemic tetany.

3.9-2: Ketosis. Ketosis occurs in dairy cattle during early lactation (10 days to 6 wk). A similar condition occurring during pregnancy rather than lactation is called pregnancy toxemia, which occurs in sheep bearing multiple fetuses. These animals are under greater metabolic stress than sheep bearing a single fetus. This metabolic disorder, characterized by elevation of ketone bodies (acetoacetic acid), BHBA, and acetone, is due to increased production of these compounds rather than reduced metabolism. A number of blood metabolites are altered during ketosis. However, the concentration of ketone bodies in body fluids is considered the most reliable indicator of the condition.

Table 3.12. Blood components of normal and ketotic cows

Component (mg%)	Normal	Ketotic
Blood		
glucose	52	28
ketones (total)	3	41
Plasma		
free fatty acids	3	33
triglycerides	14	8
free cholesterol	29	15
cholesterol esters	226	150
phospholipids	174	82

Source: Adapted from Schultz 1974.

Symptoms of this condition include decreased appetite, lethargy, decreased milk yield, increased milk fat percent, acetonelike odor of milk and of the cow's breath, and reduced body weight.

Blood metabolite changes occurring in ketotic animals are shown in Table 3.12. These changes include development of hypoglycemia; increases in concentrations of ketones and free fatty acids; and decreases in plasma triacylglycerol, free cholesterol, cholesterol esters, and phospholipids.

The sequence of events believed to lead to development of ketosis is initiated by an underlying negative energy balance, occurring in high-producing cattle in early lactation and multiple-conceptus-bearing sheep in late pregnancy. For reasons not fully understood, ketotic animals fail to maintain blood glucose concentrations, resulting in increased fat catabolism and transport of fatty acids into the liver in quantities greater than can be adequately metabolized. The result is development of fatty deposits in the liver and overproduction of ketone bodies by the liver. Most nonhepatic tissues can metabolize ketone bodies only in limited quantities. During ketosis in cattle, hepatic production exceeds capacity of nonhepatic tissues to metabolize ketone bodies, ketone bodies appear in urine (ketonuria), and there is an acetonelike odor of milk and breath. Treatment is based on increasing blood glucose concentration via glucose infusion and/or injection of glucocorticoids (or ACTH). Glucocorticoid injections stimulate gluconeogenesis and have a more prolonged effect on increasing blood glucose than glucose infusion.

Prevention of ketosis is generally centered on feeding practices during the dry period and early postpartum period. Overfeeding cattle during the dry period leads to excessive weight gain and reduced ability of animals to mobilize sufficient nutrients in early lactation. Thus, moderate feeding during the dry period is recommended. However, during the last 2–3 wk prepartum, concentrate levels should be increased to prepare animals for onset of lactation. This is termed challenge feeding. In addition, contrate levels should be increased rapidly in the postpartum period to aid animals in meeting energy requirements.

3.9-3: Parturient hypocalcemia (milk fever). Milk fever, a metabolic disease occurring in cattle during the immediate postpartum period, can be fatal if not treated promptly. Symptoms include low body temperature, unsteady gait or inability to stand, and depressed feed intake. Incidence is highest in Jersey cattle; within breeds, milk fever is usually associated with high milk production. Changes in blood constituents during milk fever include decreased plasma calcium, phosphorus, and parathormone and increased plasma calcitonin. Kinetic studies show that cattle are in negative calcium balance during lactation, due to high concentrations of calcium in milk. Ability of cattle to mobilize calcium from bone and absorb calcium from the digestive tract is essential to maintain blood calcium during this period.

Standard treatment of the disease is intravenous infusion of a calcium gluconate solution. Inflation of the udder, which greatly slows the rate of milk synthesis, is an old treatment that may be used if calcium solutions are not available. This treatment is recommended only as a last resort.

Preventive practices include feeding a low-calcium diet during the dry period to stimulate calcium mobilization, incomplete milking during the first 3 days following calving, and injection of vitamin D 3 days before expected calving date. Since gestation length is quite variable in cattle, the latter is difficult to time correctly. Numerous experiments show that overfeeding calcium during the dry period greatly increases the incidence of milk fever. Thus, dry-cow management is one of the most important factors in reducing incidence of the disease.

3.9-4: Hypomagnesemic tetany. This disease is sometimes referred to as grass tetany, since it occurs most commonly in cattle switched from hay and concentrates to lush pasture or grazing animals switched to a new pasture. Symptoms include low or normal blood magnesium and calcium, muscle spasms, excessive salivation, uncoordination, convulsions, coma, and death.

Decreased magnesium content of the diet or decreased uptake of magnesium across the gut is believed to be the primary cause of the disease. Treatment involves infusion of calcium gluconate containing magnesium. Preventive measures include magnesium supplementation of the diet. Additionally, magnesium may be increased in the feed by adding it to the fertilizer used on the soil.

REFERENCES

Allen, R. S. 1981. Lipid metabolism. In The Large Intestine, 560. See Wrong, Edmunds, and Chadwick 1981.

Bauman, D. E., and C. L. Davis. 1974. Biosynthesis of milk fat. In Lactation, 2:36, 38, 52. See Larson and Smith 1974.

Bauman, D. E., and W. B. Currie. 1980. Partitioning of nutrients during pregnancy and lactation: A review of mechanisms involving homeostasis and homeorhesis. J. Dairy Sci. 63:1514.

Bryant, M. P. 1981. Microbiology of the rumen. In The Large Intestine, 484. See Wrong, Edmunds, and Chadwick 1981.

Campbell, J. R., and J. F. Lasley. 1975. The physiology of digestion in nutrition. In The Science of Animals That Serve Mankind. 2d ed., 385. St. Louis: McGraw-Hill.

Davis, C. L., and D. E. Bauman. 1974. General metabolism associated with the synthesis of milk. In Lactation, 2:7. See Larson and Smith 1974.

Foley, R. C., D. L. Bath, F. N. Dickinson, and H. A. Tucker. 1972. Nutrient requirements. In Dairy Cattle: Principles, Practices, Problems, Profits, 208. Philadelphia: Lea & Febiger.

Heeken, M. M., R. J. Collier, D. Caton, and C. J. Wilcox. 1983. Variability of resting blood flow in nonlactating Holstein cows. J. Dairy Sci. 66:1742.

Hill, K. 1981. Digestion in the small intestine. In The Large Intestine, 391. See Wrong, Edmunds, and Chadwick 1981.

Larson, B. L., and V. R. Smith, eds. 1974. Lactation: A Comprehensive Treatise, vols. 1–3. New York: Academic.

Linzell, J. L. 1974. Mammary blood flow and methods of identifying and measuring precursors of milk. In Lactation, 1:206. See Larson and Smith 1974.

McDonald, P., R. A. Edwards, and J. F. D. Greenhalgh. 1973. Carbohydrates. In Animal Nutrition, 2d ed., 136, 216. Edinburgh, Scot.: Oliver and Boyde.

McDowell, R. 1981. Cited in Effect of Environment on Nutrient Requirements of Domestic Animals, 79. Washington, D.C.: National Research Council, National Academy Press.

National Research Council. 1975. Nutrient Requirements of Sheep. 5th ed. Washington, D.C.: National Academy of Science.

______. 1978. Nutrient Requirements of Dairy Cattle. 5th ed. Washington, D.C.: National Academy of Science.

______. 1979. Nutrient Requirements of Swine. 8th ed. Washington, D.C.: National Academy of Science.

______. 1984. Nutrient Requirements of Beef Cattle. 6th ed. Washington, D.C.: National Academy of Science.

Ortiz, D. L., D. Costa, and B. J. Le Boeuf. 1978. Water and energy flux in elephant seal pups fasting under natural conditions. Physiol. Zool. 51:166.

Phillipson, A. T. 1970. Ruminant digestion. In The Large Intestine, 424. See Wrong, Edmunds, and Chadwick 1981.

Reidman, M., and C. L. Ortiz. 1979. Changes in milk composition during lactation in the northern elephant seal. Physiol. Zool. 52:240.

Schultz, L. H. 1974. Ketosis. In Lactation, 2:320. See Larson and Smith 1974.

Swenson, M. J., ed. 1970. Dukes' Physiology of Domestic Animals. 8th ed. Ithaca, N.Y.: Cornell Univ. Press.

Wrong, O. M., C. J. Edmunds, and U. S. Chadwick, eds. 1981. The Large Intestine, 3–10. Lancaster, Eng.: MT.

CHAPTER 4

BIOSYNTHESIS AND CELLULAR SECRETION OF MILK

BRUCE L. LARSON

4.1: INTRODUCTION

The overall process of milk synthesis and secretion involves the supplying of suitable precursors to the mammary gland, their conversion into milk, and its ejection from the gland. The lactating mammary gland is a complex organ composed of specialized cells, which respond to and work in harmony with the remainder of the animal during lactation. Milk, a product containing many unique constituents not found elsewhere in nature, is synthesized in the highly specialized secretory cells of the mammary gland. The conceptual understanding of how milk synthesis occurs in these cells has been a fascinating story paralleling the development of the fields of physiology, endocrinology, biochemistry, and molecular biology. The mechanisms that remain unknown lie at the inner intricate molecular aspects of the functions of living cells.

Many species have been used to study the mechanisms of milk synthesis and secretion. Although broad generalities cover all species, caution in interpretation is necessary because of the considerable species variations in types and relative amounts of certain milk constituents. Milks of some related species contain unique proteins or high amounts of other proteins found only in traces in other species. Certain related species contain little or no lactose, and fat composition varies widely, both in total amount and in component fatty acids. The milk system studied most extensively is that of the ruminants, the bovine in particular. Synthetic mechanisms in the mammary gland have been studied principally with ruminant species and, in more recent years, with common laboratory species. Many of these studies have been extrapolated directly to other species, such as human, which in some situations has led to erroneous conclusions.

Consideration of the factors involved in the synthesis and cellular ejection of milk requires a basic understanding of the biological concepts concerning cells and their organelle components and metabolism. Some background concepts have been covered in previous chapters. If the reader encounters difficulties in understanding, reference to some basic biology and biochemistry texts on fundamental principles should be made.

4.2: LACTATING MAMMARY GLAND

4.2-1: Development. The mammary gland is an organ under complex endocrine control that proceeds through the early stages of development in the young animal, eventually into pregnancy, lactation, and the regression cycle. During pregnancy, cells of the future secretory epithelium proliferate and differentiate into secretory function with approaching parturition and onset of milk production. Various hormones, including estrogen and progesterone, are involved as mitogenic and morphogenic agents with early alveolar and lobular development. Working in harmony, particular hormones have specific effects. Corticosteroids have been implicated in the development and maintenance of cellular structures for the synthesis of the export proteins, and prolactin is necessary for the initiation and functional maintenance of the cellular apparatus for milk secretion. See Chapters 1 and 2 for further discussion.

4.2-2: Structure. The secretory tissue of the lactating mammary gland is arranged in lobules, with each containing clusters of alveoli (Fig. 4.1). The alveoli are surrounded by intertwined blood vessels, and each alveolus contains a single layer of secretory epithelial cells surrounding the central lumen into which the cells eject the synthesized milk (Fig. 4.2). These structures are shown dramatically in the scanning electron micrograph (Fig. 4.3), where the surrounding tissue of an individual alveolus has been digested away. The secretory cells comprise about one-half the total cells in the secretory tissue of the bovine mammary gland in lactation. The single-thick layer of cells is referred to as the secretory (or alveolar) epithelium and sometimes as the mammary barrier, since this cell layer stands as a barrier between materials in the blood and milk. Individual cells of the mammary secretory epithelium are most commonly referred to as secretory cells; the term alveolar cells is also used. In medical literature dealing with humans and laboratory species, the term acinus is used synonymously with alveolus; the term acinar cell also is encountered.

4.2-3: Secretory cells. Electron and light micrographs of prepartum secretory cells are shown in Figure 4.4, lactating secretory cells are in Figure 4.5, and a lactating secretory cell is shown diagrammatically in Figure 4.6. The alveolar secretory epithelial cells are approximately cuboidal in shape with about 10 μm on a side. Individual cells are joined to their neighbor cells in the sheet on all sides by a tight junctional complex struc-

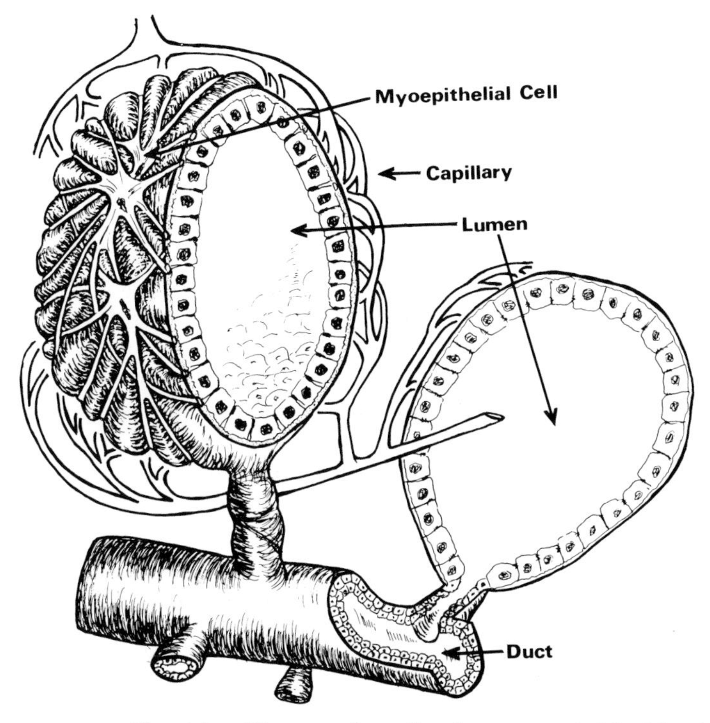

Fig. 4.1. Diagram of an alveolus surrounded by blood vessels and myoepithelial cells in the lactating mammary gland. Each alveolus contains a single layer of secretory (alveolar) cells that secrete milk into the interior lumen. Several alveoli in a group form a lobule. (Drawn by C. Andersen)

ture located around the apical portion that forms a tight barrier, which stops the passage of materials between cells under normal conditions. Blood components cross the basement membrane and are located in the interstitial spaces below and between individual cells along the basal and lateral (basolateral) membranes up to the tight junctional complex. The cells are probably also bound to adjacent cells through gap junctions, structures somewhat analogous to a sieve, which allow low molecular weight materials to pass from cell to cell. This intercellular exchange probably contributes to the observation that secretory cells in a particular alveolus are synchronized in their periodic discharge of milk into the lumen. A cross section of a myoepithelial cell process, part of the network surrounding each alveolus that responds by contraction to the hormone oxytocin, is shown in Figure 4.6 (network in Figs. 4.1 and 4.3). The resultant squeezing of the alveolus causes the flow of milk from the lumen into the ductal passages (see Chap. 2).

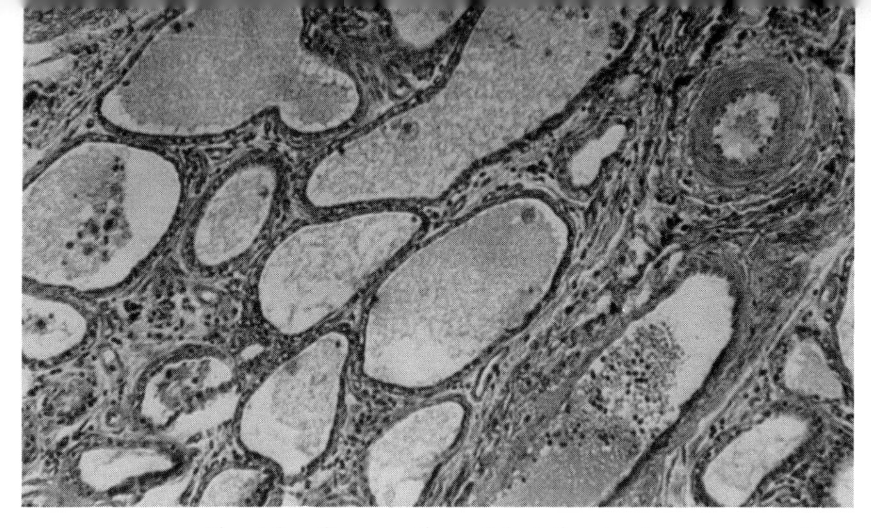

Fig. 4.2. Cross section of lactating bovine mammary tissue showing several alveoli lined with secretory cells, the interior lumen, and the stromal areas of various types of cells lying between the alveoli. A blood vessel is shown in the upper right portion of the picture. Milk in the lumen is somewhat distorted due to the fixation process in preparing the microscopic mount. About ×100 magnification.

Fig. 4.3. Scanning electron micrograph of lactating murine mammary tissue incubated in collagenase and hyaluronidase to digest away extraneous tissues. An alveolus is shown with individual secretory cells (*A*) surrounded by an encircling blood vessel (*B*) and myoepithelial cells (*C*). 1 micron (μ) = 1 micrometer (μm). (From Caruolo 1980)

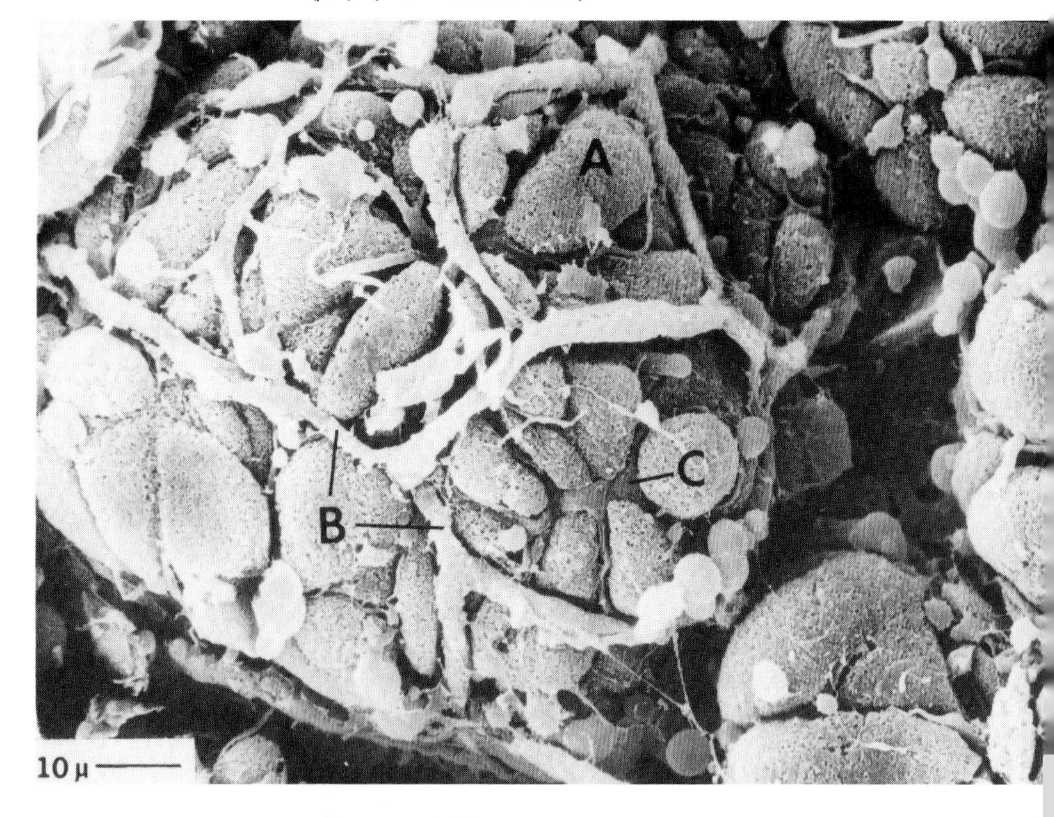

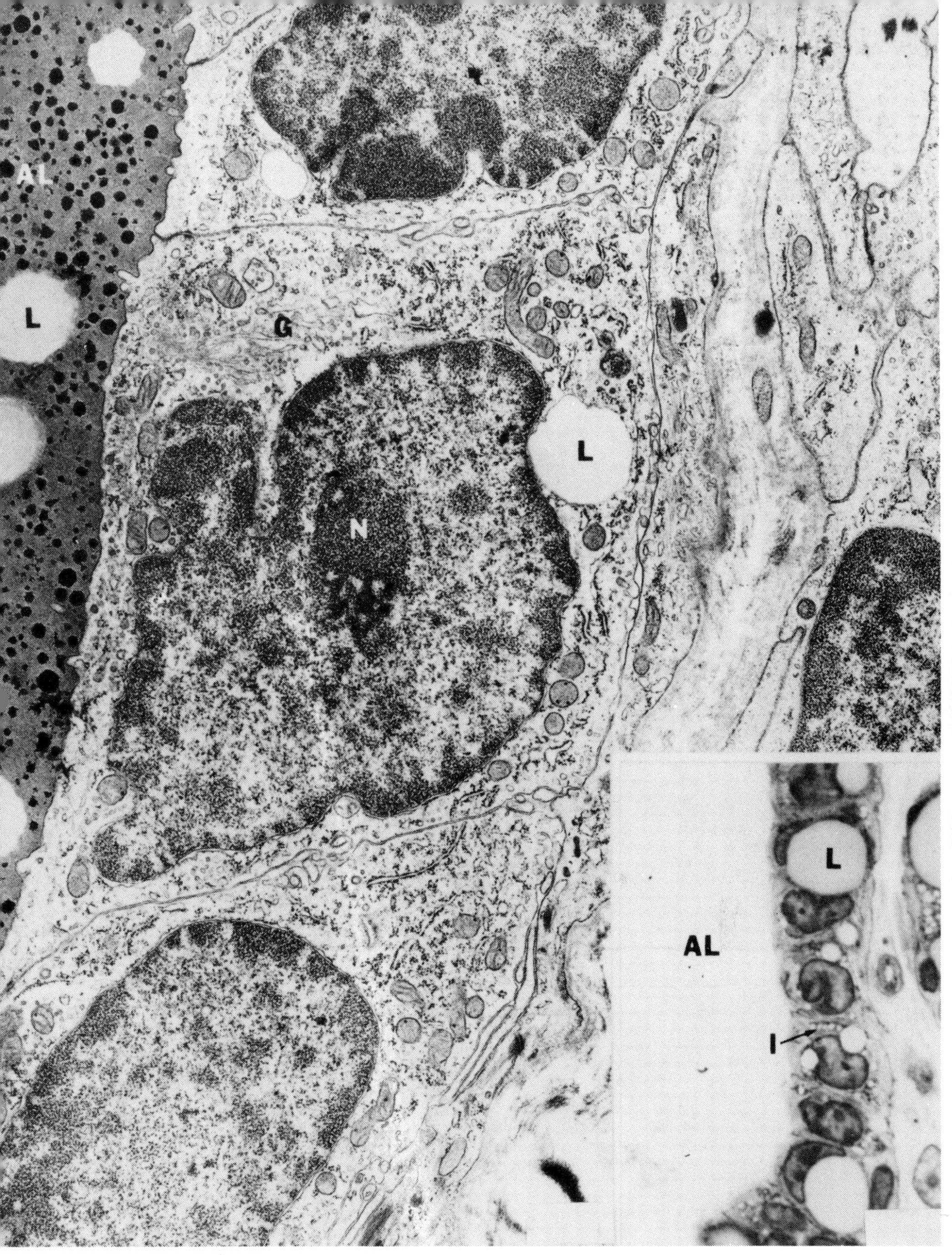

Fig. 4.4. Electron micrograph of 2-day prepartum bovine alveolar epithelium. The cells contain large irregular-shaped nuclei (*N*) and lipid inclusions (*L*). There is limited development of the Golgi (*G*) and rough endoplasmic reticulum (see Fig. 4.5). The alveolar lumen (*AL*) contains accumulated secretions with the electron-dense material, presumably protein. About ×10,000 magnification. Inset: Light micrograph of prepartum alveolar epithelium taken from a comparable region. Cells lack the polarity of fully differentiated secretory cells (see Fig. 4.5) but contain lipid droplets varying in size from large (*L*) to small (*l*). (From Saacke and Heald 1974)

Fig. 4.5. Electron micrograph of postpartum bovine alveolar epithelium. The cells contain rounded-up nuclei (*N*), a well-developed cytomembrane system characterized by Golgi (*G*) in the apical region, and rough endoplasmic reticulum (*ER*) in the basal region. The Golgi vacuoles and secretory vesicles contain secreted milk with casein micelles similar to that secreted into the alveolar lumen (*AL*). Lipid droplets (*L*) are also present in the cell and lumen. Approximately ×8,000 magnification. Inset: Light micrograph of lactating alveolar epithelium taken from a comparable region. The cells show polarity due to the distribution of the cytomembrane system with the Golgi and secretory vesicles in the apical region and the rough endoplasmic reticulum in the basal and lateral regions. (From Saacke and Heald 1974)

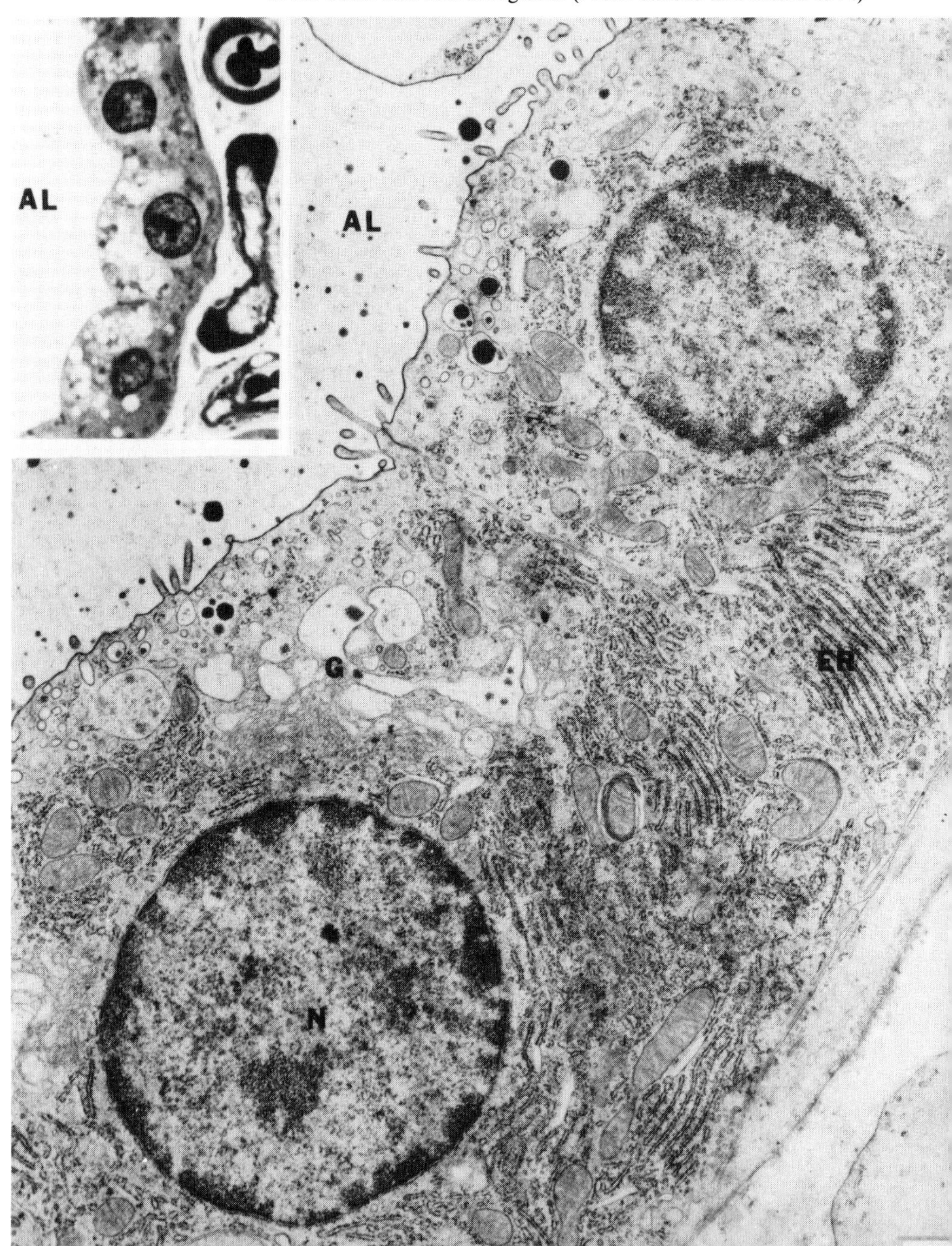

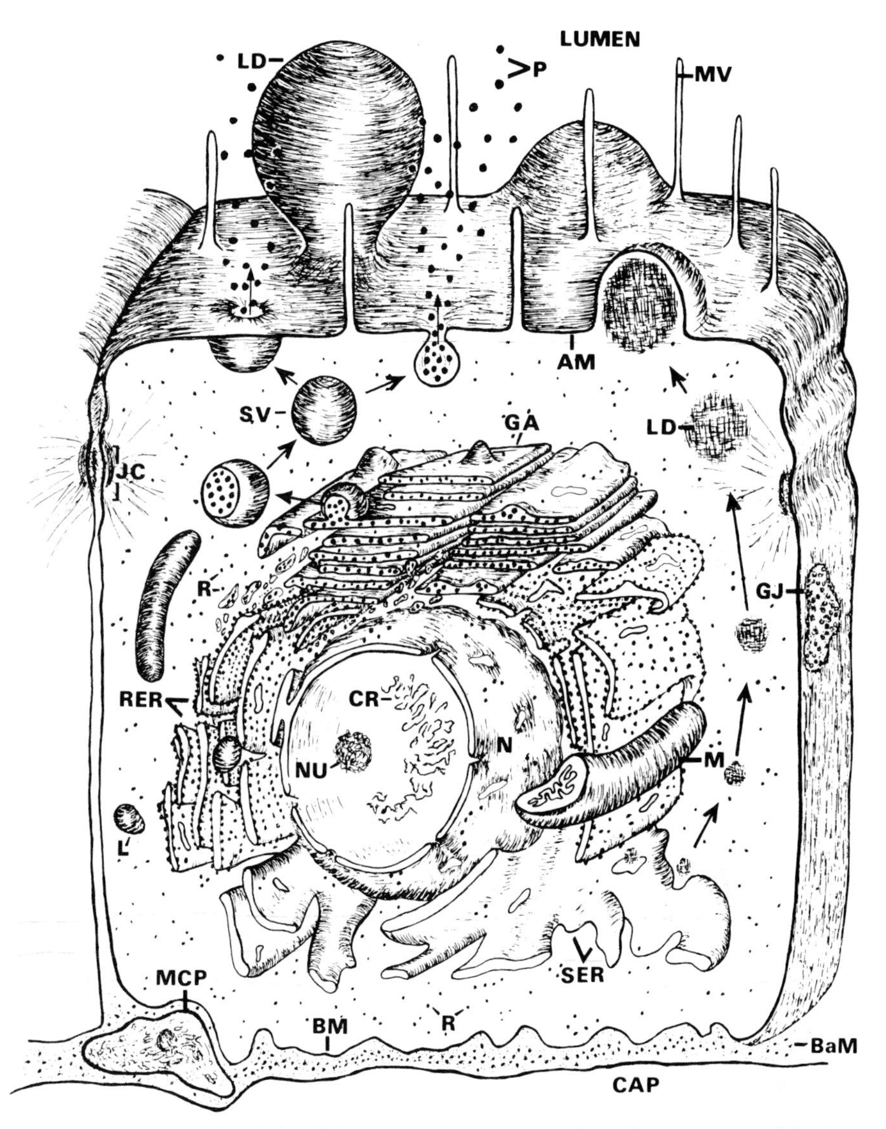

Fig. 4.6. Diagrammatic representation of a secretory cell in the alveolar epithelium of the lactating mammary gland. *AM* = apical plasma membrane; *BM* = basal plasma membrane; *BaM* = basement membrane; *CAP* = capillary; *CR* = chromosomes; *GA* = Golgi apparatus; *GJ* = gap junction; *JC* = junctional complex; *L* = lysosome; *LD* = lipid droplet (globule); *M* = mitochondrion; *MCP* = myoepithelial cell process; *MV* = microvilli; *N* = nucleus; *NU* = nucleolus; *P* = protein (casein micelle); *R* = ribosomes (free and bound); *RER* = rough endoplasmic reticulum; *SER* = smooth endoplasmic reticulum; *SV* = secretory vesicle. Precursors from the blood stream (*CAP*) enter the cell and exit into the lumen as milk constituents. (Drawn by C. Andersen)

The functions of the various organelles (Fig. 4.6) directly concerned with milk synthesis and secretion will be discussed in more detail later in the chapter. However, all cellular components are involved in one way or another with the cellular metabolism and must be considered part of the total functioning of the cell. Precursors from blood are taken into the cells through the basal and lateral membranes, and milk is discharged through the apical membrane into the lumen. The aqueous milieu within the cell forms the cytoplasm (or cytosol) in which the various internal organelles are interdispersed. The nucleus is the most prominent feature containing the genome (genes), which controls the functioning of the cell. The secretory cells have a well-developed endoplasmic reticulum (ER), a system of membrane-bound channels that begins with the nucleus and extends through the cytoplasm. Membranes comprising the ER are composed primarily of lipids and lipoproteins. They are the site of lipid synthesis and part of the flow of membranes that form inner vesicles as well as the outer plasma membrane surrounding the cell (see 4.5). Smooth endoplasmic reticulum (SER) is devoid of ribosomes, whereas the rough endoplasmic reticulum (RER) is covered with attached ribosomes. The RER in secretory cells is the site of synthesis of the polypeptide chains of export proteins, which comprise the major specific milk proteins. Unattached ribosomes exist in the cytosol, in particular in the areas surrounding the ER and Golgi, where synthesis of the cellular, or constitutive, proteins (structural and enzymatic) takes place. Mammary cells are typical secretory cells possessing a well-developed RER and Golgi apparatus, where the synthesized export proteins coming from the RER are modified and probably most of the nonfat milk constituents are added. Secretory vesicles originate in the Golgi to carry milk constituents and the vesicular membrane to the surface of the cell. The membranes of the cell, including essentially the ER, Golgi, vesicles, and plasma membranes, comprise the often referred to microsomal fraction isolated by centrifugal fractionation in mammary tissue studies.

Other essential cellular organelles include the mitrochondria, where energy is transferred from oxidizable substrates to ATP needed for the synthetic processes in the cell. Mitochondria are also the sites of synthesis of citrate and compounds used for the synthesis of nonessential amino acids. Lysosomes contain various enzymes that degrade unwanted materials and play a major role in the destruction of the cells with involution at the end of lactation. Microtubules and microfilaments also are present in many types of cells and are likely present in the mammary secretory cells in the process of milk synthesis.

4.3: METHODS OF STUDY

The biosynthesis and secretion of milk have been studied by a wide variety of techniques. Milk formation involves the transfer of some materials coming unchanged directly from blood, as well as the movement of precursors of the unique milk constituents from blood into the cell. Thus, the study of milk constituent synthesis in the mammary cell has necessarily followed development of the understanding of the origin of individual milk constituents. Changes in concentration of materials in the arterial blood supply to the mammary gland compared with the concentrations in the venous blood leaving it have been used as evidence that certain materials are removed and hence used for milk formation. While simple in concept, such arterio-venous techniques to determine the origin and amount of constituents were actually quite difficult to interpret with accuracy in the intact animal. Excision of the mammary gland and perfusion with blood under controlled conditions also has been used, allowing some better control, but eventual loss in function occurs within 24 hr. Today, these arterio-venous techniques can be conducted with reasonable accuracy for most materials. This was not true for many years through which controversy raged about the origin of certain milk constituents. For example, it was known that the mammary gland removed amino acids from blood, but it was not until the major milk proteins had been individually characterized and radioactive tracers had become available that it could be definitively established that the major milk proteins were synthesized completely from free amino acids and did not originate partly from preformed proteins removed from the bloodstream.

Methods that have provided significant insight into the functioning of secretory cells in milk synthesis include column techniques for the fractionation of proteins and other cellular compounds, use of radioactive tracer studies of metabolic pathways and precursors, enzyme assays and analysis of pathway intermediates, cell and organ cultures, isolation of cellular organelle fractions by centrifugation techniques, and electron microscopy.

4.4: PRECURSORS OF MILK AND METABOLIC PATHWAYS

Precursors of milk come from the bloodstream. The degree to which the individual milk constituents are different from or identical to those in blood and, thus, apparently pass unchanged into milk was a fertile field of investigation for many years. The predominant carbohydrate found in milk is the disaccharide lactose, composed of the two monosaccharides, glucose and galactose; only free glucose is found in blood. Some fatty acids are typical of milk fat in certain species, and the major milk proteins are not present in blood. Many materials in milk come unchanged from the bloodstream, including minerals, certain hormones, and several proteins, including some of the immunoglobulins. In ruminants, the latter pass the mammary barrier in huge amounts into colostrum just prior to parturition (see 4.8-4).

A comparison of bovine blood and milk is shown in Table 4.1, grouped according to the origin of the constituent in milk and to the precursor (or the same material) in blood. Large differences in sugar and salt concentrations are balanced since blood and milk are isotonic to each other with the same osmolality or osmotic pressure. A concentration effect is apparent for many constituents such as calcium, potassium, lactose, and the major proteins, with their precursor level in blood many times smaller than that found in milk. The reverse is true for others such as sodium, chloride, and serum albumin, where the blood amount is much larger than that found in milk. These observations of concentration differences in a constituent between blood and milk do not give much indication of whether there are special transfer mechanisms involved. Such observations also do not state unequivocally that the source of a constituent found in both places came from the blood. For example, the major source of citric acid, phospholipids, and orotic acid in bovine milk arises by synthesis in the secretory cell, not from blood. Many materials supply the mammary cell with the precursors necessary for milk synthesis; their identity depends to some degree on whether the animal is a ruminant or nonruminant.

Nutritional requirements for the general metabolism of the secretory cells and for the synthesis of the milk constituents, derived from feed consumed by the animal, are extracted from the blood. Animals require dietary

Table 4.1. Comparison of some bovine milk constituents with their precursor (or similar material) in blood

Constituent	Blood	Milk
	% (g/100 ml)	
Water	91	86
Glucose	0.05	tr
Lactose	0	4.6
Amino acids (free)	0.02	tr
Caseins	0	2.8
β-Lactoglobulin	0	0.32
α-Lactalbumin	0	0.13
Immunoglobulins	2.6	0.07[a]
Serum albumin	3.2	0.05
Triacylglycerols	0.06	3.7
Phospholipids	0.25	0.035
Citric acid	tr	0.18
Orotic acid	0	0.008
Calcium	0.01	0.13
Phosphorus	0.01	0.10
Sodium	0.34	0.05
Potassium	0.025	0.15
Chloride	0.35	0.11

Source: Data represent approximations from various sources. See Chapter 5 for more precise milk values.

[a]Colostrum may contain over 20% IgG.

sources of carbon and energy-producing materials, along with certain minerals including calcium, phosphorus, sodium, potassium, magnesium, chloride, copper, cobalt, manganese, iron, zinc, molybdenum, iodine, fluorine, selenium, and sulfur, together with the fat-soluble vitamins A, D, and E. Nonruminants also must be supplied with essential amino acids. Ruminants must extract all these essential materials from plant materials, composed primarily of cellulose, starch, fat, and protein. They undergo extensive degradation and resynthesis in the digestive process to provide the source of carbon for the major precursors, including essential amino acids synthesized by microorganisms in the rumen. Large amounts of water are also necessary. See Chapter 3 for further details on nutritional requirements.

The primary substrates extracted from blood by the lactating mammary gland are glucose, amino acids, fatty acids, and the mineral constituents. For ruminants, acetate and β-hydroxybutyrate (BHBA) are also prime substrates. Glucose is the precursor of lactose, citric acid, and most of the glycerol portion of the triacylglycerols synthesized in the cell. All essential amino acids and some nonessential amino acids required for milk protein synthesis come from blood. All purine and pyrimidine nucleotides required for DNA and RNA synthesis and involvement in lactose synthesis and other cellular functions are most likely synthesized in the cells. The energy source for synthetic processes in the cell is oxidation of glucose and acetate in the citric acid cycle and respiratory chain of reactions to oxygen. Reduced nicotinamide adenine dinucleotide phosphate (NADPH) provides the reducing power equivalents required for fatty acid synthesis, and it is produced from glucose through the pentose-shunt pathway and by the oxidation of isocitrate formed in the citric acid cycle.

An appreciation of the characteristics of the metabolic pathways from which the precursors of milk are assembled into milk constituents and which provide the energy to carry out these processes is fundamental to a general understanding of the processes of milk synthesis and secretion. The general concepts of these pathways and the specific compounds involved (see Chap. 3) include (1) the adenosine triphosphate (ATP) molecule and high-energy anhydride phosphate bonds, (2) reduced nicotinamide adenine dinucleotide (NADH) and NADPH and their role in electron transport, (3) the general pathway of oxidative phosphorylation, (4) the Embden-Meyerhoff glycolytic pathway, (5) the citric acid cycle, and (6) the pentose-monophosphate-shunt pathway.

There are many additional metabolic pathways operative in the cells. Two of note are those concerned with the synthesis of the purine and pyrimidine nucleotides present in DNA and RNA and some other important compounds. A fairly rapid turnover of certain RNAs is involved in the synthesis of the milk proteins. The pyrimidine nucleotide, uridine triphos-

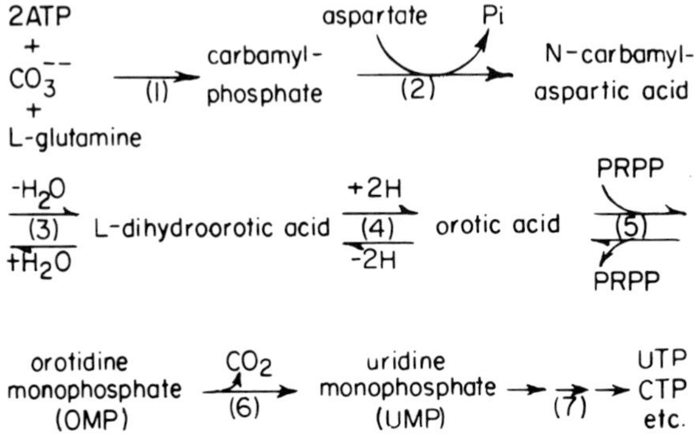

2ATP + CO_3^{--} + L-glutamine →(1) carbamyl-phosphate →(2) [aspartate → Pi] N-carbamyl-aspartic acid

$\underset{+H_2O}{\overset{-H_2O}{\rightleftharpoons}}$ (3) L-dihydroorotic acid $\underset{-2H}{\overset{+2H}{\rightleftharpoons}}$ (4) orotic acid $\rightleftharpoons$ (5) [PRPP / PRPP]

orotidine monophosphate (OMP) →(6) [CO_2] uridine monophosphate (UMP) → → (7) → UTP, CTP etc.

Fig. 4.7. Enzymatic steps of the pyrimidine synthesis pathway. The enzymes are (*1*) carbamyl phosphate synthetase, (*2*) aspartate transcarbamylase, (*3*) dihydroorotase, (*4*) dihydroorotic acid dehydrogenase, (*5*) orotate phosphoribosyl-transferase, (*6*) orotidine monophosphate decarboxylase, (*7*) other enzymes catalyze further steps past uridine monophosphate to uridine and cytidine triphosphates and the corresponding deoxyribonucleotides.

phate (UTP), plays a direct role in the synthesis of lactose. An intermediate on the pyrimidine synthesis pathway, orotic acid, also is found in elevated amounts in certain milks, particularly that of the bovine. For a better understanding of these roles, the pyrimidine synthesis pathway is shown in Figure 4.7, starting with the precursors to uridylic acid (uridine monophosphate or UMP), which upon successive phosphorylations yields uridine diphosphate (UDP) and UTP.

4.5: MILK FAT BIOSYNTHESIS

4.5-1: Background. The amount of fat in milk shows large species differences ranging from less than 1 or 2% to over 50%. The fat content of milk produced by the dairy cow is subject to wide variation between and within breeds. The same cow may show large differences depending on alterations in diet and environment.

Triacylglycerols (also called triacylglycerides and triglycerides) primarily comprise the lipids found in milk (97–98%); the remaining 2–3% are phospholipids and other minor constituents. Over half the milk lipid phosphorus is in the fat globule membrane with the remainder in the skim milk phase. Fat soluble constituents existing in association with the lipid fraction include various hydrocarbons and vitamin A; sterols, including vitamin D and cholesterol; tocopherols and vitamin E; sphingolipids; mono- and diacylglycerols; some alkylglyceryl ethers; and vitamin K (trace).

The biosynthesis of some of the fatty acid precursors occurs in the mitochondria, especially in nonruminants. The biosynthesis of fatty acids, glycerol, and other related intermediates occurs in the cytosol, and the biosynthesis of triacylglycerols takes place in or near the endoplasmic reticulum.

Pathway diagrams for the synthesis of fatty acids and triacylglycerols from their precursors and other related pathways have been presented in detail in Chapter 3. Detailed fatty acid analyses of milk lipids from different species are shown in Chapter 5. This present discussion will capsulize those presentations, along with relevant information concerning lipid synthesis in the total context of milk synthesis.

4.5-2: Origin of fatty acids and glycerol. The early use of the arterio-venous technique provided useful but often conflicting information on the precursors of milk fat. Following the advent of radioactive tracers and studies on their incorporation into metabolic intermediates, the molecular pathway for the synthesis of lipids in the mammary gland has become reasonably well delineated. The distribution of fatty acids of different chain lengths found in milk are dependent to a large degree on species and diet.

There are three sources for the origin of fatty acids present in milk triacylglycerols. The first source is glucose through glycolysis to pyruvic acid, which then goes into the citric acid cycle with the formation of acetyl CoA and oxaloacetate from citrate (see Figs. 3.9–3.12). This is a major source of fatty acids in nonruminants, but not in ruminants, which cannot utilize acetyl CoA formed from glucose in the mitochondria.

The second source is triacylglycerols consumed in the diet, or formed by bacteria in the rumen, that are absorbed intestinally as triacylglycerols and are present in the blood as chylomicra and low-density lipoproteins. These triacylglycerols are apparently hydrolyzed at the capillary wall/cell surface with the aid of lipoprotein lipase; fatty acids, glycerol, and some monoacylglycerols are then carried into the secretory cell. These fatty acids are generally more than 14 carbons in length and chiefly C_{16} (palmitic) and C_{18} (stearic, oleic, and linoleic) acids, a major source of fatty acids in all species. Estimates in ruminants are that about half or more of the fatty acids in milk are derived directly from the blood, including about one-third of the C_{16} acids and most of the C_{18} acids.

The third major source of milk fatty acids, and of prime importance for ruminants, is from fatty acids synthesized in the mammary gland from acetate and BHBA carried to it in blood from the rumen where they were produced in the bacterial fermentation. BHBA is used primarily for the first four carbons of most of the fatty acids synthesized in the gland and part is cleaved into C_2 units to be utilized as acetyl CoA for fatty acid synthesis. Acetate contributes to all the shorter (C_4–C_{14}) fatty acids and to a portion of the C_{16} fatty acids. The NADPH required for each reductive step on the pathway comes from the breakdown of glucose on the pentose-phosphate-shunt pathway and the oxidation of isocitrate to α-ketoglutarate in the citric acid cycle. The malonyl CoA pathway, with successive additions of two carbons in building up the carbon chain, is the major pathway for the synthesis of fatty acids in the ruminant mammary gland. The enzyme complex involved in this stepwise synthesis is fatty acid synthetase.

Species specificities shown in the relative prevalence of certain of the longer chain fatty acids synthesized in the malonyl CoA pathway apparently reflect some differences in the mechanism by which fatty acids are removed from the fatty acid synthetase complex. Also, the presence of butyric acid (C_4) is a characteristic of ruminant milks. See Table 5.5 for species analysis of fatty acids.

Fatty acids ingested in plant foods tend to be unsaturated and are altered to a considerable degree by rumen microorganisms that hydrogenate double bonds to produce the more saturated fatty acids. To increase the unsaturated fatty acid content of milk fat, there have been many studies in recent years in which cows were fed unsaturated fatty acids encapsulated in a coat of material resistant to rumen degradation, such as formaldehyde-treated casein. This coat is subsequently digested after leaving the rumen, releasing the unsaturated fatty acids, which are absorbed as such into the blood and pass into the milk fat. The mammary cells of ruminants possess some enzymatic activity that desaturates stearic acid (C_{18}) to oleic acid.

The primary source of glycerol for triacylglycerols in most species is glycerol-3-phosphate, formed either from glucose in the Embden-Meyerhoff glycolytic pathway or in the phosphorylation of glycerol originating from the lipolysis of triacylglycerols during uptake by the mammary gland. A much smaller source is from free glycerol taken up from the bloodstream.

4.5-3: Biosynthesis of triacylglycerols. Two major pathways for the synthesis of triacylglycerols are known; the α-glycerol phosphate pathway appears to predominate almost exclusively in mammary tissue. Free fatty acids are activated in the α-glycerol phosphate pathway by the formation of esters with CoA to form long-chain (fatty) acyl CoA. Two such molecules react with α-glycerol-3-phosphate to form phosphatidic acid, which, upon removal of the phosphate, leaves a 1,2-diacylglycerol. An additional long-chain acyl CoA adds the final fatty acid, with the formation of the triacylglycerol and CoA.

The placement of three fatty acids on the glycerol molecule does not occur in a random manner. Rather, the positions are characterized by the presence of certain predominant fatty acids. The short-chain fatty acids C_4 and C_8 found in ruminant milks are essentially in the 3-position of the glycerol. This location of the short-chain fatty acids resulting from de novo synthesis in the mammary gland suggests that they are esterified to a diac-

SCFA - Sn-3
C16 Sn-2
C18 Sn1 Sn-3

ylglycerol, which is already occupied in the 1- and 2-positions. The 2-position is characterized as the site of preferential esterification of palmitate (C_{16}) in higher molecular weight triacylglycerols and in the 1- and 3-positions in lower molecular weight triacylglycerols. Studies with bovine milk have indicated that the C_{18} fatty acids tend to be on the terminal 1- and 3-positions. These apparent consistencies in the location of fatty acids on glycerol strongly indicate the presence of some mechanism capable of differentiating between fatty acids of different chain lengths in the esterification process.

The generalized scheme of pathways for the origin and synthesis of triacylglycerols in milk indicating the major differences between ruminants and nonruminants is shown in Figure 4.8. It should be appreciated that while the major features of these pathways are well defined, there are yet extensive areas of incomplete knowledge, especially as concerns species differences. See Chapter 3 for detailed pathways.

4.5-4: Biosynthesis of other lipids. Phospholipids comprise as much as 1% of the total milk lipids, with about one-half or less in the skim milk fraction and the remainder associated with the fat globule membrane. Varieties of phospholipids include phosphoglycerides, phosphatidylcholine, phosphatidylserine, phosphatidylethanolamine, and phosphatidylinositol, and the sphingolipids, including sphingomyelins, glucosylceramides, and lactosylceramides. All appear to be synthesized de novo in the mammary cells. Phospholipids are taken up by the secretory cells from blood but metabolized into their components with the glycerol and fatty acids utilized for triacylglycerol synthesis. All of the phosphorus components of various milk constituents synthesized in the cells are formed from a common phosphate pool, including phospholipids, phosphate esterified on casein, and inorganic phosphate.

The origin of other materials associated with the lipid fraction of milk is not well delinated. Cholesterol in milk apparently arises both from synthesis within the mammary cells and by uptake from blood. Certain hydrocarbons, sterols (and vitamin D), tocopherols (and vitamin E), carotenoids (and vitamin A), and vitamin K are plant products found in milk; the content varies widely depending on the diet. See Chapter 5 for further discussion.

4.6: LACTOSE BIOSYNTHESIS

4.6-1: Background. Lactose (milk sugar), the principal carbohydrate found in milk, is a disaccharide composed of one molecule of glucose and one molecule of galactose joined in a 1-4 carbon linkage as a β-galactoside, specifically 4-*O*-β-D-galactopyranosyl-D-glucopyranose. Lactose is found in the milks of all species studied with but one exception (see Chap.

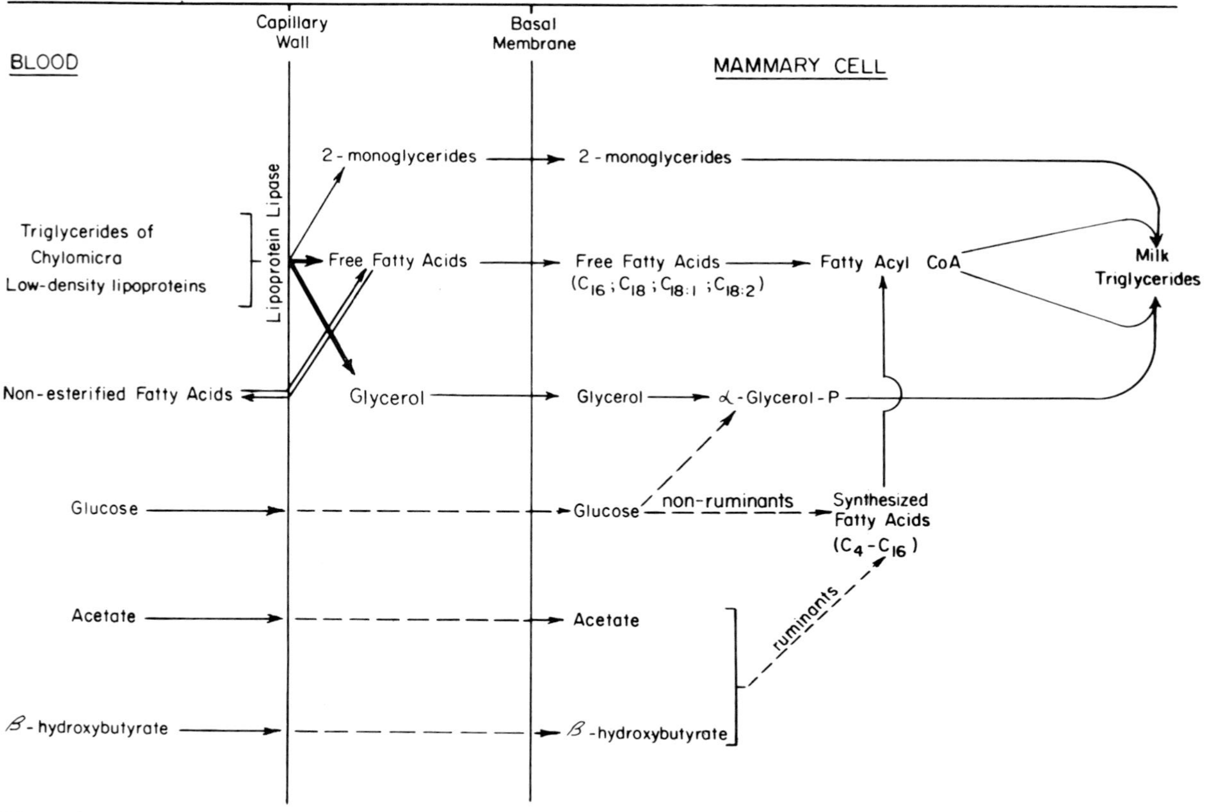

Fig. 4.8. Pathways for the origin of milk triglycerides (triacylglycerols). (From Bauman and Davis 1974)

5). Its concentration ranges from only traces in some aquatic species to around 7% in humans. In bovine milk, it is around 4.6%, the most constant constituent, and is related to its role in maintenance of the osmolality of the milk in the formation and secretion process.

4.6-2: Synthetic pathway. The pathway for lactose biosynthesis was considered for many years to involve a single enzyme, lactose synthase (formally called lactose synthetase), but the mechanism of its action remained elusive. It is now known that lactose synthase is composed of two proteins that must be together in performing the critical step in lactose synthesis. The synthetic pathway is as follows:

$$\text{UTP} + \text{glucose-1-P} \xrightarrow{(1)} \text{UDP-glucose} + \text{P-P}$$

$$\text{UDP-glucose} \xrightarrow{(2)} \text{UDP-galactose}$$

$$\text{UDP-galactose} + \text{glucose} \xrightarrow{(3)} \text{lactose} + \text{UDP}$$

where UTP = uridine triphosphate, UDP = uridine diphosphate, UDP-glucose = uridine diphosphoryl glucose, UDP-galactose = uridine diphosphoryl galactose, P-P = pyrophosphate, (1) = uridine diphosphoryl glucose pyrophosphorylase, (2) = uridine diphosphoryl galactose-4-epimerase, and (3) = lactose synthase (composed of galactosyl transferase and α-lactalbumin).

UTP is a product of the pyrimidine synthesis pathway, through progressive phosphorylations of UMP, with the UDP recycled back into UTP. UDP-galactose-4-epimerase (2) is an enzyme catalyzing inversion of the hydroxyl group on the number 4 carbon of UDP-glucose. It appears before parturition and its specific activity increases dramatically at the onset of copious milk synthesis with lactation. UDP-glucose pyrophosphorylase (1) is present in mammary as well as many other tissues; its specific activity also increases greatly at the onset of lactation.

The enzyme lactose synthase (3) demonstrates a dramatic change in enzymatic function with the onset of lactation. Composed of two components, the basic unit is a galactosyl transferase found both in mammary cells and various other tissue cells. This enzyme catalyzes the transfer of galactosyl groups from UDP-galactose to *N*-acetylglucosamine residues present in oligosaccharides attached to glycoproteins. In the presence of the milk protein α-lactalbumin, the action of the galactosyl transferase is modified so that it transfers a galactosyl group to free glucose with the formation of lactose. This discovery was an early example of an allosteric enzyme exercising control over an enzymatic reaction by cooperative interaction between the subunits. Glucose is a very poor acceptor of galactosyl residues ($K_m = 1.5$ M), but in the presence of α-lactalbumin, the galactosyl transferase is so altered that glucose becomes an acceptable substrate ($K_m = .001$ M). (K_m, the Michaelis constant, is equal to the molar substrate concentration that results in one-half the numerical maximum velocity of the enzymatic reaction.) The site of synthesis is in the membranes of the Golgi, where the galactosyl transferase is chiefly bound on their inner surfaces. The rate of synthesis is controlled by various factors, foremost of which is the availability of α-lactalbumin from synthesis in the RER and transfer to the Golgi. The lactose synthase system requires the presence of Mn^{2+} and is a complex stepwise reaction modified by the specifier protein α-lactalbumin.

4.6-3: Other carbohydrates in milk. In addition to small amounts of free glucose and galactose, there is a wide variety of carbohydrate-containing compounds that exist in milk and colostrum. Wide species differences exist in type and amount. These carbohydrates are almost completely in the combined state as oligosaccharides, glycopeptides, and glycoproteins and components of the nucleotide sugars. The presence of many of these components reflects in part the complexity of the milk synthesis and secretion processes, with some being by-products of these processes. Others represent the degradation of cells and cellular components.

4.7: MILK PROTEIN BIOSYNTHESIS

4.7-1: General origin of proteins. Milk proteins arise from several different origins. The majority represent specific proteins unique to lactation, whose polypeptide chains are synthesized under genetic control from free amino acids in the RER of the secretory cells. Cell culture studies have shown that bovine mammary cells require the usual essential amino acids for milk protein synthesis. Rat mammary cells do not require cysteine. The other nonessential amino acids are synthesized in the mammary cells of both species.

Certain blood proteins and similar proteins synthesized in plasma cells lying adjacent to the secretory epithelium are also transferred preformed into the lacteal secretions; large amounts are found in colostrum. Sources of additional proteins present in milk in small amounts include sloughed-off secretory cells, parts derived from these cells, and various types of other whole cells and their components. Centrifugation of milk (10,000 × *g*) removes most of the minor protein constituents associated with the fat globule membrane, intact cells, and larger cellular fragments. Proteins from these sources possess a host of immunological, enzymatic, and other functional properties and collectively contribute to the complex protein system in milk.

This section will discuss the biosynthesis of the major milk proteins synthesized in the mammary secretory cell for export in milk. These proteins in bovine milk include all the major casein proteins (α_s-caseins, β-casein, κ-casein and γ-casein), β-lactoglobulin, and α-lactalbumin. Proteins analogous to most of these are found in milks of all species in varying amounts (see Chap. 5). Proteins entering the lacteal secretions from blood and cells and their fragments are discussed in 4.8.

4.7-2: Genome. Milk proteins for export are synthesized according to predetermined plans encoded in the genes. The genome is composed of deoxyribonucleic acid (DNA) and comprises the essential portion of the chromosomes present in the nucleus. Each cell contains a complete genome, and the DNA exists as a long-chain, double-strand molecule composed of two purine bases (guanine and adenine) and two pyrimidine bases (cytosine and thymine) bonded with the sugar deoxyribose and phosphate. DNA has the ability to direct the synthesis of enzymes that results in its own replication.

4.7-3: Protein biosynthesis pathway. The overall mechanism by which proteins are synthesized according to the encoded genetic plan is shown in Figure 4.9. Several types of ribonucleic acids (RNA) are involved. The RNAs are composed of the sugar ribose and phosphate plus three of the same purine and pyrimidine bases found in DNA, but the pyrimidine base, uracil, replaces thymine. In the presence of DNA-dependent RNA polymerase (transcriptase) and the appropriate nucleotide precursors, guanosine triphosphate (GTP), adenosine triphosphate (ATP), cytidine triphosphate (CTP), and uridine triphosphate (UTP), synthesis of a long-chain RNA molecule takes place along certain specified portions of one strand of the DNA chain. This transcription process results in the formation of a strand of messenger RNA (mRNA), complementary to the DNA from which it was formed through cross–hydrogen bonding of adenine to thymine (or uridine) and guanine to cytosine. The mRNA formed now carries the encoded message from the gene.

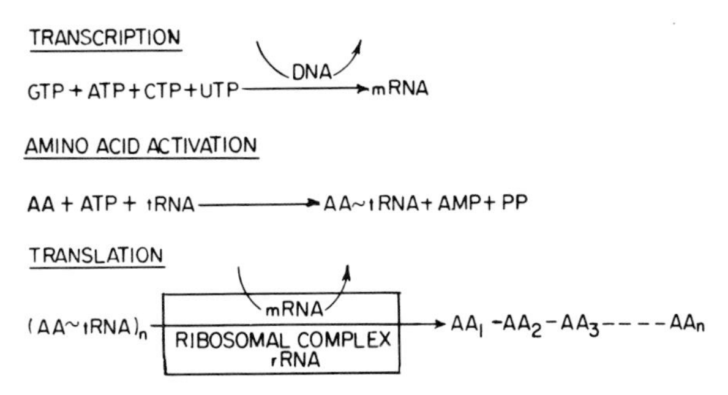

Fig. 4.9. Pathway for the synthesis of proteins from amino acids.

The mRNA moves from the nucleus to the ribosomes, located in the RER and cytoplasm. Ribosomes are composed of ribosomal RNA (rRNA) and several proteins in a ribonucleoprotein complex and are synthesized under direction from DNA but serve in the synthesis of many different proteins. Amino acids are first activated by reaction with ATP and attachment to transfer RNA (tRNA), forming aminoacyl-tRNA compounds. The tRNAs are specific for each amino acid, are small in molecular size, and are synthesized under direction from DNA.

The protein polypeptide chain is actually synthesized in the ribosomal complex in the translation process (Fig. 4.9). A ribosome attaches to the end of the mRNA chain, which moves through it similar to a computer tape. Each trinucleotide sequence within the mRNA chain codes an amino acid and is called a codon. Located in the tRNA is a trinucleotide anticodon sequence that recognizes it. As each codon on the mRNA comes into position, the appropriate aminoacyl-tRNA for which it codes moves in and the amino acid is joined to the previous one, resulting in a chain of amino acids moving out of the ribosome. Several ribosomes may be on a mRNA chain, collectively called a polysome. In the synthesis of export proteins in the RER, ribosomes are attached to the RER, and the protein polypeptide chain is synthesized with an additional initial chain of 10–20 amino acids. This initial signal peptide sequence mediates the passage of the start of the amino acid chain through the membrane of the RER into the inner passages and is clipped off in the process. The polypeptide chain inserted into the RER folds up in a configuration as a function of the physical forces in the amino acid sequence. Depending on the protein, certain other materials may be added later, such as a phosphate or certain types of sugar molecules. The final three-dimensional structure of the protein molecule determines its function and properties.

Secretory cells contain mitochondria, which also possess a small amount of DNA that genetically codes for some of the proteins and enzymes involved with mitochondrial function. Plants also contain mitochondria and chloroplasts that possess small amounts of DNA. Some bacteria have plasmids that contain DNA. These less-complicated sources of DNA have been the site of intense interest in genetic engineering advances. Specific animal genes have been inserted into DNA in bacterial plasmids, for example, which are passed on to daughter cells and carry on the inserted gene function.

4.7-3a: Control mechanisms. All cells in an organism contain a complete set of genes, and any one, such as a mammary secretory cell, at a given time only manufactures a small proportion of the proteins whose structures are encoded in its genome. Cells possess control mechanisms for turning on and off and controlling the rate of synthesis of specific proteins. Mammalian cells contain many times the amount of DNA necessary to encode all the functional proteins produced by the cell, and much of this DNA appears to be superfluous, not encoding anything. In the transcription process, mRNAs with functional (exons) as well as intervening nonfunctional (introns) regions are produced. Nuclear RNAs reflect not only RNAs involved in control mechanisms but also mRNA that has been produced, but as yet unprocessed, to remove the introns. Various inhibitors of protein synthesis operate at different points in the synthetic pathway. Some of these are useful antibiotics. For example, actinomycin D inhibits mRNA formation by inhibiting DNA-dependent RNA synthesis. Puromycin inhibits the incorporation of the aminoacyl-tRNA complexes into the ribosomes.

4.7-3b: Genetic code and mutations. The nucleotide sequence that specifies a certain amino acid could be expressed either as the trideoxynucleotide sequence in DNA or as the trinucleotide sequence in the complementary RNA; the RNA sequences are usually used. Certain amino acids, especially those with the largest amounts in proteins, have several trinucleotide codons in mRNA, coding for the same amino acid.

Mutations occur if an event changes the structure or order of the nucleotide base sequence in the DNA chain of the gene. This may be caused by a host of factors including certain mutagenic chemicals and physical forces such as ultraviolet light, radiation from X rays, radioactive isotopes, and cosmic rays, producing free radicals. Most changes are in a single base and may not be expressed if it still codes for the same amino acid. Even if expressed, an alteration in one amino acid may be of little consequence. If the mutation should add, delete, or alter one or more of the amino acids in a critical position important to the physical configuration of the protein, or in the active site of an enzyme, the protein may change its characteristics and no longer be functional. Conversely, new enzymes and functional proteins can arise in this manner.

Several genetic variants of the major milk proteins, derived from mutations, are known. For example, α-lactalbumin B, found in western cattle, differs from α-lactalbumin A, found in eastern cattle, in that one arginine in the former has been replaced by a glutamine in the latter. Similarly, α_{s1}-casein B is more prevalent in western cattle, particularly in Holsteins, Ayrshires, and Shorthorns. It differs from α_{s1}-casein C, which is more prevalent in eastern cattle, such as Zebu (India), Boran (Africa), Guernsey, and Jersey, in that one glutamic acid in the former has been replaced by a glycine in the latter. One particular blood line of Holstein cattle produces α_{s1}-casein A, which represents a deletion of 13 amino acids from the polypeptide chain.

These genetic polymorphs of the milk proteins differ from each other, with the variants of the genes occurring in an animal either singly in homozygotes (AA or BB for α-lactalbumin) or together in heterozygotes for a specific milk protein (AB for α-lactalbumin). The genetic variants of the milk proteins produced by an animal can serve as a useful index of the origin of that animal and may help explain differences in the physical properties of milk proteins isolated from different animals. See Chapter 5 for further discussion.

4.7-3c: Posttranslational modifications. After synthesis in the RER, the export milk proteins are transported to the Golgi apparatus of the cell in membrane-bound vesicles that break away from the RER. Modifications of the milk proteins, as well as synthesis and addition of most of the other nonlipid constituents of milk, occur in the Golgi region.

Phosphorylation of threonine and serine residues in the caseins occurs in the Golgi region catalyzed by protein kinases. Only certain threonyl and seryl hydroxyl groups are phosphorylated, depending on their location in the polypeptide chain. Glycosylation of certain proteins, including κ-casein and part of the α-lactalbumin molecules, also occurs in the Golgi. Glycosyl transferases first attach an *N*-acetylglucosamine to either the amide N of an asparaginyl residue or the hydroxyl oxygen of a seryl or threonyl residue. Additional galactosyl or *N*-acetylneuraminyl residues then attach to the *N*-acetylglucosamine.

Other posttranslational modifications can also have a great effect on the structure of the resultant protein. The formation of disulfides by joining two cysteinyl residues in both α-lactalbumin and β-lactoglobulin does not occur at random. The folding of the protein occurs so that the two critical cysteinyl residues, which may be far apart on the polypeptide chain, are brought into a position next to each other. In the presence of calcium and inorganic phosphate in the Golgi, the casein molecules aggregate into micelles. It is not until the individual caseins have been glycosylated and phosphorylated and calcium and inorganic phosphate added that the casein components assume their final three-dimensional structure in the complex micelle as it exists in secreted milk.

4.7-3d: Study of protein synthesis. The study of protein biosynthesis in the secretory cell on a molecular basis is extremely difficult; many of the mechanisms involved lie at the very heart of the most intricate aspects of molecular biology. For example, it is known that proteins synthesized in the cell are under hormonal control, but it is not known how this occurs on a molecular basis from the time a hormone or combination of hormones is picked up by a cell to the production within the nucleus of specific mRNAs that code for the synthesis of milk proteins and enzymes involved with the synthetic pathways of lactation. Considerable interest has centered around the mammary secretory cells as a model system for studying endocrine control and fundamental mechanisms of gene expression in protein synthesis. Undoubtedly, there will be a continuing advance in sophisticated techniques in this area. In vitro protein-synthesizing systems that will synthesize milk proteins have been established in the laboratory, and purified mRNAs that code for only certain milk proteins have been isolated.

Complementary DNA (cDNA) probes have been synthesized in the presence of mRNAs found in the lactating cell using the enzyme reverse transcriptase. Subsequent isolation and insertion of the cDNA into the plasmids of certain bacteria have already resulted in the in vitro production of these milk proteins by the bacteria. Studies with cDNA probes have shown that neither gene amplification (more than one copy of the gene in a cell for a specific protein present) nor accumulation of mRNAs for milk protein biosynthesis occurs prior to the onset of copious milk production at parturition. Further advances in the area of genetic understanding and engineering undoubtedly will occur, with the future holding promise for genetic manipulation of the dairy cow for more efficient milk production.

4.7-4: Biological significance of milk proteins. The concept of milk as a food and of the milk proteins as a nutritional source for the young animal dominated thought for many years. Milk proteins are not as easily considered functional compared to constitutive enzymes and other proteins with apparent specific cellular roles. The discovery that α-lactalbumin forms a part of the enzyme lactose synthase suggests that other major milk proteins also may have some specific intracellular function. Many investigators have looked without success for a major function for β-lactoglobulin, also synthesized in the RER and exported similarly to α-lactalbumin in ruminants and related species.

It may be speculated that the evolutionary precursors of caseins had some biological function, perhaps of a structural nature in the cell, that has been lost through evolution. The rather loose and open structure of casein argues against a specific biological function in the usual sense. The ability of casein to incorporate large amounts of phosphate (and associated calcium), which results in an easily digestible protein with a high essential amino acid content, argues for an evolutionary biological advantage for its presence in the secretory product available to the young animal.

A host of other proteins found in milk with defined enzymatic or other functions may represent either by-products of the synthetic processes or possibly products imparting an advantage to the young. Bovine milk has considerable xanthine oxidase, a major component of the fat globule membrane; it is difficult to explain why there is so much. Components such as lysozyme and lactoferrin are found in milk. Human milk contains quite high levels of each. Lactoferrin concentration is high in the dry bovine mammary gland. The antibacterial properties of these materials, lysozyme digesting bacterial polysaccharides and lactoferrin sequestering iron required by bacteria, argues for the evolutionary development of their beneficial role in reducing mastitic infections. The comparative location of similar amino acids in the polypeptide chains of lysozyme and α-lactalbumin demonstrates considerable homology, indicating that both are descended from a common evolutionary ancestor. Both proteins are enzymes concerned with carbohydrates, one with synthesis and the other with breakdown. As more sequence analysis of proteins is accomplished, ancestral relationships will become more apparent (see Chap. 5).

4.8: CELLULAR SECRETION OF MAJOR MILK CONSTITUENTS

The development of transmission electron microscopy has been a powerful tool in furthering the understanding of organelle components and pathways taken by precursors and constituents of milk in the secretory processes within the cell. In concert with cytological studies and the development of detailed centrifugal methods for the isolation and characterization of specific cellular organelles, it is now possible to understand the generalized secretion processes in the lactating cell. Mechanisms of the synthetic and secretory processes bear strong similarities in all types of secretory cells of exocrine glands that have been studied, especially those of the pancreas and salivary glands.

4.8-1: Pathway for export proteins and most nonfat constituents. The major milk proteins synthesized in the RER pass to the Golgi complex, where the other major nonfat constituents including lactose and salts are incorporated into the Golgi vesicles. Lactose is formed inside the vesicles and cannot diffuse out, thus drawing in water because of the differing osmotic pressure. The secretory vesicles, containing essentially the nonfat milk constituents, bud off from the Golgi and move toward the apical region of the cell (Fig. 4.6). Evidence from electron micrographs shows that the casein-protein complex in the secretory vesicles undergoes a maturation process as it passes to the apical membrane. Newly formed vesicles contain long stringy filaments, which in the more mature vesicles are more densely stained, rounded-up particles, similar to the casein micelles observed in secreted milk. The secretory vesicles move to the apical surface where the membrane surrounding each vesicle fuses with the plasma membrane, and the vesicular contents are discharged into the lumen (exocytosis).

4.8-2: Pathway for lipid globules. A second separate secretion pathway is taken by lipids, essentially triacylglycerols, which are synthesized in the vicinity of the ER. Lipid droplets increase in size as they move from the ER and through the cytoplasm toward the apical membrane, where they push through and bud off as globules encased in an envelope of apical plasma membrane. The apical membrane is composed primarily of lipids and related materials, which come from the walls of the secretory vesicles carrying the nonfat constituents of milk to the apical surface.

4.8-3: Membrane flow. The movement of essential materials leading to the synthesis and discharge of the milk constituents occurs in a sequential manner in the cell. The membranes involved in these processes contain many constituent types of lipids and proteins; the latter include both intrinsic proteins anchored in the lipid matrix as well as extrinsic proteins bound to the surface through ionic interactions.

The origin and flow of membranes and their constituent proteins form an essential part of the understanding of the processes of milk synthesis. It is believed that all of the membranes, starting with the nuclear envelope, ER, Golgi apparatus, secretory vesicles, and the plasma membranes, are functionally connected. Other membranes, including the outer mitochondrial and lysosomal, also may be connected. Constituent membrane proteins and complex lipids are synthesized and inserted into the membranes of the nuclear envelope and the ER. The membranes, or selected portions of them, are transported to the Golgi from the ER, probably in vesicles, where new membrane lipids and proteins are added and existing ones modified and/or deleted in a highly selective process. A significant concentration of free ribosomes (and polysomes) is observed in the Golgi area of the cell, indicating that active protein synthesis is occurring. These new proteins include enzymes and other proteins involved in the alteration of milk proteins, synthesis and incorporation of other milk constituents, and secretion of the secretory vesicles.

The Golgi apparatus is arranged in groups of platelike membranes (cisternae) into which the membranes and enclosed products move from the RER (Fig. 4.6). The membrane plates are progressively displaced across the stack in the cisterna, while alteration of the export proteins is occurring, along with the synthesis and incorporation of most of the other nonfat milk constituents. Secretory vesicles bud off from the opposite face of the cisterna to move to and fuse with the apical plasma membrane. The topological orientation of the complex lipid and protein constituents in the membranes is an important consideration, since the outer layer of the apical membrane and the fat globule membrane formed from it are derived from the inner membrane layer of the Golgi and secretory vesicles.

There are many aspects of membrane flow and secretion in the secretory cell that have not yet been adequately explained. Considerably more membrane is inserted into the apical membrane, with the secretion of the nonfat constituents, than is removed with the secretion of the fat globules. The source of the basal and lateral membranes of the cell also is likely from Golgi vesicles, which do not contain secretory products. The possible role of microtubules in the milk secretion process needs better definition. Inhibitors of microtubule function, such as colchicine, inhibit cellular secretion but not milk synthesis.

4.8-4: Pathway for blood immunoglobulins. The transport of blood immunoglobulins (Igs) into the lacteal secretions occurs by a specific intracellular transport mechanism that goes through the secretory cells, not between them. On the surfaces, the secretory cells possess specific receptor groups for both of the subclasses of IgG, IgG_1 and IgG_2. Those for IgG_1 are the most plentiful and increase in binding affinity at the time of maximum transport just before parturition. This results in about 5–20 times more IgG_1 than IgG_2 being transported through the secretory cell into colostrum. The mechanism of transport for IgG_1 (and probably IgG_2) involves the binding of the IgG_1 to receptor groups concentrated on the cell surface in certain areas that form coated pits, so called because of their electron-dense characteristic under electron microscopy. These pits on the basolateral membranes below the tight junctions further invaginate by pinocytosis to form vesicles (endocytosis) that travel through the cell, discharging their contents at the apical membrane (exocytosis). Electron micrographs of cells transporting large amounts of IgG_1 just before parturition are shown in Figure 4.10 (a, b).

Other Igs, notably IgA and IgM, also pass through the secretory cells by a somewhat different mechanism. Instead of being directly derived from blood, all, or most of the IgA and IgM, appear to be synthesized in plasma cells lying adjacent to the secretory epithelium. The pathway for IgA transport involves the synthesis of IgA and a small molecule called J chain in the plasma cell. These move from the plasma cell to the surface of the secretory cell, where the IgA binds to a protein receptor called secretory component (SC). Two IgA molecules, the J chain, and SC join into a complex called secretory IgA (sIgA), which moves through the secretory cell to the apical surface and is discharged into the colostrum or milk as sIgA. Some free SC also exists in the lacteal secretions. The pathway for IgM transport probably is similar to that for IgA.

In ruminants, IgG (and particularly IgG_1) is the predominant Ig found in milk and colostrum, with massive quantities transported just before parturition into the colostrum. Upon ingestion by the neonate and absorption into its own blood system, these Igs provide immunity to the neonate. In species such as the human and rabbit, the transport of IgG occurs across the placenta to the developing embryo, and the concentration of Igs in colostrum is much smaller and composed chiefly of IgA and IgM. Other species, including dogs, cats, and rodents, transfer Igs by both routes. See Chapter 7 for more details.

4.8-5: Pathway for blood leukocytes. Many types of white blood cells (leukocytes) are found in colostrum and milk. Their numbers are dependent to a considerable extent on the health of the animal and level of any infection or inflammation of the mammary gland. Macrophages, polymorphonuclear neutrophils (PMNs), lymphocytes, plasma cells, and other types of cells cross the mammary barrier, either by passing between

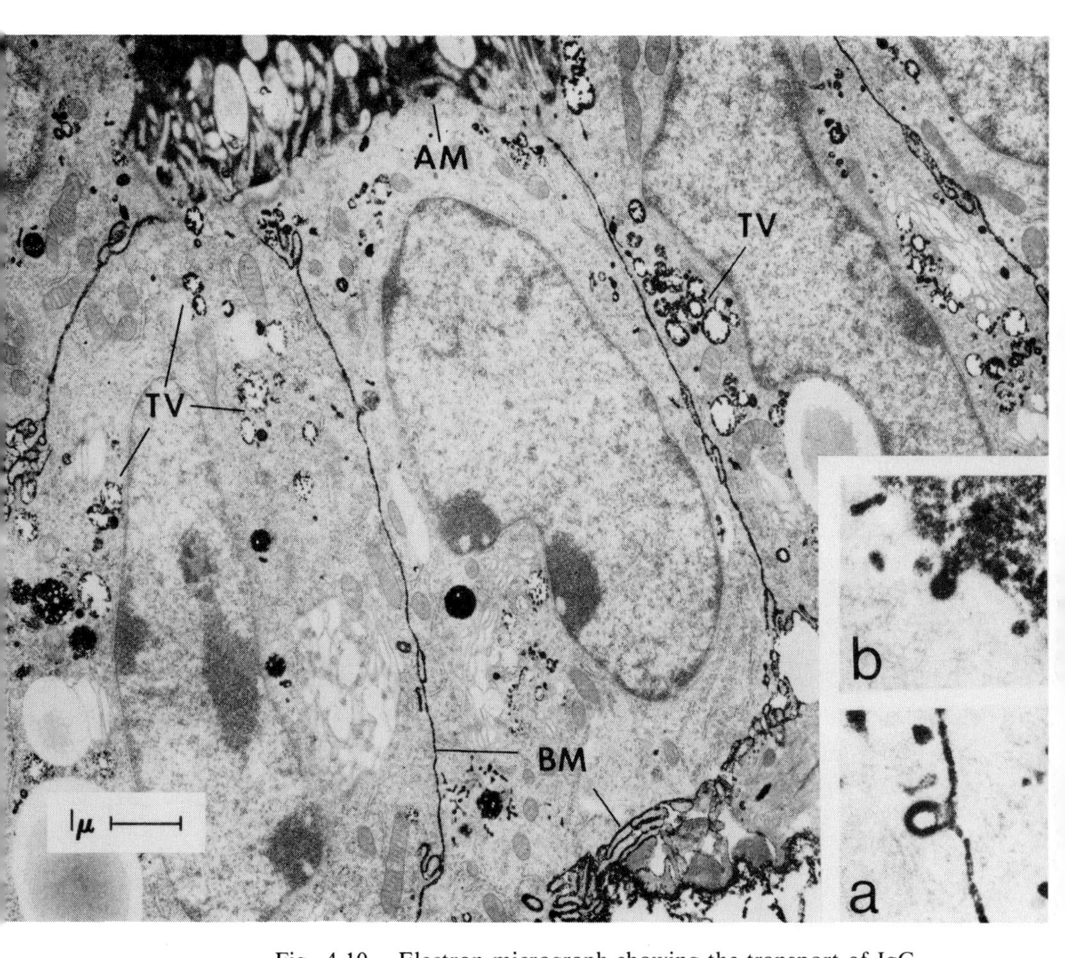

Fig. 4.10. Electron micrograph showing the transport of IgG_1 through the bovine mammary secretory cell a few days before parturition. IgG_1 coupled to horseradish peroxidase (HRP), as an enzymatic marker, was fed to mammary tissue explants in a culture medium. The electron-dense areas show the location of IgG_1-HRP in the cells. The secretory cells at this time of maximum IgG_1 transport from blood to colostrum contain numerous electron-dense transport vesicles (*TV*) lined with IgG_1-HRP, moving from the basolateral plasma membrane (*BM*) to the apical plasma membrane (*AM*). This pathway is distinctly separate from that involved with the synthesis and discharge of the major export proteins of milk. Inset *a:* The formation by endocytosis of a transport vesicle from a coated pit at the basolateral plasma membrane. Same conditions as above but higher magnification. Inset *b:* The fusion of a transport vesicle with the apical plasma membrane to discharge its contents into the lumen by exocytosis. Same conditions as in (*a*) above. (From Leary and Larson 1985)

the secretory cells through the tight junctional complex, or by pushing a secretory cell out of the epithelial sheet into the lumen.

4.9: TRANSPORT OF VARIOUS MATERIALS INTO MILK

4.9-1: Introduction. An almost infinite variety of other materials may be found in milk in addition to the major fat, lactose, and export protein constituents synthesized in the secretory cells. The fourth largest category is the different salts and minerals that contribute collectively to the ash content. Many additional materials in small to minute amounts in milk, related to the metabolic processes occurring in the cells, include enzymes and several trace minerals that are part of some metabolic functions, pathway intermediates, and structural components of cellular organelles. Milk contains many large pieces of cells and whole cells representing secretory cells, as well as blood leukocytes, which continue their metabolic processes after the milk has been secreted. Fat globules in milk may have attached pieces of cytoplasm ripped from the cell; thus, milk may contain virtually any component normal to living cells. Abnormal environmental contaminants also are found.

The mechanisms by which many of the materials coming from blood pass into milk are not known. Some involve only a simple passive transport process by diffusion. Other materials, especially those of larger size that travel through the cell by an intracellular (transcellular) pathway, may involve an active transport process where energy is required.

4.9-2: Tight junctions. The tight junctions held together by the junctional complex between the secretory cells form before parturition, and in normal lactation, they do not allow blood constituents other than some small ions to pass between the cells. Some seepage (transudation) of other materials by this paracellular pathway through leaky junctional complexes probably occurs in the dry gland and in abnormal situations, such as severe infection with microorganisms. Milk constituents may move in the other direction with induced involution at the end of lactation. High intramammary pressure, induced by the cessation of milking, breaks down the tight junctions of the secretory epithelium, and lactose and milk proteins may be forced back into the bloodstream at this time.

4.9-3: Major salts and minerals. Differences in ion concentrations across a membrane suggest that active transport with an energy-requiring pump to concentrate the material is operative. The high potassium and low sodium content of milk compared to blood (Table 4.1) is indicative that a Na^+,K^+-pump is operative in the basal membrane of the secretory cells. The hydrolysis of ATP in Na^+,K^+-ATPase provides the energy for this pump, which simultaneously moves potassium into the cell with the removal of sodium. This is shown diagrammatically in Figure

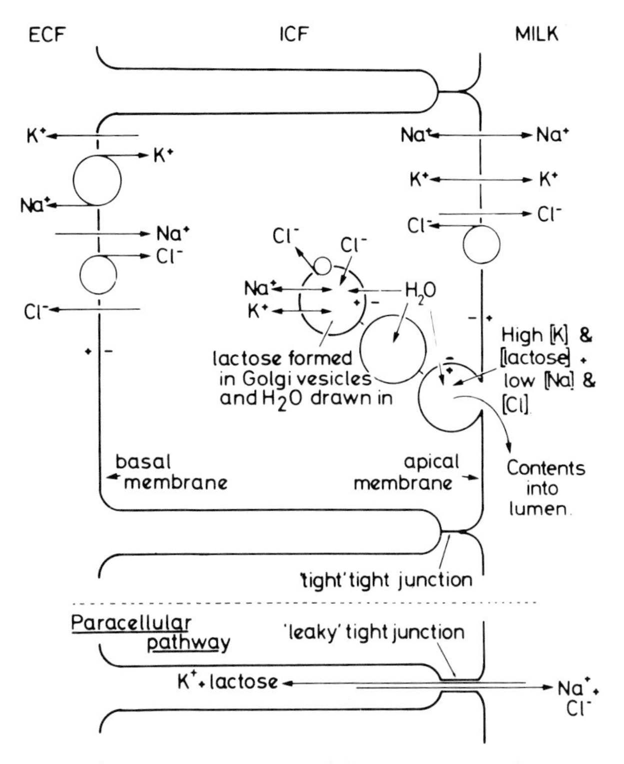

Fig. 4.11. Lactose and ion movements between extracellular fluid (*ECF*), intracellular fluid (*ICF*), and milk in the mammary gland. A circle represents an ion pump, known to be operative for sodium and potassium. The movements of chloride are not well defined. A pump also probably exists to transport calcium into Golgi vesicles. The paracellular pathway between the cells is shown. The directions of the charged potential difference are shown by the plus and minus signs. (From Peaker 1978)

4.11, along with the movements of some other ions and lactose on the transcellular and paracellular pathways.

The apical membrane is considered to be more or less impervious to ionic movement, but an anomaly to this concept exists in the perplexing possible reason for the many microvilli present. In most other cellular systems with many microvilli, they are considered to be involved with ion transfer and transport.

Movements of ions and synthesis of lactose are regulators of water intake into the Golgi and secretory vesicles. Lactose is the chief regulator, and ultimately, its availability is the major factor in determining the volume of milk secreted.

Minerals enter the cells both from passive and active transport. Calcium probably requires an active transport system. It is almost certain that its high concentration in the Golgi vesicles involves a calcium pump, probably a Ca^{2+}-stimulated ATPase. Recent evidence indicates that the protein calmodulin regulates a wide spectrum of enzymes that control a variety of cellular processes in many types of cells, including the metabolism of cyclic nucleotides, glycogen synthesis, muscle contraction, cell mobility, and microtubule disassembly; it is now believed to be the major intracellular receptor and carrier of Ca^{2+} in the cell.

Little is known about the mechanism by which phosphate enters the cell and the Golgi vesicles. Synthesis of all phosphate compounds in the cells, derived from a common pool of phosphate, indicates rapid equilibrium in the intracellular pool across the internal cytomembranes.

4.9-4: Miscellaneous materials.

4.9-4a: Citric acid. Citrate is a product of the citric acid cycle in the mitochondria from which it diffuses into the cytosol. Ruminants cannot split citric acid; it is found at rather high concentrations in their milks, where it forms a stable soluble ion with calcium. This lowers the Ca^{2+} activity, which helps elevate the concentration of calcium in milk. The mechanism by which citrate passes into milk is not known; it is likely that it is incorporated in the Golgi region (see Chap. 5).

4.9-4b: Purines and Pyrimidines. The milk and colostrum of different species contain various amounts of a large number of purine and pyrimidine bases and related compounds, which are both intermediates and end products of the purine and pyrimidine synthesis pathways. These compounds include the free bases, nucleosides (base plus ribose), and nucleotides (mono-, di-, and triphosphates of nucleosides). Ruminant milks tend to contain a significant amount of orotic acid, an intermediate on the pyrimidine synthesis pathway. Bovine milk contains about 80 μg/ml orotic acid, with some cows producing up to ten times that amount. Orotic acid fed to rats produces fatty livers but this effect is species specific to the rat. The reason for the accumulation of orotate in bovine milk is not known. It is synthesized in the secretory cells and probably is incorporated into the milk in the Golgi region. The accumulation in some cows at extreme levels may be due to a depressed ability to convert orotate to orotidine monophosphate in the pathway and represents a genetic defect (Fig. 4.7).

4.9-4c: Pesticides, drugs, and antibiotics. Many materials may be found in milk resulting from treatment for various conditions, disease, or environmental exposure. Entrance to the animal may be through the skin, lungs, alimentary tract (most common), or the mammary gland itself, such as antibiotics through the teat. The pathways into milk are varied.

Fat-soluble materials, such as the organochlorine insecticides and polychlorinated (and brominated) biphenyls, tend to be persistent and become incorporated into lipid materials in the body, including milk fat.

Lactation reduces the body load of these materials, but in so doing, they are passed into the milk. Other pesticides, such as the organophosphate compounds and the carbamates, are more readily biodegraded and usually do not appear in milk.

Almost any chemical compound (drug) administered to an animal can appear in milk. The transfer of administered drugs to milk is dependent on many factors, including the solubility and chemical properties of the material and the extent of any transport mechanism that may be present for some related material. Certain drugs, such as some of the barbiturates, may be partially fat soluble and found primarily in the lipid phase; others are in the aqueous phase or bound to the protein fraction of milk. Many drugs apparently enter the milk by diffusion of the free unionized portion across the mammary barrier. The pH of ruminant milks (bovine, 6.7) tends to be lower than blood (7.4), so drugs of an acid nature have a higher concentration in blood than in milk; the reverse is true with alkaline drugs.

The presence of antibiotics in milk resulting from treatment for mastitis or some other type of infection has posed dairy industry problems. Some people are allergic to certain antibiotics. If an antibiotic is used that appears in milk, the milk and subsequent milkings, by law, must be removed from the market until the antibiotic has cleared. If it is injected intramuscularly or subcutaneously, the pathway of the antibiotic into milk will be similar to that of drugs, and several days may be required before the milk level falls to insignificance. If administered directly into the mammary gland via the teat, absorption into the tissues takes place, and while the initial voiding of the antibiotic may be large, several days may still be required before the antibiotic has effectively disappeared from the milk. Milk from untreated as well as treated quarters will contain the antibiotic and should be discarded.

4.9-4d: Toxic elements. Naturally-occurring toxic materials and elements also enter milk and pose health problems. Arsenic is similar in some properties to phosphorus and probably is incorporated into the same types of compounds in the body. However, only small amounts of fed arsenic appear in milk. Mercury, lead, and cadmium also are transferred into milk in minute amounts. In general, the mammary gland screens out unusual toxic metals and does not pass significant amounts into milk until the animal itself begins to show outward signs of severe poisoning. Some minerals are essential nutrients in trace amounts, but too much can be deleterious. See Chapters 3 and 5 for further information.

4.9-4e: Discrimination and radionuclides. The transport pathway for some trace minerals may involve a discrimination in favor of some related mineral. Such is the case for strontium, which is associated with calcium in its metabolism. Both are alkaline earth elements forming divalent ions. Too much strontium in the diet can result in bone abnormalities.

The amount of strontium found in body organs and tissues is a function of the relative strontium:calcium (Sr:Ca) ratio in the diet, not just the absolute amount of strontium consumed. If the Sr:Ca ratio in the total feed a cow consumes is taken as 1, the Sr:Ca ratio depositing in its bones is only one-fourth that amount and the Sr:Ca ratio appearing in its milk is only one-tenth that amount. This occurs because in the passage of calcium across membranes in the body, including the intestine, kidney, mammary gland, and other cellular barriers, there is a discrimination against strontium in the transport process that favors the body retention of calcium and exclusion or elimination of strontium.

An unexpected need for appreciation of this discrimination against strontium in synthesizing milk came into the forefront rather suddenly in the late 1950s, with the testing of nuclear devices. This testing was spreading radioactive materials around the world; the heaviest fallout was occurring in the temperate regions of the northern hemisphere, which include the major food-growing areas of the world. Radionuclides being deposited on plant materials that found their way into milk included strontium (^{90}Sr), iodine (^{131}I), barium (^{140}Ba), and cesium (^{137}Cs). Of these, ^{90}Sr initially received the most attention. Milk readily served as an index for monitoring worldwide spread of these radioactive materials since it is harvested daily in all parts of the world, in contrast to other foods harvested regionally and infrequently during the year. The use of milk for testing cast aspersions on the safety of milk consumption. The ^{90}Sr appeared in foods because it is similar to calcium and is found in the same places. Over 70% of the dietary consumption of calcium in the United States comes from milk and dairy products.

Research studies soon indicated, however, that the ^{90}Sr:Ca ratio found in milk was considerably lower than that found in the average of other foods being consumed by humans. This was due to the discrimination by the cow in producing milk against ^{90}Sr in favor of calcium. Removal of milk with the majority of the total dietary calcium from the human diet would actually increase, instead of decrease, the bone deposition level of ^{90}Sr. Also, it should be noted that the amounts of ^{90}Sr in milk and other foods were quite small and represented a very minute risk. The general nutritional implications of removing dairy products from the diet could be considerably more serious.

Another radionuclide of importance in milk from radioactive fallout is ^{131}I, where the situation is quite different. Iodine in the diet is readily transferred without discrimination across the mammary gland into milk. Even though ^{131}I has a short half-life (8 days) compared to ^{90}Sr (28 yr), it is now considered the most important radioisotope contaminant in dairy products resulting from nuclear detonations. The body concentrates iodine in the thyroid gland, creating a high local level of radiation in thyroid tissue if the iodine is a radioactive isotope. Storing cattle feed under cover to reduce fresh fallout contamination or storing dairy products made from contaminated milk to allow time for significant decay of the ^{131}I are means of reducing the amount of human exposure. In severe situations, the consumption of elevated amounts of nonradioactive iodine to dilute out the ^{131}I is also a technique to reduce exposure of the thyroid gland to radiation. However, exposure to high nonradioactive iodine levels may have other deleterious side effects.

4.9-4f: Other materials. The mechanisms by which various hormones and certain blood constituents get into milk are probably many, with some virtually unknown. One route for lipid-soluble hormones and their derivatives is the same as for other lipid-soluble materials, such as drugs and pesticides. However, hormones affecting the cell bind to specific receptors on the basolateral membrane of the secretory cells and then are carried to the site of their action, most likely the nucleus. From there the pathway to excretion from the cell is unknown, but for the lipid-soluble ones, it is likely related to the flow of the lipid-containing membranes through the ER, Golgi, and secretory vesicles.

In the early stages of hoof-and-mouth disease in cattle, the virus is found in the interface between the lipid droplets and the cytosol in the secretory cells. Similarly, the blood protease plasmin, which is found in small amounts in milk, is present in the secretory cells at the lipid-cytosol junction of the droplets. Apparently, certain materials find the lipid-cytosol interface a compatible location for moving in and through the cell.

4.10: ASPECTS OF GLANDULAR SECRETION

4.10-1: Continued synthesis. The synthesis of milk by secretory cells is a continuing process that does not necessarily cease for some constituents when secreted from the cell; cells and pieces of cells in the milk may still be functional. If pathogenic bacteria are present in the ductal system, such as in mastitis, degradation of the milk constituents will occur. The ductal system itself appears impervious to resorption of milk constituents or adding further ingredients. Changes that occur in normal milk after secretion include the continued synthesis of a low level of triacylglycerols, desaturation of saturated fatty acids, the cleavage by plasmin of β-casein to form γ-casein, and changes in composition and orientation of materials in fat globule membranes.

4.10-2: Mastitis effects. Infection of the mammary gland with microorganisms that produce mastitis can have a profound effect on the synthesis of milk and its composition. In severe mastitis, with breakdown of the secretory epithelium, blood components can appear in milk. Mastitic milk is characterized by high amounts of sodium and chloride, lower lactose, and high leukocyte (or somatic cell) counts. Blood constituents appear to enter the milk directly by passing between the cells with the breakdown of the junctional complexes that normally hold the secretory cells together. Secretory areas, following severe breakdown, form scar tissue and do not recover completely, severely diminishing the potential for future milk production.

4.10-3: Rate of cellular synthesis and milk production. It has been estimated that to produce 1 l milk, the dairy cow requires 500 l blood moving through the mammary gland to provide the precursors. One gram of active bovine mammary secretory tissue can secrete about 1–2 g milk per day and contains about 1×10^8 cells. Estimates are that a cow producing about 25 l milk per day possesses about 400 m^2 secretory epithelium, with each cell within it producing about $0.5–1 \times 10^{-8}$ g milk per cell per day. Thus, a cow producing about 25 kg milk per day possesses about 5×10^{12} secretory cells.

There is, at present, limited evidence that individual secretory cells from high- and low-producing cows differ in their innate capacity to synthesize milk. Nevertheless, it is likely that genetic differences between cows exist in critical components of cellular pathways concerned with milk synthesis and discharge, which affect the ability to carry out those functions. In addition to these possible cellular factors, the amount of milk produced by a cow is dependent on many other considerations: the size of the mammary gland as related to the number of secretory cells present, the nutritional status of the cow and her ability to mobilize and transfer nutrients for the maintenance of milk production, the presence and balance of hormones, the frequency of milk collection, and a host of other factors that collectively operate in the lactating animal.

REFERENCES

Baldwin, R. L., and Y. T. Yang. 1974. Enzymatic and metabolic changes in the development of lactation. In Lactation, 1:349. See Larson 1978.

Bauman, D. E., and C. L. Davis. 1974. Biosynthesis of milk fat. In Lactation, 2:31. See Larson and Smith 1974.

Caruolo, E. V. 1980. Scanning microscope visualization of the mammary gland secretory unit and of myoepithelial cells. J. Dairy Sci. 63:1987.

Craig, R. K., and P. N. Campbell. 1978. Molecular aspects of milk protein biosynthesis. In Lactation, 4:387. See Larson 1978.

Davis, C. L., and D. E. Bauman. 1974. General metabolism associated with the synthesis of milk. In Lactation, 2:3. See Larson and Smith 1974.

Ebner, K. E., and F. L. Schanbacher. 1974. Biochemistry of lactose and related carbohydrates. In Lactation, 2:77. See Larson and Smith 1974.

Jenness, R. 1974. The composition of milk. In Lactation, 3:3. See Larson and Smith 1974.

Johke, T. 1978. Nucleotides of mammary secretions. In Lactation, 4:513. See Larson 1978.

Jones, E. A. 1978. Lactose biosynthesis. In Lactation, 4:371. See Larson 1978.

Keenan, T. W., D. J. Morre, and C. M. Huang. 1974. Membranes of the mammary gland. In Lactation, 2:191. See Larson and Smith 1974.

Keenan, T. W., W. W. Franke, I. H. Mather, and D. J. Morre. 1978. Endomembrane composition and function in milk formation. In Lactation, 4:405. See Larson 1978.

Larson, B. L. 1979. Biosynthesis and secretion of milk proteins: A review. J. Dairy Res. 46:161.

______. ed. 1978. Lactation: A Comprehensive Treatise, vol. 4. New York: Academic.

Larson, B. L., and G. N. Jorgensen. 1974. Biosynthesis of the milk proteins. In Lactation, 2:115. See Larson and Smith 1974.

Larson, B. L., and V. R. Smith, eds. 1974. Lactation: A Comprehensive Treatise, vols. 1–3. New York: Academic.

Leary, H. L., Jr., and B. L. Larson. 1985. Intracellular transport pathway of IgG1 through the bovine mammary secretory cell. In preparation.

Lengemann, F. W., R. A. Wentworth, and C. L. Comar. 1974. Physiological and biochemical aspects of the accumulation of contaminant radionuclides in milk. In Lactation, 3:159. See Larson and Smith 1974.

Linzell, J. L. 1974. Mammary blood flow and methods of identifying and measuring precursors of milk. In Lactation, 1:143. See Larson and Smith 1974.

Mepham, T. B., ed. 1983. Biochemistry of Lactation. Amsterdam-New York: Elsevier/North-Holland.

Peaker, M. 1978. Ion and water transport in the mammary gland. In Lactation, 4:437. See Larson 1978.

Saacke, R. G., and C. W. Heald. 1974. Cytological aspects of milk formation and secretion. In Lactation, 2:147. See Larson and Smith 1974.

Smith, E. L., R. L. Hill, I. R. Lehman, R. J. Lefkowitz, P. Handler, and A. White. 1983. Principles of Biochemistry. 7th ed. New York: McGraw-Hill.

Turner, C. W. 1952. The Mammary Gland, vol. 1. The Anatomy of the Udder of Cattle and Domestic Animals. Columbia, Mo.: Lucas Bros.

CHAPTER 5

BIOCHEMICAL AND NUTRITIONAL ASPECTS OF MILK AND COLOSTRUM

ROBERT JENNESS

5.1: INTRODUCTION

The biological function of milk is to supply nutrition and immunological protection to the young mammal. In some species, milk is the sole food consumed for weeks or months and, thus, it must furnish all nutritive requirements (energy, amino acids, minerals, and vitamins) for maintenance and growth. In other species, the composition of milk is not so critical because the young soon begin to consume other food. Some species, such as ruminants, rely almost exclusively on milk to transfer antibodies from mother to young. Others, such as primates, transfer antibodies via the placenta; thus, they are not dependent on milk for this function. Milk performs its nutritional and immunological functions with a wide array of compounds, many of which are distinctive products of the mammary gland, occurring nowhere else in nature. Large interspecies differences occur in the quantitative composition of milk. Furthermore, milks of some species contain distinctive components not found in all milks, reflecting the metabolic processes of the species. In some particulars, they are correlated with differences in nutritive requirements of the young.

Milks of various species of mammals are referred to frequently in this chapter. In general, English vernacular species names are used, but, in Table 5.1, Latin binomials are given for nearly all species encountered in the chapter. There is no completely unambiguous English name in common use for domestic cattle. In this chapter they are considered as two species, *Bos taurus* and *Bos indicus,* even though many taxonomists regard them as conspecific. The terms bovine and cow will refer to either species, western cattle to *B. taurus,* and Indian cattle and zebus to *B. indicus.*

The composition of milk is greatly influenced by the type of diet and the digestive processes of the lactating animal. As pointed out in Chapter 3, mammalian digestive tracts can be classified into four major groups, one of which is herbivores with a foregut fermentation chamber; ruminants are in this group. Animal scientists often designate mammals belonging to the other three groups as nonruminants. Such lumping obscures differences among the three groups and should be avoided.

5.2: COMPOSITION OF MILK

5.2-1: Gross composition. Gross composition refers to the proportions of water, fat, proteins, carbohydrates, and mineral constitutents in milk. Water content is determined as loss in weight by drying under conditions that minimize decomposition of organic constituents. Fat consists of materials extractable by defined methods; milk fat consists largely of triacylglycerols.

Protein content is the aggregate of all the proteins, including enzymes, present. Often it is determined by analyzing milk for nitrogen and multiplying by a factor, usually 6.38, representing the reciprocal of the nitrogen content of the proteins. Frequently, protein is calculated as crude protein (total N $\times$ 6.38), thus overestimating protein by including nitrogenous nonprotein constituents. Such constituents account for 5–6% of the total nitrogen in cows' milk and up to 20% in milks of some other species. Obviously, nonprotein nitrogen should be subtracted in calculating true protein content. A modern, rapid, semiautomated method determines milk protein by its capacity to bind certain cationic dyes. Milk proteins are often subdivided into two classes (caseins and whey proteins) representing, respectively, the insoluble and soluble fractions at, or about, pH 4.6.

Milk carbohydrates are usually expressed as lactose, based on calculation of the lactose equivalent of reducing power or optical rotation. Such methods may include other carbohydrates that, in milks of some species, represent a considerable portion of the total. Caution must be exercised in comparing published lactose contents because sometimes they have been calculated as lactose monohydrate and, therefore, are about 5% too high. A rapid method for determining fat, protein, and lactose, successively in a single sample, is based on their respective absorbances of infrared light at 5.8, 6.5, and 9.6 μm.

The aggregate of milk minerals, usually expressed as ash, is calculated from the weight of residue remaining after incineration. Ash does not truly represent milk salts or even milk minerals because (1) organic ions, such as citrate, are destroyed on incineration; (2) some of the phosphate in ash is from protein and phospholipid phosphorus; (3) carbonate, chloride, sodium, and potassium are volatilized to varying extents in ashing; and (4) some oxidation of metals to oxide occurs.

Variations in gross composition of milk arise from differences in relative rates of synthesis and secretion of milk components by the mammary gland. Variations are due to differences among species, between genetic strains within a species, between individuals within a strain, and between conditions affecting an individual.

5.2-1a: Variation among species. Analytical data are available for milks of about 200 (in 17 orders) of the more than 4,000 species of extant mammals. The data range from comprehensive and systematic surveys of milk of domestic cattle to analyses of single opportunistically collected samples for some species. Thus, adequate interspecies statistical comparisons are not possible.

Table 5.1 gives gross composition of milks of 30 species, including at least one for each order that has been sampled, and including all whose milks are consumed by humans. Interspecies variations in concentrations of constituents are great; fat varies from a trace to 50%, lactose from 0–10%, protein from 1–20%, and ash from 0.2–2%.

Several correlations can be noted among contents of constituents when milks of various species are compared. Highly significant negative correlations are found between lactose and the sum of sodium and potassium and between lactose and chloride. This is due to the fact that the rate of synthesis of lactose differs among species, and milk is maintained virtually isoosmotic, with the constant mammalian blood osmolality of about 0.3 *M*. Milks, like those of certain seals, that contain little or no carbohydrate at all have osmolalities of about 0.3 *M;* presumably this is maintained by the concentration of salts. Synthesis of lactose in the Golgi vesicles is the primary regulator of the amount of water that dilutes the protein to its final concentration. Hence, a highly significant negative correlation exists between the protein and lactose contents. The relation is approximately

$$P = 20 - 2.8L \tag{5.1}$$

where L and P, respectively, are grams of protein and lactose/100 ml fat-free skim milk.

The concentrations of protein and fat are strongly correlated in milks of ungulates (hoofed mammals). For 20 species of ungulates

$$P = 1.05 + 0.57F \tag{5.2}$$

where F and P are percentages of fat and protein. The correlation between the rates of synthesis of protein in the Golgi and fat in the cytosol of the cell is not clear. In many species other than ungulates, the protein content is

Table 5.1. Composition of milks of various species

Species	Percentage by Weight						Energy
	Water	Fat	Casein	Whey protein	Lactose	Ash	(kcal/100 g)
Echidna (*Tachyglossus aculeatus*)		19.6	8.4	2.9	2.8	0.8	233
Opossum (*Didelphis virginiana*)	76.8	11.3	8.4[a]		1.6	1.7	142
Red kangaroo (*Macropus rufus*)	80.0	3.4	2.3	2.3	6.7	1.4	76
Hedgehog (*Erinaceus europaeus*)	79.4	10.1	7.2[a]		2.0	2.3	100
Fringed bat (*Myotis thysanodes*)	59.5	17.9	12.1[a]		3.4	1.6	223
Tree shrew (*Tupaia belangeri*)	59.6	25.6	10.4[a]		1.5		278
Human (*Homo sapiens*)	87.1	4.5	0.4	0.5	7.1	0.2	72
Sloth (*Bradypus variegatus*)	83.1	2.7	6.5[a]		2.8	0.9	62
Rabbit (*Oryctolagus cuniculus*)	67.2	15.3	9.3	4.6	2.1	1.8	202
Gray squirrel (*Sciurus carolinensis*)	60.4	24.7	5.0	2.4	3.7	1.0	267
Rat (*Rattus norvegicus*)	79.0	10.3	6.4	2.0	2.6	1.3	137
Guinea pig (*Cavia porcellus*)	83.6	3.9	6.6	1.5	3.0	0.8	80
Dolphin (*Tursiops truncatus*)	58.3	33.0	3.9	2.9	1.1	0.7	329
Dog (*Canis familiaris*)	76.4	10.7	5.1	2.3	3.3	1.2	139
Black bear (*Ursus americanus*)	55.5	24.5	8.8	5.7	0.4	1.8	280
Fur seal (*Callorhinus ursinus*)	34.6	53.3	4.6	4.3	0.1	0.5	516
Aardvark (*Orycteropus afer*)	68.5	12.1	9.5	4.8	4.6	1.4	184
Indian elephant (*Elephas maximus*)	78.1	11.6	1.9	3.0	4.7	0.7	143
Manatee (*Trichechus manatus*)	87.0	6.9	6.3[a]		0.3	1.0	88
Horse (*Equus caballus*)	88.8	1.9	1.3	1.2	6.2	0.5	52
Donkey (*Equus asinus*)	88.3	1.4	1.0	1.0	7.4	0.5	44
Pig (*Sus scrofa*)	81.2	6.8	2.8	2.0	5.5	1.0	102
Camel (*Camelus dromedarius*)	86.5	4.0	2.7	0.9	5.0	0.8	70
Reindeer (*Rangifer tarandus*)	66.7	18.0	8.6	1.5	2.8	1.5	214
Cow (*Bos taurus*)	87.3	3.9	2.6	0.6	4.6	0.7	66
Zebu (*Bos indicus*)	86.5	4.7	2.6	0.6	4.7	0.7	74
Yak (*Bos grunniens*)	82.7	6.5	5.8[a]		4.6	0.9	100
Water buffalo (*Bubalis bubalis*)	82.8	7.4	3.2	0.6	4.8	0.8	101
Goat (*Capra hircus*)	86.7	4.5	2.6	0.6	4.3	0.8	70
Sheep (*Ovis aries*)	82.0	7.2	3.9	0.7	4.8	0.9	102

[a]Percentage of combined protein.

lower in relation to fat than indicated by Equation 5.2; in a few, such as rabbits, it is higher. The proportions of casein to whey protein vary greatly among species. The data in Table 5.1 show casein:whey protein ratios ranging from 0.6 for elephant to 4.7 for cow. Artiodactyls, in general, and ruminants, in particular, characteristically have high casein:whey protein ratios. Both calcium and phosphorus in milks are highly correlated with casein and with each other (see 5.3).

The energy available from each milk in Table 5.1 was calculated in the usual way (4 kcal/g for protein and lactose and 9 kcal/g for fat). In general, sugar and protein furnish 30–60 kcal/100 g milk and additional energy, up to as much as 500 kcal/100 g, is supplied by fat. The proportion of total energy supplied by protein and the ratio of sugar energy to fat energy vary greatly among species. Milks of high fat contents are characteristic of arctic and aquatic species, whose young require much energy for metabolism and fat for insulation.

For 19 species for which milk yield has been determined, the maximum output of milk energy has been shown to be rather constant, about 127 $kcal \cdot W^{0.69} \cdot day^{-1}$, where W is body weight of the lactating female in kg. Only one arctic and no aquatic species were included in this calculation; undoubtedly, such species have higher energy outputs.

5.2-1b: Intraspecific genetic variation. Genetically controlled variation in milk composition is best known from differences among the breeds of dairy cattle. Table 5.2 gives data obtained from sampling herd milk from five breeds in a single geographic area (Manitoba) over a period of two years. This is one of very few extensive studies in which total solids, fat, protein, lactose, and ash were all determined independently. Similar breed differences have been found in other studies, but there is some variability in compositions obtained for a given breed at different times and geographic locations. For example, the fat content of the milk of Friesian cattle (called Holstein-Friesians in the United States for many years but now simply Holsteins) averaged 3.62, 3.70, 3.80, 4.00, and 4.54% in extensive surveys in Canada, United States, United Kingdom, Netherlands, and New

Table 5.2. Composition of milks of five breeds of dairy cattle

		Mean % by Wt[a]					
Breed	Samples[b]	Total solids	Fat	Casein	Whey protein	Lactose	Ash
Ayrshire	70	12.69	3.97	2.68	0.60	4.63	0.72
Brown Swiss	23	12.69	3.80	2.63	0.55	4.80	0.72
Guernsey	23	13.69	4.58	2.88	0.61	4.78	0.75
Holstein	75	11.91	3.56	2.49	0.53	4.61	0.73
Jersey	72	4.15	4.97	3.02	0.63	4.70	0.77

Source: Adapted from Reinart and Nesbitt 1956.
[a]All determined independently.
[b]Monthly herd samples collected over 2-yr period.

Zealand, respectively. Milk of this breed averaged 3.35% fat in the United States in 1933 and 3.70% in 1960, 3.10% in the Netherlands in 1900 and 4.00% in 1970. These geographic and temporal differences likely reflect the effects of both genetic segregation and changes in husbandry practices.

Breed differences in milk composition, particularly in fat content, have been documented in Indian cattle, water buffaloes, and goats, although not so definitively as for western cattle. In general, the average for fat and protein contents of all breeds of these species falls close to the relationship in Equation 5.2. Many analyses of human milk have been made, but sampling schemes have been inadequate to reveal whether any distinctive ethnic differences in composition occur.

Intrabreed variability in fat and protein contents and yields among five breeds of dairy cattle are shown in Table 5.3. These data represent over 22,000 lactation records for cows milked twice a day for 305 days in 22 states of the United States. The standard deviations include variances from genetic and environmental sources. (In this particular survey, some variance is also due to differences in methods used to determine fat and protein.) By considering only differences among cows of the same breed, kept in the same herd, calving at the same age in the same month of the year, the standard deviations in Table 5.3 are reduced by about 25% for the yield parameters and by 12–18% for the fat and protein contents. Substantial phenotypic variances still remain.

By comparing phenotypic variances for half-sibling progeny of a given bull and for daughters with their dams, estimates may be made of the fraction of variance assignable to heredity. Heritability, h^2, is the ratio of genetic variance, σ_G^2, to total phenotypic variance, σ_P^2. Heritabilities of fat and protein contents average 0.58 and 0.49, respectively, for the data in Table 5.3; those of milk yield, fat yield, and protein yield average 0.27, 0.25, and 0.26, respectively. Several other studies of heritability of milk fat and protein have been made, and a few have included lactose, as well. Mean heritabilities calculated from all data are about 0.60 for the contents

Table 5.3. Yields and concentrations of fat and protein in milks of five breeds of dairy cattle

	Yield						Content			
	Milk		Fat		Protein		Fat		Protein	
Breed	Mean	S.D.	Mean	S.D.	Mean	S.D.	Mean	S.D.	Mean	S.D.
	(kg/lactation)[a]						*(g/100 ml)*			
Ayrshire	5,247	1,061	211	45	177	38	3.99	0.33	3.34	0.29
Brown Swiss	5,812	1,421	244	63	210	52	4.16	0.35	3.53	0.26
Guernsey	4,809	1,095	236	56	177	42	4.87	0.45	3.62	0.29
Holstein	7,073	1,425	264	58	226	47	3.70	0.39	3.11	0.25
Jersey	4,444	1,130	230	62	175	44	5.13	0.54	3.80	0.30

Source: Adapted from Wilcox et al. 1971.
[a]Means of twice-a-day, 305-day lactation averages.

of fat and protein and 0.55 for lactose. Thus, the concentrations of all three major components are genetically controlled to a considerable extent. The evidence for genetic control has been derived by statistical methods and, to date, there is virtually no indication as to what specific aspects of the synthetic and secretory mechanisms of the mammary gland are inherited. One small clue is the fact that cows homozygous for β-lactoglobulin A produce this protein at a considerably greater rate than those homozygous for β-lactoglobulin B (see 5.2-3b).

Genetic correlations between fat and protein contents of milk are of the order of 0.45 (range in five breeds, 0.20–0.69); between lactation yields of fat and protein, they are about 0.83. Thus, there is some room for selectively increasing protein content, without likewise increasing fat content, by identifying and using breeding animals that transmit the potential for higher than average protein:fat ratios.

5.2-1c: Variation during lactation. Colostrum, the initial mammary secretion after parturition, differs greatly in composition from milk. Details of its composition and of the transition to normal milk, with successive milkings, have been studied in only a few species (cows, goats, humans, pigs), although the changes in immunoglobulin (Ig) concentrations have been determined in several more.

Cows' colostrum contains more mineral salts (ash) and protein and less lactose than milk; fat content is often, but not always, higher than that of milk. Composition of colostrum differs more among individual cows than does the composition of their milk. Of the individual minerals, calcium, sodium, magnesium, phosphorus, and chloride are present in higher concentrations in colostrum, but potassium content is lower. The most remarkable difference between colostrum and milk is the extremely high Ig content of colostrum. The Igs accumulate in the mammary gland before parturition and transfer immunity to the neonate. The kinds and concentrations of Igs in colostra of several species and their transfer to the young are discussed in Chapter 7.

Figure 5.1 shows the change in concentration of some of the principal constituents in cows' colostrum and milk in the first few milkings after parturition. Similar patterns have been observed for goats and humans. In cows, the changes in composition occurring during the first few days continue, although at reduced rates, for approximately 5 wk of lactation. Following this, the fat and protein contents rise gradually and may increase more sharply near the end of the period. Calcium, phosphorus, and chloride also tend to follow this pattern; lactose contents may diminish gradually as lactation progresses. Figure 5.2 shows the pattern usually observed with dairy cows. The increase in protein content after 6 mo seems to be associated with pregnancy, as it does not occur in nonpregnant cows.

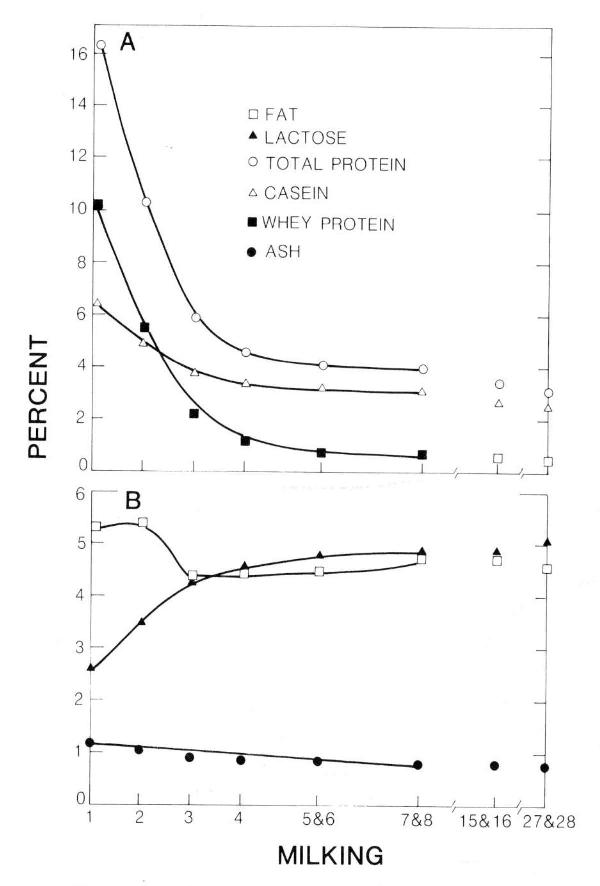

Fig. 5.1. Change in composition of milk at successive milkings after parturition. (Modified from Parrish et al. 1948, 1950)

The limited data available on the composition of goats' milk through lactation indicate that both fat and solids-not-fat contents fall to a minimum at about 4 mo and gradually increase thereafter. In humans, lactose content increases sharply for about the first week and very slightly during the ensuing 20 wk. Protein reaches mature milk levels at about 3 wk and then decreases slightly.

In some species of kangaroos, much greater changes in milk composition occur during lactation than in any placental animal yet observed. Total solids content increases from about 12 to 40% during 40 wk of lactation, total carbohydrate increases to a maximum of over 11% at about 26 wk and then falls to under 1%; salt concentration changes inversely to carbohydrate, and protein remains at about 4% for 18 wk and then increases

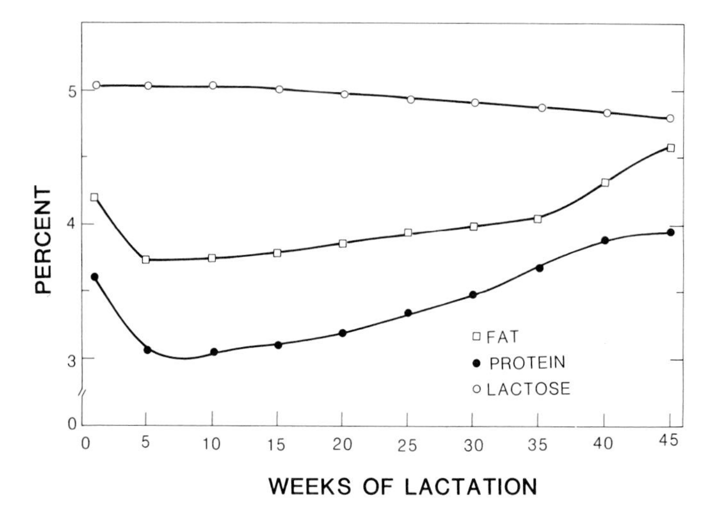

Fig. 5.2. Changes in fat, protein, and lactose contents of milk from dairy cows over the lactation period. (Modified from Bonnier 1946)

sharply to about 12%. Furthermore, the composition of fat, protein, carbohydrate, and lactose changes markedly during lactation. When two young of different ages are being suckled, the two glands produce milk of quite different composition. It is not known whether similar changes occur in marsupials other than kangaroos.

5.2-1d: Other sources of variation. Decreases in fat content of about 0.2% and in solids-not-fat of 0.4% over five lactations have been observed in dairy cows. The decrease in solids-not-fat seems to be due entirely to casein. It has been suggested that the change in milk composition in successive lactations may be due to deterioration of udder tissue, increased incidence of mastitis, or to selective culling for high production. No consistent changes in composition of human milk have been found to be associated with age or with number of lactations (parity).

The plane of nutrition and the composition and physical state of the ration fed to dairy cows materially influences the gross composition of milk produced. The ration also influences the composition of milk fat considerably (see Chaps. 3 and 4). Effects of dietary levels of minerals, vitamins, and contaminants are discussed later in this chapter. In humans, inadequate protein intake reduces the quantity of milk produced but does not appear to affect its fat, protein, or lactose contents.

Seasonal variations in milk composition commonly are observed with dairy cattle in temperate regions. In summer, the fat content may average 0.4% lower and protein content 0.2% lower than in winter. The possibility that differences in day length may contribute to the compositional difference seems to be ruled out by experiments in which the ratio of light and dark was varied. Increased exposure to light increased feed consumption and milk yield but did not influence milk composition. Conflicting results have been reported on the possible influence of temperature on milk composition. Some workers have found increases in fat and chloride contents and decreases in milk yield, solids-not-fat, protein, and lactose at temperatures above 30°C; others have not observed such effects. Very likely, the observed seasonal differences in milk composition are attributable mostly to pasture vs. dry feed and to stage of lactation.

Variations in milk composition also occur due to peculiarities of the milking procedure. Fat content increases continuously during the milking process; the first milk drawn is low and strippings are high in fat. Solids-not-fat, calculated as percentage of fat-free skim milk, does not change during the milking process. The increase in fat content apparently results from the tendency of the fat globules to cluster and be trapped in the alveoli. Thus, at an incomplete milking, fat content will be lower than normal, but at a subsequent complete milking, fat content will be higher than normal. Furthermore, when intervals between milkings are unequal, the milk yield is greater and fat content lower following the longer interval. The effects of incomplete milking on milk composition and of varying the intervals on milk and fat yields are discussed further in Chapter 6 (see 6.6 and Tables 6.4, 6.5, and 6.6). For intervals longer than about 15 hr, the rate of milk secretion decreases; concentrations of fat, whey protein, sodium, and chloride increase; and solids-not-fat, lactose, and potassium decrease.

Infection of the udder greatly influences the composition of milk. Concentrations of fat, solids-not-fat, lactose, casein, β-lactoglobulin, α-lactalbumin, and potassium are lowered, and concentrations of blood serum albumin, Igs, sodium, and chloride are increased. The ability of the cells to synthesize lactose and the specific milk proteins is impaired, salts enter the milk to offset the osmotic pressure deficiency caused by the lowered lactose level, and the tight junctions between cells become more permeable to blood constituents. In severe mastitis, the casein content may fall below the normal limit of 78% of total protein, and the chloride content may rise above the normal maximum of 0.12%. Mastitis is undoubtedly responsible for many of the reported differences in composition of milk from different quarters of a cow's udder. Effects of disease of the mammary gland on the lactation process are discussed more fully in Chapters 3 and 7.

5.2-2: Lipids. Milk lipids, or fats, consist of a mixture of compounds having the common property of solubility in nonpolar solvents and nearly complete insolubility in aqueous liquids. The principal classes are triacylglycerols, diacylglycerols, monoacylglycerols, phospholipids, cere-

Table 5.4. Composition of milk lipids of three species

Lipid	Wt % of Lipids		
	Cow	Human	Rat
Triacylglycerols	97–98	98.2	87.5
Diacylglycerols	0.25–0.48	0.7	2.9
Monoacylglycerols	0.02–0.04	T	0.4
Free fatty acids	0.1– 0.4	0.4	3.1
Phospholipids	0.6–1.0	0.25	0.7
Cholesterol	0.2–0.4	0.25	1.6
Cholesterol esters	T	T	

Note: T = trace.

brosides, gangliosides, sterols and sterol esters and derivatives, carotenoids, tocopherol, vitamin A, and free fatty acids. A comparison of the proportions of these classes in milks of the cow, human, and rat are given in Table 5.4.

5.2-2a: Triacylglycerols. The most abundant class of lipids in milk fat, as in most other fats, is triacylglycerols, which contain a great diversity of fatty acids. As many as 437 different ones have been identified in cows' milk fat. There is great variation in chain length, number, position, and geometric isomerism of double bonds. Some branched-chain acids and some keto- and hydroxy-acids also occur in small amounts. The complete fatty acid composition has been approached only for bovine and human milk fats, but the patterns of principal fatty acids (those present to the extent of 0.2% or more) have been determined for a large number of species. Table 5.5 gives data for 16 species, including one of each of 15 orders and both a ruminant and a nonruminant for artiodactyls. Fatty acid

Table 5.5. Fatty acid composition (wt %) of milk fats

Species	6:0	8:0	10:0	12:0	14:0	16:0	16:1	18:0	18:1	18:2	18:3	Other
Echidna			T	0.3	2.5	23.2	5.0	9.1	44.6	12.1	1.1	2.0
Opossum			T	T	2.6	32.2	3.3	12.2	39.0	T–18.7	T–3.0	
Hedgehog	T	T		1.3	4.4	29.1	5.0	10.5	39.6	4.4	3.1	2.6
Human	T	T	1.3	3.1	5.1	20.2	5.7	3.0	46.6	13.0	1.4	
Domestic rabbit	T	22.4	20.1	2.9	1.7	14.2	2.0	3.8	13.6	14.0	4.4	0.9
Laboratory rat	T	2.5	8.7	9.5	11.9	30.1	2.2	3.0	18.9	11.4	1.3	0.5
Little brown bat				4.1	3.3	21.0	11.6	5.4	24.7	12.0	11.0	7.0
Armadillo			0.7	2.6	12.2	32.2	5.3	9.4	28.6	3.6	1.1	5.3
Aardvark					5.5	30.9	4.2	7.5	35.8	10.1	1.3	4.7
Right whale	T				5.0	14.7	23.6	6.3	23.3	T		27.1[a]
Dog			0.8	0.5	4.0	27.3	6.4	4.4	41.8	12.6	1.9	
Northern fur seal					5.8	22.0	10.0	1.7	33.6	2.4	8.3	16.2[b]
Indian elephant	0.4	5.8	43.4	21.5	3.5	9.1	1.9	0.5	9.8	2.3	0.5	1.3
Horse	T	1.8	5.1	6.2	5.7	23.8	7.8	1.1	20.9	14.9	12.6	
Pig			0.7	0.2	4.0	32.9	11.3	3.5	35.2	11.9	0.3	
Cow	1.6	1.3	3.0	3.1	9.5	26.3	2.3	14.6	29.8	2.4	0.8	5.3[c]

Source: Data from Glass and Jenness 1971; Glass et al. 1967.

Note: Fatty acids are designated by number of carbons and number of double bonds; thus 6:0 signifies six carbons and no double bonds. T = trace.

[a]Mostly 3 long-chain components.

[b]11.7% 3 long chains.

[c]3.3% 4:0.

composition appears to be a blend of acids synthesized by the mammary gland with those transferred from the diet (see Chaps. 3 and 4). The relative proportions from the two sources vary among species and the composition varies somewhat with stage of lactation.

Distinctive patterns of fatty acid composition characterize the milk fats of each order. Palmitate (16:0) and oleate (18:1) are usually, but not always, prominent. Most of the acids of milk fats of carnivores, swine, and the aardvark have 16 or 18 carbons. These probably are derived principally from the diet, and little synthesis of fatty acid occurs in the mammary gland. Linoleate (18:2) very likely comes entirely from diet, since mammals cannot synthesize it. The high concentrations of long-chain polyunsaturated acids in milk fats of whales, seals, and polar bears are very likely derived from dietary fat. In herbivores, mammary synthesis is prominent, and saturated fatty acids of varying chain length are incorporated into the fat. The patterns differ between ruminants and caecum fermenters, like rabbits and horses. Butyrate (4:0) seems to be a hallmark of ruminant milk fat. Some, but by no means all, rodents produce milk fat with considerable short-chain acids (Table 5.5, laboratory rat). This is probably related to the high activity of ATP-citrate lyase in their mammary cells, which enables them to split citrate to acetyl CoA, and thus to synthesize fat from carbohydrate.

Kangaroos, though having a digestive tract somewhat like that of ruminants, produce milk fat devoid of short-chain acids; the fatty acid composition changes markedly from early lactation (45% palmitic, 25% oleic) to late lactation (25% palmitic, 45% oleic).

The distribution of fatty acids in the triacylglycerol molecules of milk fat is not random, and it differs markedly among species. Milk fats of ruminants can be separated, by distillation or chromatography, into long-chain and short-chain fractions, having, respectively, 40–58 and 26–44 acyl carbons per molecule. Nearly all the butyrate is in the short-chain fraction. Milk fats of species other than ruminants cannot be separated into such distinct fractions. The distribution of acyl carbon numbers differs widely among species. Ruminant milk fats have significant amounts of all components with even acyl carbon numbers from 32–54. In horse milk fat, there are considerable concentrations of molecules with 40, 42, 44, and 46 carbons; in rabbits, molecules with 24, 26, 28, 30, 32, 34, 36, 38; in humans, molecules with more than 46; and in rats, molecules with a broad spectrum from 40–52.

Differences in the synthetic and assembly processes result in characteristic positional arrangements of the acyl groups in the triacylglycerols of different species (see Chap. 3). In ruminant milk fat, butyrate is located almost exclusively in the sn-3 position, palmitate is equally divided between the sn-1 and sn-2 position, and oleate is rather evenly divided among all three positions. In milk fats of placental mammals other than ruminants, and in those of marsupials, palmitate is heavily concentrated in sn-2 and oleate in sn-1 and sn-3. This positional arrangement differs greatly from that in tissue lipids, where palmitate is found principally in sn-1 and is virtually excluded from sn-2. The milk fat of the echidna (an egg laying, or monotreme mammal) differs from all others yet described in that oleate is concentrated at sn-2 and palmitate is nearly entirely excluded from that position.

5.2-2b: Other lipids. Small amounts of mono- and diacylglycerols and free fatty acids are always found when milk fat is examined. It is difficult to decide if these are present in the milk as secreted, are produced by lipolysis in the cisterns, or after the milk is drawn. The contents of these classes of compounds, given in Table 5.4, for cow and human lipids are about the minimum observed. It is questionable whether a rat milk fat, free of postsecretion lipolysis, has been examined.

Phospholipids include phosphoglycerides, plasmalogens, and sphingomyelins. Phosphoglycerides are derivatives of phosphatidic acid, which consists of glycerol with fatty acids esterified in positions 1 and 2 and phosphoric acid in position 3. The four classes of phosphoglycerides are phosphatidylcholine (PC), phosphatidylethanolamine (PE), phosphatidylserine (PS), and phosphatidylinositol (PI), each having the indicated compound esterified to the phosphate. Plasmalogens are similar to PC and PE except that they have long-chain alk-1-enyl or alkyl groups linked by ether linkages at positions 1 and 2 of glycerol. Sphingomyelins (Sphs) consist of a long-chain 2-amino-1,3-dihydroxy base, with an amide-linked fatty acid and a phosphocholine esterified with the C_1 hydroxyl. The proportions of these classes of phospholipids in milks of six species are shown in Table 5.6; there is little species variation. Small portions of the PC and PE are undoubtedly plasmalogens in each case. About two-thirds of the phospholipids are in the fat globule membrane and one-third in the milk plasma. Fatty acid composition of the phosphoglycerides is similar to that of triacylglycerols except that saturated acids containing fewer than ten carbons are conspicuously lacking, even in ruminants, and the proportion of long-chain, polyunsaturated acids is greater. Saturated acids with 16–24

Table 5.6. Composition of milk phospholipids of several species

	Mol % of Total Phospholipid					
Species	PE	PC	PS	PI	Sph	Other[a]
Cow	31.8	34.5	3.1	4.7	25.2	
Goat	33.3	25.7	6.9	5.6	27.9	
Pig	36.8	21.6	3.4	3.3	34.9	
Donkey	32.1	26.3	3.7	3.8	34.1	
Rat	31.6	38.0	3.2	4.9	19.2	3.1
Human	25.9	27.9	5.8	4.2	31.1	5.1

[a]Lysophosphatidylcholine and lysophosphatidylethanolamine.

carbons and 16:0, 16:1, 18:0, and 18:1 (sphingosine) bases predominate in the Sphs.

Another class of lipids is glycosylceramides (cerebrosides), which are similar to Sphs but have a carbohydrate instead of phosphocholine attached to the C_1 of the base; both glucosyl and lactosyl ceramides have been found in bovine milk fat. Their bases and fatty acids are similar to those of the Sphs. Gangliosides are glycosyl ceramides in which the carbohydrate moiety consists of an oligosaccharide, including at least one *N*-acetylneuraminic acid (NANA, or sialic acid) residue.

Bovine milk fat contains 0.3–0.4% cholesterol; most of it is free, but a small portion consists of esters with various fatty acids. About 80% of the cholesterol is dissolved in the fat, 10% is in the fat globule membrane, and the remainder in the plasma. Milk fats of the goat, sheep, pig, horse, and human have cholesterol contents similar to those of the bovine. Detectable amounts of sterols, other than cholesterol, and some preformed vitamin D also are present in milks.

Small amounts of hydrocarbons such as pristane, phytane, and squalene are found in milk fat, but the principal hydrocarbons of interest are carotenoids because of their vitamin A potency (see 5.4).

5.2-3: Proteins. Milk proteins fall into several families of polypeptide chains, which were delineated first, and to date most completely, in the milk of domestic cattle (*Bos taurus*); a system of nomenclature was developed for that species. Almost all milk proteins of other species defined to date appear to be homologs of those of *B. taurus* and are named accordingly. The principal kinds of milk polypeptides are: α_{s1}-, α_{s2}-, β- (and γ-) and κ-caseins (abbreviated α_{s1}-cn, β-cn, etc.); β-lactoglobulins (β-lg); α-lactalbumins (α-la); blood serum albumin (Alb); immunoglobulins IgG_1, IgG_2, IgA, IgM, and IgE; secretory component (SC); β_2-microglobulin (β_2m); lactoferrin (Lf); transferrin (Tf); fat globule membrane proteins (MFGM); whey phosphoproteins (WPP, so far, found only in milks of certain rodents); and enzymes (named according to the recommendations of the International Union of Biochemistry). With the exception of the immunoglobulins, in normal usage the full names of these proteins are used. The abbreviations are most commonly encountered when referring to genetic variants and other genetic implications. Each kind is considered to be coded for by a single gene, or in the case of the immunoglobulins (Igs), by multigene complexes. Within each homologous family of polypeptides, intra- and interspecies variants occur as a result of both genetic polymorphism and posttranslational modification. The first is due to mutations in the cistrons coding for particular proteins and the second to many different reactions, including phosphorylation, glycosylation, and proteolytic cleavage.

The best criterion for establishing homology among proteins is congruence of amino acid sequences. Homology may also be inferred, but not as definitively, from biological function and from immunological cross-reactivity. Similarity of amino acid composition gives some indication of homology but is not an entirely reliable guide. An index sometimes used to compare protein composition is

$$S\Delta Q = \Sigma_j(X_{i,j} - X_{k,j})^2$$

where i and k identify proteins being compared and X_j is the content of amino acid j in mol/100 mol. Glutamic acid (Glu) residues are not differentiated from glutamine (Gln), nor are aspartic acid (Asp) residues from asparagine (Asn) in this calculation. Pairs of homologous proteins generally have values of SΔQ well below 100.

For purposes of analysis and isolation of components, milk proteins are sometimes fractionated into three classes: caseins present in micelles (see 5.3), whey proteins present in solution, and fat globule membrane proteins on the surface of fat globules (see 5.3). These categories are not quite exclusive; few individual proteins are found in more than one. In analytical fractionations, the fat globule membranes are often simply included in the casein category. Enzymes are present in the casein micelles, in solution, and in the fat globule membrane, but a given enzyme is usually in only one location. Table 5.7 lists the principal proteins of bovine and human milk, together with their concentrations and some of their properties.

5.2-3a: Caseins. Caseins designate a group of milk-specific proteins characterized by ester-bound phosphate, high proline contents, few or no cysteine (Cys) residues, and low solubility at pH 4.0–5.0. It is impossible to define caseins, either on the basis of composition or properties, in

Table 5.7. Properties and content of some milk proteins

		Residues/mole[a]							Content (g/l)	
Protein	Mol Wt[a]	Total	Pro[b]	Cys[c]	-S-S-[d]	P[e]	pI[f]	A_{280}[g]	Bovine	Human
α_{s1}-Casein	23,614	199	17	0	0	8	5.0	10.1	10.0	3.3 (for all caseins)
α_{s2}-Casein	25,230	207	10	2	?	11	5.3	14.0	2.6	
β-Casein	23,983	209	35	0	0	5	5.2	4.5	9.3	
κ-Casein	19,023	169	20	2	?	1	5.5	10.5	3.3	
α-Lactalbumin	14,176	123	2	8	4	0	5.4	20.9	1.2	1.5
β-Lactoglobulin	18,363	162	8	5	2	0	5.3	9.5	3.2	neg.
Serum albumin	66,267	582	34	35	17	0		6.6	0.4	0.4
Lactoferrin	ca 90,000	ca 700	28						<0.1	1.5
Lysozyme	14,701	130	2	8	4	0			neg.	0.4
Immunoglobulins	See text								See Table 7.2	

[a]For most common variant.
[b]Proline.
[c]Cysteine.
[d]Disulfide.
[e]Phosphorus.
[f]Isoionic pH.
[g]Absorbance at 280 nm.

such a way as to include all proteins belonging to the group and to exclude all others. The most widely used operational definition of caseins, as proteins that precipitate from milk at pH 4.6 and 40°C, includes most of them.

In cows' milk, α_{s1}-casein is the casein present in highest concentration. It is a chain of 199 amino acid residues with either 8 or 9 phosphate groups. Five genetic variants are known of which one has a deletion of 13 residues. Water buffalo and sheep milks certainly appear to contain α_{s1}-casein homologs. Protein components isolated from dog and rabbit milks also may possibly be α_{s1}-casein homologs. It is a minor and variable casein component in goat milk.

The α_{s2}-caseins consist of polypeptide chains of 207 residues of which 2 are Cys. Variants have 10, 11, 12, and 13 phosphates, and at least 1 disulfide-linked polymer occurs commonly. Homologs have been found in milks of the guinea pig, water buffalo, and goat.

Bovine β-caseins are chains of 209 residues, including 5 phosphoserines (except in 1 variant) and no Cys residues. Homologs have been found in milks of all ten species checked for it. Their SΔQ values vs. cow β-casein A^2 range from 2.3 for water buffalo to 79 for rat. Pig β-casein has 8 phosphates and the β-casein of the horse and rabbit each have 6. The horse β-casein is the only one in which a Cys residue has yet been found. Human β-casein is particularly interesting in that it consists of a single polypeptide chain with 0–5 phosphorylated residues.

A protein component, designated γ-casein and known for a long time in bovine milk, was ultimately shown to consist of fragments resulting from posttranslational cleavage of about 10% of the β-casein by the indigenous protease plasmin. These fragments consist of residues 29-209, 106-209, and 108-209; they are included in casein separated by acid precipitation. The smaller complementary fragments 1-28, 28-105, 28-107, 1-105, and 1-107 are found in the acid whey when casein is precipitated. They constitute part of a fraction, long designated the proteose-peptone fraction of whey. Proteins resembling bovine γ-caseins have been isolated from sheep and horse milks and, undoubtedly, are present in milks of other species.

Bovine κ-caseins consist of polypeptides of 169 residues having Cys at positions 11 and 88, phosphoserine (Ser P) at 149 and sometimes at 127, and variable degrees of glycosylation, mostly at threonine (Thr) 133. The κ-casein stabilizes the casein micelles of milk and loses this power when cleaved at linkage 105/106 by proteolytic enzymes. The enzyme chymosin (rennin), secreted by the gastric mucosa of sucklings, has high specificity for cleavage at this particular linkage. Fragment 1-105 is termed para-κ-casein and 106-169, glycomacropeptide, or caseinomacropeptide.

The caseinomacropeptides from seven species and the entire κ-caseins from cows, sheep, and goats have been sequenced. Sequence differences among species are small in the para-κ-casein and much greater in the caseinomacropeptides. The chymosin-sensitive bond is phenylalanine (Phe) 105-methionine (Met) 106 in ruminant κ-caseins and isoleucine (Ile) 105-Met 106 in those of humans and pigs.

5.2-3b: Whey proteins. When casein is precipitated from milk by acid, the resulting whey contains the soluble proteins, including the proteose-peptone fragments derived by cleavage of β-casein. Whey produced by the action of rennin also includes the caseinomacropeptide from the splitting of β-casein. Two of the principal whey proteins (α-lactalbumin, β-lactoglobulin) are specific products of the mammary gland; most of the others, including enzymes, are synthesized elsewhere.

The α-lactalbumin plays an essential role in the biosynthesis of lactose (see Chap. 4) and is secreted along with lactose in milk. It has been found in all milks checked except that of certain seals, which contains no lactose. Milks of some species have a lactose:α-lactalbumin molar ratio of about 1,000. The α-lactalbumins have been isolated from milks of 20 species, several of which are shown in Table 5.8. All 20 promote the formation of lactose when incubated with glucose, UDP-galactose, and bovine galactosyl transferase. Sequence and compositional differences show a gradation of relationship (Table 5.8). All but two consist of 123 residues; rabbit α-lactalbumin lacks 1 residue at the C-terminus, and rat α-lactalbumin has an extended C-terminal segment of 17 residues. All but mouse α-lactalbumin have 4 disulfide linkages; mouse α-lactalbumin has 3. The α-lactalbumins of ruminants exhibit varying degrees of immunological cross-reaction with antibovine α-lactalbumin, but the α-lactalbumins of nonruminants do not cross react as readily with it. The only clearly documented case of genetic polymorphism in α-lactalbumin involves position 10; α-lactalbumin B, occurring in western breeds of cattle (*B. taurus*), has arginine (Arg), whereas α-lactalbumin A from zebus (*B. indicus*) has glutamine at this position.

Table 5.8. The α-lactalbumins of various species

	Difference vs. Cow α-la B	
Species	SΔQ	Sequence[a]
Cow (western)	0	0
Zebu	1.3	1
Water buffalo	1.3	2
Goat	3.9	12
Sheep	21	
Pig	19	
Horse	21	14/30
Rat		45
Mouse	84	
Guinea pig	29	45
Rabbit	17	53
Human	52	32
Grey kangaroo	51	26/42

Source: From Jenness 1982.
[a]Substitutions in chain of 123 residues except in two cases in N-terminal portion of chain.

Table 5.9. β-Lactoglobulins of various species

Species	No. Variants	Cys/mol	Difference vs. Cow β-lg B	
			SΔQ	Sequence
Cow	4[a]	5		
Water buffalo	1	5	1.3	2
Goat	1	5	2.7	6
Sheep	2	5	2.3	6
Red deer	2	5	5.5	
Pig	2[b]	4	32	
Horse	1	4	44, 46	
Dog	1	5	57	

Source: From Jenness 1982.
[a]An additional variant occurs in yak and two more in banteng.
[b]Possibly a third variant occurs.

Other variants in several species appear to involve differences in glycosylation.

The β-lactoglobulin is the most abundant protein in bovine whey and has been isolated from milks of several other species (Table 5.9) but is present in only tiny concentrations, if at all, in some others (e.g., human); its biological function is unknown. It consists of a chain of 162 residues of which either 4 or 5 are Cys. Ruminant β-lactoglobulins associate to form noncovalently-linked dimers at pH 3–7, but those of the pig and horse do not so dimerize.

Blood serum albumin, characteristic of a species, always seems to be present in milk and is synthesized in liver; its concentration in blood is 30–40 g/l. It is transported into milk through the mammary cells and, probably, in the case of mastitis, via leaky junctions between cells as well. It has been isolated from milks of two species, cow and human; such isolates appear to be identical to the albumins isolated from blood. Its concentration is about 0.4 and 0.6 g/l in cow and human milks, respectively.

Two iron-binding proteins, transferrin and lactoferrin, are found in milk. Transferrin is a common blood plasma protein, and lactoferrin is secreted by several other organs besides the mammary gland. Both are large, single-chain proteins of 600–700 residues of which about 4 mol% are Cys, carry covalently-linked carbohydrate, and bind 2 atoms of Fe^{3+}/mol. They differ markedly from each other in composition and electrophoretic mobility and do not cross react with each other immunologically. Transferrins have been isolated from bloods of many species but only from milks of the cow and rabbit. Lactoferrins have been isolated from milks of the human, mouse, guinea pig, cow, goat, and sheep. Both can be determined quantitatively by techniques of immunodiffusion using specific antisera. Their concentrations and ratios in milk differ markedly among species and with stage of lactation. Human milk is rich in lactoferrin but contains little transferrin. Rat and rabbit milks, on the other hand, contain much transferrin and little lactoferrin. Milks of the mouse, guinea pig, horse, pig, cow, goat, and sheep have intermediate contents of both, but dog milk contains little of either.

Immunoglobulins are antibodies synthesized by the animal in response to foreign antigens to which it has been exposed. The structures of these proteins and their concentrations in milk and colostrum are discussed in Chapter 7; their transport into the mammary secretions are dealt with in Chapter 4.

A protein of 98 residues, of which two are Cys, is β_2-microglobulin. It is present in several body fluids and in membranes of various types of cells. Its amino acid sequence indicates homology with the constant regions of light and heavy chains of Igs. In 1977, a protein previously isolated from bovine milk and designated lactollin was shown to be β_2-microglobulin. Its concentrations in bovine colostrum and milk are about 6 and 2 mg/l, respectively. Concentrations in human colostrum and milk are much higher, 100 and 10–20 mg/l, respectively.

The proteose-peptone fraction of bovine whey proteins consists of four principal components that are not rendered acid insoluble by previous heating of the milk. One of these is probably derived from a fat globule membrane constituent, and the others are fractions derived by proteolysis of β-casein (see 5.2-3a). The aggregate of these components is about 1 g/l. It is likely that similar components occur in milks of other species, but they have not been looked for.

A group of whey phosphoproteins isolated from rat milk appears to consist of a polypeptide chain of 118 residues of which 0, 1, 2, and 3 are phosphorylated. These proteins may amount to as much as 5 mg/ml in rat whole milk (about 6% of the total protein). An acid whey protein isolated from mouse milk is about the same molecular size as the whey phosphoproteins of rat milk, but it has not been demonstrated to be phosphorylated, and its amino acid composition is somewhat different. Proteins similar to these in rat and mouse milks have not been detected in milks of other species.

Specific proteins that bind folate, vitamin B_{12}, and corticosteroids have been isolated from milks of a few species. Cow, goat, and human milks contain, respectively, about 50, 6, and 50 μg folate and 8, 12, and <1 mg/l folate-binding proteins (FBPs). The FPBs have molecular weights of 35,000–38,000 and bind around 10 mg folate/g. They are heavily glycosylated proteins. The concentrations of vitamin B_{12}-binding proteins vary greatly among milks of different species. Cow, goat, human, rat, and pig milks bind about 0.5, 2.7, 80, 126, and 245 μg vitamin B_{12}/l. Human and rat milks have been found to contain a protein similar to the corticosteroid-binding globulin present in blood serum.

Milk and colostrum contain several not very well defined glycoproteins in addition to the ones already mentioned. Concentrations of these components usually are much greater in colostrum than milk and vary greatly among species.

5.2-3c: Fat globule membrane proteins. The membranes enclosing fat globules of milk consist of plasma membrane of the secretory cells that envelops the fat globule as it is secreted (see Chap. 4) and is later somewhat modified and rearranged. About half the membrane is protein and it accounts for about 1% of the total milk protein. The fat globule membrane protein is included as casein when the usual methods of acid precipitation for analytical purposes are applied to whole milk. The great majority of attempts to resolve and characterize the mixture of fat globule membrane proteins have been done with bovine milk. As many as 40 electrophoretically distinguishable components have been observed and a few fairly homogeneous entities isolated, but the mixture is far from being resolved on a molecular basis. The two components present in greatest concentrations are the enzyme xanthine oxidase and a distinctive protein, sometimes called butyrophyllin.

5.2-4: Enzymes. Approximately 50 enzymatic activities have been detected in bovine milk and many of them in milks of a few other species, as well. Some are constituents of leukocytes and some may gain access from blood. Most, however, are constituents or products of the mammary cells that enter milk during the secretory process; a few (e.g., galactosyl transferase) have known functions in the biosynthetic processes of the cells. Some (e.g., plasmin, lipase) act on substrates that are present as normal constituents of milk and may play either beneficial or deleterious roles in dairy processes and products. There is no well-documented case of a milk enzyme being of direct nutritional value to the consumer of the milk.

Concentrations and activities of milk enzymes vary greatly among species, and large variations occur among individual animals. Activities are generally higher in colostrum than in midlactation milk. Any disease condition that allows increased concentrations of leukocytes or blood constituents to enter the milk will increase certain enzymatic activities.

Activities of 15 enzymes in bovine milk are compiled in Table 5.10, and, in cases where intralaboratory comparisons are possible, the ratio of activities in bovine and human milks is given. Milks of these two species differ enormously in their profile of enzyme activities; lactoperoxidase, xanthine oxidase, ribonuclease, and alkaline phosphatase are all high in cows' milk and low in human milk. On the other hand, amylase and lysozyme activities are much greater in human than in bovine milks.

5.2-5: Carbohydrates. The predominant and distinctive carbohydrate of milks of many species is lactose (4-*O*-β-D-galactopyranosyl-D-glucopyranose). It is synthesized in the mammary cells (see Chap. 4) and occurs scarcely anywhere else in nature. Milks of certain seals contain very low concentrations of lactose and one, the California sea lion, appears to

Table 5.10. Activities of some milk enzymes

Enzyme	E.C. No.[a]	Activity	
		Cow[b]	Human: Cow
Lactate dehydrogenase	1.1.1.27	40	3.5
Malate dehydrogenase	1.1.1.37	40	1.8
Xanthine oxidase	1.2.3.2	175	0[c]
Catalase	1.11.1.6	300	10
Lactoperoxidase	1.11.1.7	22,000	0.03
Superoxide dismutase	1.15.1.1	0.1–0.5	
Galactosyl transferase	2.4.1.38	50	
Lipoprotein lipase	3.1.1.34	600	
Alkaline phosphatase	3.1.3.1	500	0.02
Phosphoprotein phosphatases	3.1.3.16	13	1.2
Ribonuclease	3.1.27.5	11 mg[d]	0.3
α-Amylase	3.2.1.1		36[e]
Lysozyme	3.2.1.17	130 μg[d]	3,000
Aldolase	4.1.2.13		4.7[e]
Glucose phosphate isomerase	5.3.1.9	155	2.1

[a]Number assigned by Enzyme Commission, International Union of Biochemistry.
[b]In μmol • min^{-1} • l^{-1} except as noted.
[c]Activity close to zero in human milk.
[d]Weight/l.
[e]Ratio calculated from arbitrary units of activity.

lack it entirely. Lactose is present in milks of marsupials (pouched mammals) and monotremes (egg-laying mammals) but is generally not the major carbohydrate (as described later). Published reports of lactose contents of milks of various species must be taken with reservation because many of the analyses have been made by methods not specific for lactose. Those in Table 5.1, for example, are merely the lactose equivalents of the total reducing power or optical rotation or color intensity upon reaction with H_2SO_4 and a phenolic compound. The discrepancy is small in the case of ruminant milks because concentrations of other carbohydrates are small, but it is large, and in many cases not yet determined, in milks of many other species.

Milk carbohydrates, other than lactose, are monosaccharides, sugar phosphates, nucleotide sugars, free neutral and acid oligosaccharides, and glycosyl groups of peptides and proteins. Free glucose (Glc), galactose (Gal), *N*-acetylglucosamine (GlcNAc 2-acetamido-2-deoxy-D-glucose), *N*-acetylneuraminic acid (NANA, or sialic acid), and the sugar alcohol *myo*-inositol all are present in milk. Free Glc and Gal are readily detected in bovine milk, but there is lack of agreement on their concentration. Analyses made by gas liquid chromatography have indicated concentrations of 100–150 mg/l for each of them, but specific enzyme assays have detected only about 20 mg/l Glc and 40 mg/l Gal. Free *myo*-inositol has been found in milks of several species (in addition to that bound in phosphatidyl inositols, Table 5.6). Cow milk contains only about 40–50 mg/l *myo*-inositol, but human milk contains over 300 mg/l; milks of rodents and rabbits may contain as much as 900 mg/l. In rat milk, the content depends on dietary intake and is depressed to only about 100 mg/l, when none is fed. Rat milk also contains up to 125 mg/l 6-*O*-β-D-galactopyranosyl *myo*-inositol; synthesis of this disaccharide in the mammary gland from lactose and *myo*-inositol is catalyzed by β-galactosidase. Both *myo*-inositol and another isomer, *scyllo*-inositol, have been detected in dolphin milk.

Small concentrations of sugar phosphates (e.g., Glc-1-P, Glc-6-P, fructose [Fru]-6-P, Fru-1,6-diP, GlcNAc-1-P, and lactose phosphorylated in various positions) are detectable in bovine milk. Many nucleotide sugars (e.g., UDP-Glc, UDP-Gal) have been found in the milks of the few species examined; human milk contains much lower concentrations than do cow, goat, pig, or horse milks.

Oligosaccharides in milk consist of various polymers, about thirty of which have been isolated and identified, and are mostly from human colostrum and milk. They range up to 14 saccharide units per molecule. Units that have been found in oligosaccharides are D-glucose, D-galactose, L-fucose (Fuc), *N*-acetylglucosamine (GlcNAc), and NANA. All milk oligosaccharides yet isolated and characterized contain a lactose, or lactosamine (Gal-[β1,4]-Glc, or Gal-[β1,4]-GlcNAc) in the reducing terminal position. Some simple ones are sialyllactose (*O*-NANA-[2,6]-Gal-[β1,4]-Glc), fucosyllactose (Fuc-[1,2]-Gal-[β1,4]-Glc), and difucosyllactose (same as previous but with a second fucosyl residue-linked α-1,3 to the glucose). Others contain the tetrasaccharide sequence Gal-GlcNAc-Gal-Glc with Fuc, NANA, or additional Gal or GlcNAc units attached to it in various ways.

Bovine milk contains only 1–2 g/l oligosaccharides, human milk, 10–25 g/l. Colostrums of both species have higher concentrations. Milks of some monotremes contain more fucosyllactose or difucosyllactose than lactose itself. Kangaroos exhibit an interesting pattern of change in content and composition of carbohydrates during the lactation period. In one study, the total content (expressed as hexose) rose gradually from about 7% at 2 wk to over 11% at 26 wk postpartum, after which it fell rapidly to less than 1%. Up to 26 wk, the carbohydrates consisted of no monosaccharides, a small amount of lactose, and oligosaccharides of 3–6 units composed of Glc, Gal, GlcNAc, and NANA, with Gal predominating (70–80%). The proportion of oligosaccharides of larger size increased up to 26 wk and declined thereafter. Also, in late lactation, monosaccharides became prominent. When two young of different ages were being suckled, the milk supplied to the younger had high total hexose and much oligosaccharide, while that supplied to the older had a low content of carbohydrate consisting mostly of monosaccharides.

Glycopeptides isolated from bovine and human colostrums contain Gal, GlcNAc, GalNAc, and NANA. Those from human colostrum also contain Fuc. In 5.2-3, several glycosylated milk proteins were mentioned: κ-casein, some variants of α-lactalbumin and β-lactoglobulin, immuno-

Table 5.11. Principal salt constituents in bovine and human milks

	Bovine		Human	
Constituent	Total	Diffusible	Total	Diffusible
		(mmol/l)		
Sodium	25.2	25.2	6.5	6.5
Potassium	35.3	35.3	14.0	14.0
Calcium	30.1	10.4	6.7	4.0
Magnesium	5.1	3.3	1.4	1.2
Inorganic phosphate	22.3	12.4	2.1	1.2
Phosphate esters	3.4	2.6	2.4	1.6
Chloride	28.0	28.0	12.1	12.1
Citrate	10.6	9.3	1.6	1.5
Other organic acids	2			
Carbonate	2			
Sulfate	1			

globulins, lactoferrin and transferrin, and the fat globule membrane proteins. The carbohydrate moieties of these glycoproteins are composed of most of the same units found in the free oligosaccharides.

5.2-6: Salts. Salts in milk consist of ions and ion complexes; principal cations are Na^+, K^+, Ca^{2+}, and Mg^{2+}, and anions are Cl^-, inorganic phosphate (P_i), citrate (Cit^{3-}), HCO_3^-, SO_4^{2-}, and proteins. The concentrations and proportions of these constituents differ enormously among milks of different species. Table 5.11 gives analyses of the salt system of bovine and human milks. The salt system is regulated to a large extent by the relative rates of synthesis of carbohydrate, casein, and citrate and by the extent of paracellular leakage of blood constituents into milk. In general, the total concentration of salt constituents varies inversely with both inter- and intraspecies variations in carbohydrate content in keeping with the principle of isoosmolarity. The molar ratio of K^+:Na^+ is 2.0 or higher in normal milks of most species investigated; in colostrum and in milk from late lactation or from mastitic glands, the ratio is lower. The K^+:Na^+ ratios of kangaroo milk are very different from those of placental mammals. In the early stages, it is about 0.66 but rises to 1.0 at about 23 wk, to about 2.0 at about 31 wk, and then drops to about 1.0 for the remainder of lactation. It appears that considerable leakage of Na^+ occurs through the junctions between cells. Possibly, the kidneys of the very immature marsupial young cannot regulate urinary losses of Na^+ and K^+, so these ions must be supplied in a suitable ratio via the milk.

The milk salt system can be partitioned readily into a diffusible fraction of low molecular weight constituents and a nondiffusible, or colloidal, fraction of proteins and ions bound to them. The Na^+, K^+, and Cl^- are almost entirely in the diffusible fraction; Ca^{2+}, Mg^{2+}, P_i, and citrate are distributed between both; and protein is entirely nondiffusible. In the diffusible salt fraction, the monovalent ions Na^+, K^+, Cl^-, and $H_2PO_4^-$ form relatively weak complexes and, thus, are present largely as free ions; Ca^{2+},

Mg^{2+}, Cit^{3-}, and HPO_4^{2-} complex much more strongly. Only about 20% of the diffusible calcium and 40% of the diffusible magnesium of bovine milk are present as the free ions, Ca^{2+} and Mg^{2+}. Most of the diffusible citrate is present as $CaCit^-$ and $MgCit^-$ and nearly half of the phosphate as undissociated complexes with the cations. Diffusible calcium is highly correlated with citrate, and the concentration of the latter varies greatly among species and, in some, during the course of lactation. Milk citrate depends, in part, on the mammary cell activity of ATP-citrate lyase. Some rodents, having high activities of this enzyme, secrete virtually no citrate in milk; others (e.g., cow, goat, rabbit) have low activities of this enzyme, and their milks have a citrate concentration of 150–300 mg/100 ml.

In the nondiffusible fraction, a small amount of Ca^{2+} is bound specifically to α-lactalbumin (2 atoms per molecule), but most of this fraction consists of the casein micelles in which Ca^{2+}, Mg^{2+}, P_i, and a little citrate are complexed with casein (see 5.4 for description of these micelles). The distribution of these constituents, between diffusible and nondiffusible fractions in milks of two species, is shown in Table 5.11.

Total calcium (Ca) and total phosphorus (P) (sum of inorganic phosphate esters and organically bound phosphorus in casein) are closely correlated. Milks of about 40 species with Ca contents from less than 10 to 140 m*M* have an average Ca:P molar ratio of about 1.25; both Ca and P are closely correlated with casein. For the same 40 species as above, the slope of plots indicates that 1 g casein micelles contains about 0.9 mmol Ca and 0.8 mmol P. The casein content of milks of these species is 0.5–10 g/100 g milk. The proportions of individual kinds of casein vary greatly, but the average overall amounts of Ca and P carried per gram are approximately constant. Milks of some seals have somewhat lower contents of Ca and P in relation to casein than those just mentioned.

5.2-7: Miscellaneous components. Milk contains a large number of compounds in concentrations generally less than 100 mg/l; many do not fit unequivocally into any of the classifications of the previous sections. Here, they will be grouped into the categories of natural components and contaminants, the latter including radionuclides.

5.2-7a: Natural components. Natural components are compounds generally detectable in all, or nearly all, samples in which they are sought. Many of them are intermediate products of the metabolic processes occurring in the mammary gland: gases, trace elements, alcohols, aldehydes, ketones, carboxylic acids, nonprotein nitrogenous compounds, sulfur-containing compounds, phosphate esters, nucleotides and nucleic acids, hormones, and vitamins.

The gases CO_2, N_2, and O_2 are present in anaerobically-drawn milk in concentrations of about 6, 1, and 0.1% by volume, respectively. Carbon dioxide is in equilibrium with the bicarbonate ion; its concentration falls rapidly in milk exposed to air, and virtually the entire CO_2-HCO_3^- system can be removed by heating or vacuum treatment. Both the oxygen and nitrogen contents increase upon exposure of milk to air. Raw commercial milk contains about 1.3% N_2 and 0.5% O_2, by volume.

The elements listed in Table 5.12 have been detected in normal milk by spectrographic and chemical methods. Data on concentration and form of occurrence are rather scanty, although molybdenum (Mo) appears to be exclusively in xanthine oxidase and cobalt (Co) exclusively in vitamin B_{12}. Iron (Fe) is an essential component of xanthine oxidase, lactoperoxidase, and catalase. Zinc (Zn) is the metal present in highest concentration; in bovine milk, most of it is bound in the casein micelles but, in human milk, probably to citrate. Copper (Cu) and Fe are bound to some extent by the fat globule membrane. Trace elements may enter milk either through the cow or by contamination, subsequent to milking. Concentrations of some of these elements in milk, such as boron (B), Co, iodine (I), manganese (Mn), Mo, and Zn can be increased by increasing their level in the ration of the cow. Metal containers and equipment coming in contact with milk are an important source of contamination with Cu, Fe, nickel, (Ni), and tin (Sn).

Ethanol and a long array of aldehydes and ketones are detectable in milk. Many aliphatic carboxylic acids have been reported: saturated C_1-C_{10} and lactic, pyruvic, and α-ketoglutaric acids. Very variable concentrations of these acids have been reported, but the total is generally 1–3 mmol/l, compared to 10 mmol/l for citrate.

Nonprotein nitrogen (NPN) compounds are of low molecular weight and are not precipitated by 12% trichloroacetic acid; some small peptides may be included. The NPN compounds aggregate, perhaps 1 g/l in bovine milk, and contain 250–350 mg/l N (6% of total N). Human milk contains

Table 5.12. Trace elements in bovine and human milks

	Content			Content	
Element	Bovine	Human	Element	Bovine	Human
	($\mu g/l$)			($\mu g/l$)	
Aluminum	100–2,100	700	Lithium	tr–29	
Arsenic	30–100	50	Manganese	5–370	30
Barium	tr–110		Mercury	≤0.1	
Boron	30–800	80	Molybdenum	5–150	2
Bromine	60–25,000		Nickel	0–130	8–80
Cadmium	≤0.5	20	Rubidium	100–3,400	
Chromium	5–82	40	Selenium	4–1200	20
Cobalt	0–20	10	Silicon	1,300–7,000	880
Copper	10–1,200	60–1300	Silver	tr–54	
Fluorine	≤50		Strontium	40–2,000	
Iodine	5–400	25–470	Tin	0–1,000	
Iron	100–2,400	1000	Titanium	20–500	24
Lead	≤5	tr–280	Vanadium	tr–311	
			Zinc	ca 4,000	2,500

Table 5.13. Principal nonprotein nitrogen (NPN) compounds in milk

	Recent Report[a]	Range in Literature
	(mg/l)	
Total NPN	296.4	229–308
Urea-N	142.1	84–134
Creatine-N	25.5	6–20
Creatinine-N	12.1	2–9
Uric acid-N	7.8	5–8
Orotic acid-N	14.6	12–13
Hippuric acid-N	4.4	4
Peptide-N	32.0	
Ammonia-N	8.8	3–14
α-Amino acid-N	44.3	29–51

[a]Adapted from Wolfschoon-Pombo and Klostermeyer 1981.

considerably more (375 mg/l, 22% of total). Table 5.13 gives analyses for the principal NPN constituents in bovine milk. Urea accounts for about half the NPN. Orotic acid is a particular hallmark of ruminant milks; milks of other species have little, if any.

Nonprotein sulfur occurs in milk in the compounds methyl sulfide ($[CH_3]_2S$), implicated in the "cowy" flavor, dimethylsulfone ($[CH_3]_2SO_2$), indoxyl sulfate, lipoic acid, thiocyanate (SCN^-), and taurine (NH_2CH_2-CH_2SO_3H). The concentration of taurine is 1–7 mg/l in bovine milk and much higher in colostrum and human milk. It may be of nutritional importance for newborn humans.

Bovine milk contains about 100 mg/l phosphorus in the form of soluble organic compounds, which are mostly esters of orthophosphoric acid, including various sugar phosphates, phosphoglycerolethanolamine, and phosphoethanolamine.

The list of nucleotides detected in milk has grown rapidly, as more sensitive methods have been developed. The common mono- and dinucleotides, 3′, 5′ cyclic AMP, and ATP are all present; ATP is located entirely in the casein micelles. Several nucleotide sugars, doubtless intermediates in glycoprotein synthesis, are found in milk, and both RNA and DNA have been detected and quantitated.

Hormones present in milk are discussed in 2.7 and vitamins in 5.4.

5.2-7b: Contaminants. Contaminants are materials that are not normally secreted in milk but enter it accidentally or by design. Three routes of entry can be distinguished: (1) materials inhaled or eaten may pass into milk via the blood and the mammary gland, (2) materials infused into the mammary ducts will be washed out in the milk, and (3) materials can fall into the milk during milking or enter it from air or equipment to which it is exposed after being drawn. Only the first two routes will be considered here. Most interest centers, of course, on materials that are potentially harmful to the consumer of the milk.

Various pesticides, herbicides, and fungicides, especially of the organochlorine type and the widely dispersed polychlorobiphenyls, have been found in milk. Because of their lipophilic nature, they tend to accumulate in the fat. Although concentrations in excess of accepted maximums were sometimes reported in the past, use of these materials has been restricted, and levels are now generally much below limits. Organophosphates and carbamates do not accumulate in the fat and primarily are broken down by the cow in the digestive tract.

Heavy metals, such as selenium, lead, mercury, and cadmium, are extremely toxic, but the cow serves as an effective filter and toxic levels have not been reported in milk. The radionuclides strontium (^{89}Sr), ^{90}Sr, iodine (^{131}I), cesium (^{137}Cs), and barium (^{140}Ba) from fallout may enter milk via the cow and, thus, potentially constitute a hazard to the consumer. Of these, ^{90}Sr and ^{131}I are the most serious, as they accumulate in bone and thyroid, respectively. The cow acts as a filter and discriminator for some radionuclides. Of the total quantities of I and Cs ingested daily, roughly 1% is secreted in each kg of milk produced. For Ba and Sr, the proportion is less. Furthermore, the cow discriminates against Sr and in favor of Ca in milk secretion. The Sr:Ca ratio is reduced by a factor of about 10 from feed to milk. Radionuclides in milk are discussed further in 4.9.

Drugs consumed by or administered to the lactating female may gain access to the milk. Antibiotics infused into the udder may cause problems in the manufacture of fermented milk products.

5.3: PHYSICAL STRUCTURE OF MILK

Physically, milk consists of a solution of salts, carbohydrates, and miscellaneous other compounds in which protein molecules and aggregates, casein micelles, and fat globules are dispersed.

The proportions of dissolved constituents of low molecular weight vary greatly among milks of different species, but their aggregate osmolality is about 0.3 *M* in every case, so that milk is isoosmotic with blood. The ionic strength of bovine milk is approximately 0.08; milks of other species certainly vary in ionic strength because of differences in salt content, but specific values have not been calculated. The pH of milk varies from about 6.2 for many carnivores to around 7.0 for primates. Normal bovine and human milks have a pH of 6.6 and 7.0, respectively.

Some individual proteins, such as α-lactalbumin, are dispersed in milk as individual molecules. Others, such as some β-lactoglobulins, form non-covalently-linked dimers. The polymeric form of the Igs was described previously. In bovine milk, caseins aggregate to form micelles with a size range of 0.02–0.3 μm in diameter and contain from 20,000–150,000 casein molecules. Virtually all the casein is present in micelles, although β-casein leaves them to some extent at low temperature. The calcium phosphate content in micelles is about 8 g/100 g casein; the voluminosity is about 2ml/g. The micelles appear to be stabilized (kept from aggregating indefinitely and precipitating) by the κ-casein component, some of whose molecules are located in the periphery of the micelles with their highly glycosylated C-terminal region projecting, resulting in the present concept of a hairy micelle structure. Proteolytic cleavage of the C-terminal caseinomacropeptide portion of the κ-casein hairs destabilizes the micelles so they precipitate. Casein micelles of species other than bovine have not been analyzed very thoroughly.

Milk fat is almost entirely in the form of globules ranging from 0.1–15 μm in diameter. Size distribution is an inherited characteristic and varies both among species and breeds of cattle. Bovine milk contains many small globules that comprise only a small fraction of the total fat. The total number is about 15×10^9/ml, 75% of which are smaller than 1 μm in diameter. The number average diameter ($\Sigma nd/\Sigma n$) is very small, about 0.8 μm. Much more meaningful is the volume:surface average diameter ($\Sigma nd^3/\Sigma nd^2$) of about 3.4 μm, which is that of a globule having the average volume:surface ratio calculated for the entire array of globules. The total surface area of the fat is 1.2–2.5 m^2/g fat, or about 80 m^2/l milk.

Fat globules are surrounded by a thin protective layer, the fat globule membrane, which protects them from flocculation and coalescence. This membrane is derived from the outer membrane of the apical part of the secretory cell and probably from some Golgi membrane, as well. These membranes surround the fat globule as it leaves the cell and are undoubtedly somewhat modified after secretion by part of the material dissolving into the core of the globule, by loss of polar substances to the plasma, by adsorption of materials from the plasma onto the globules, and possibly by enzyme action. In general, the membrane material is about 1.5 g/100 g fat (9 mg/m^2); it consists of approximately 60% protein and nearly 40% phospholipids, together with small amounts of other lipids. Several of the enzymes in milk (xanthine oxidase, alkaline phosphatase) are located in the fat globule membrane.

5.4: NUTRITIVE VALUE OF MILK

The nutritive value of a foodstuff is due to (1) the energy that it supplies; (2) its content of essential fatty acids, amino acids, minerals, and vitamins; (3) the digestibility and absorbability of its nutrients; (4) its content of allergens, protease inhibitors, and toxins; and (5) its content of antimicrobial factors, such as immunoglobulins, lactoferrin, lysozyme, and lactoperoxidase. Items in the last category are discussed in Chapter 7 in relation to protection of the udder; they may also influence the flora of the digestive tract of the suckling.

This section deals with the nutritive value of milk for a species' own young and briefly assesses the value of certain milks in the nutrition of human infants and adults.

5.4-1: Nutritive value of milk for sucklings of the species. Newborn mammals of different species differ greatly in (1) the stage of development at birth, (2) growth rate after birth, (3) proportions of nutritive requirements from birth to weaning obtained from milk, and (4) frequency of nursing. With so many variables and such wide ranges of variability within each of them, it is difficult to discern general patterns of relationship between milk composition and nutritive requirements of the young.

No general correlation has been adduced between milk composition and physiological maturity of the young at birth. In fact, examples to the contrary can be cited. Rabbits of different genera are born at widely different stages of maturity, yet their milks are similar. Artiodactyls (cattle) and perissodactyls (horses) are born at a similar stage of maturity, yet their milks differ greatly.

Since a great deal of the growth of sucklings involves formation of protein and deposition of bone, one might expect a relation between growth rate and protein and mineral contents of the milk. For a few species for which such comparison can be made, a reasonably linear correlation holds between percentage of milk energy derived from protein and logarithm of days required to double birth weight. The species range from humans, with 125 days to double birth weight and 7% of milk energy as protein, to rats, rabbits, and carnivores, with 7 days and 30%. This relation does not hold for aquatic and arctic mammals, whose milk energy is derived largely from fat and the growth of whose young consists largely of deposition of fat.

One might expect the concentration of nutrients to be greater in milks of small rather than large animals because metabolic rate is proportional to body surface area and capacity of the digestive tract is proportional to body weight. Such a relationship is valid in comparisons of milks of rats and mice, but few other comparisons can be made of closely related animals of different size.

In general, species that nurse their young on demand tend to furnish milk of lower solids and caloric content than those that nurse at scheduled intervals. In some species, especially kangaroos, whose young are solely dependent on milk for a long period over which they increase manyfold in weight, the total milk solids increase markedly during the course of lactation.

The distinctive arrays of nutritive components of milk of various species presumably result from processes of evolutionary selection, but their selective nutritive advantages are not entirely clear. The ability of caseins to form micelles carrying a great deal more calcium and phosphate than could be maintained in solution seems to constitute a distinct selective advantage, particularly for species whose young grow rapidly. The high contents of lysozyme and lactoferrin in human milk may function in controlling flora in the digestive tract. No specific nutritive roles or advantages have been suggested for proteins such as α-lactalbumin and β-lactoglobulin.

The specific evolutionary advantage of lactose, the distinctive milk sugar, remains conjectural. Certainly, a disaccharide has the advantage over a monosaccharide of nearly twice the caloric value for a given osmotic increment, but any disaccharide would do as well. A specific β-galactosidase is needed to cleave it, and, thus, it cannot be diverted until it reaches the locus of activity of such an enzyme. No doubt it avoids flora that would attack glucose and thus influences the composition of digestive tract flora. It seems to favor calcium absorption across the intestinal mucosa. Some of the oligosaccharides, which occur in such varying concentrations in milks, have been found to promote the growth of particular digestive tract organisms (e.g., *Bifidobacterium bifidus*). It is not known how significant or extensive a role these compounds play in this regard.

Milk supplies all necessary mineral elements for growth and metabolic functions of the young. The high requirements for calcium and phosphate are met by calcium complexing with citrate and the formation of casein micelles. Iron may be limiting because of difficulty with absorption, which is enhanced by lactoferrin, lactose, and ascorbate; indeed, this may constitute part of the nutritive role of these compounds.

Milks carry all the vitamins known to be required by mammals (Table 5.14); only vitamin K is present in negligible concentrations. Even though the young of most species appear to be able to synthesize L-ascorbic acid (vitamin C) in the liver, it is present in the milk of all species checked for it. For those that do not synthesize ascorbate (humans), milk appears to provide a sufficient supply for the needs of the young.

5.4-2: Nutritive value of milks for human infants. Cows' milk is used frequently, and milks of some other species less frequently, as the sole or major component of the diet of human infants. In this section, the compositions of bovine and human milks are related to the nutritive requirements of such infants. Requirements have been established in several countries; the ones used here are those of the Food and Nutrition Board, National Academy of Sciences (USA).

In spite of large differences in composition, bovine and human milks have similar total caloric content: about 70–75 kcal/100 g. In human milk, fat, protein, and lactose account for about 55, 5, and 40% of the energy,

Table 5.14. Vitamins in bovine and human milks

Vitamin	Concentration	
	Bovine	Human
	(*mg/l*)	
Vitamin A[a]	0.5	0.7
Vitamin D (cholecalciferol)	0.0004	0.0005
Vitamin E (α-tocopherol)	0.98	6.64
Thiamin (B_1)	0.44	0.16
Riboflavin (B_2)	1.75	0.36
Niacin	0.94	1.47
Pyridoxine (B_6)	0.64	0.10
Pantothenic acid	3.46	1.84
Biotin	0.031	0.008
Folic acid	0.050	0.03
Cobalamin (B_{12})	0.0043	0.0003
Ascorbic acid	21	43
Choline	121	90
Myo-inositol	50	330

Source: Data mostly from Hartman and Dryden 1974.
[a]Sum of retinol and 1/6 β-carotene.

and in cows' milk, they furnish 52, 20, and 28%, respectively. Growth rates of human infants are approximately equal when human, cow, goat, or vegetable (synthetic) milk is fed in isocaloric quantities.

The nutritive adequacy of milk for human infants can be presented as a profile relating the content of various constituents to requirements with energy as a common denominator. The quotient thus obtained is called nutrient density. For example, human infants require about 1.8 g protein/100 kcal. Cows' milk furnishes 3.2 g protein and 66 kcal/100 g and, thus, 4.8 g protein/100 kcal. Consequently, it provides 4.8/1.8, or 2.7 times the amount of protein needed in relation to energy. The profile shown in Table 5.15 was calculated in this way. Obviously, if requirements are set high, as they probably are in many cases for safety's sake, such profiles underestimate the ability of milk to meet requirements. Comparison of the profiles for human and cows' milks in the table indicates the great excess of protein, calcium, and phosphorus in cows' milk over the human infant requirement.

The nutritive value of proteins depends on digestibility and the content of the nine essential amino acids that humans cannot synthesize. Although the proportions of various proteins are very different in cows' and human milk (Table 5.7), the mixture in either species is highly digestible, and both adequately fulfill the pattern of requirements for the essential amino acids. The principal drawback of cows' milk protein for human infants is the toughness of the casein curd formed in the stomach, which slows gastric emptying and protein digestion. This can be overcome by diluting and preheating the milk. A few (perhaps 0.1–0.5% of the population) infants exhibit allergic responses to ingested cows' milk proteins. When tested separately, casein, α-lactalbumin, β-lactoglobulin, and bovine serum albumin have elicited such reactions in individual infants.

Human milk fat is superior to cows' milk fat for human infants in two respects. First, the content of dietary essential fatty acids, such as linoleic in cows' milk fat, is only about 20–25% that of human milk fat; this may be a limiting nutritional factor. Second, very young infants digest and absorb human milk fat better, probably because the predominance of palmitic acid in the sn-2 position favors these processes.

Mineral and vitamin requirements of infants are met adequately by both cows' and human milk (Table 5.15) except that both are deficient in iron and vitamin D. In some cases, cows' milk more adequately meets the requirement.

5.4-3: Nutritive value of milks for human adults. Some societies rely heavily on milks of cows or other domesticated species to supply certain nutrients to adults. Cows' milk furnishes excesses of protein, calcium, phosphate, thiamin, and riboflavin over energy. The protein is of high biological quality; occasional allergic responses have been observed.

The most widely discussed drawback of milk for adult humans is lactose intolerance, resulting from deficiency of intestinal β-galactosidase (lactase), necessary for hydrolysis of lactose. Lack of the enzyme permits lactose to pass into the large intestine, where it osmotically hinders withdrawal of water and is subject to degradation by microorganisms. Abdominal cramps, bloating, flatulence, and diarrhea result. Lactase deficiency may result from gastroenteritis or, rarely, from a congenital defect. The more common pattern is one of satisfactory lactose metabolism in infancy fol-

Table 5.15. Nutrients in milk in relation to energy

		A	B	C	Nutrient Density	
Nutrient	Unit	Cow	Human	Required[a]	A/C	B/C
Energy	kcal	100	100			
Protein	g	4.8	1.2	1.8	2.7	0.7
Vitamin A	RE[b]	66	140	42	1.6	3.3
Vitamin D	μg	0.08	0.08	1.0	0.08	0.08
Vitamin E	mg	0.15	0.9	0.4	0.35	2.2
Ascorbic acid	mg	3.2	6.0	3.7	0.9	1.6
Thiamin	mg	0.07	0.02	0.05	1.4	0.4
Riboflavin	mg	0.27	0.05	0.06	4.5	0.8
Niacin	NE[c]	1.00	0.25	0.83	1.2	0.3
Vitamin B_6	mg	0.10	0.012	0.06	1.6	0.2
Folic acid	μg	7.5	6.7	4.6	1.6	1.4
Vitamin B_{12}	μg	0.65	0.04	0.16	4.1	0.3
Calcium	mg	188	42	56	3.3	0.7
Magnesium	mg	20	5.4	7.3	2.7	0.7
Iron	mg	0.07	0.14	1.6	0.04	0.08
Zinc	mg	0.59	0.35	0.50	1.2	0.7
Phosphorus	mg	150	21	38	4.0	0.6
Iodine	μg	6.5	14.0	4.2	1.6	3.3

[a]Daily requirement per 100 kcal for infant 0.5–1 yr weighing 9 kg.
[b]Retinol equivalent (μg retinol + g carotene/6).
[c]Niacin equivalent (mg niacin + mg Trp/60). Trp in excess of 189 mg required daily by 9 kg infant. Trp = tryptophan.

lowed by loss of lactase between ages 1 and 4. Other species of mammals exhibit similar decreases in lactase activity during maturation. In humans, the degree of loss varies among ethnic groups. Descendants of groups in which adults have consumed milk for generations have much lower incidence than those from nondairy-consuming societies. For example, incidences of 10% and 70% have been reported in American white and black adults, respectively. It is not entirely clear whether lactase is induced or constitutive. Present thinking favors the idea that it is constitutive, and, thus, the loss is genetically controlled and the low incidence of lactose intolerance in some groups has resulted from a selective process.

Another defect in lactose metabolism is galactosemia, due to hereditary lack of the liver enzyme galactose-1-phosphate uridyl transferase, which catalyzes the formation of Glc-1-P from Gal-1-P. In the absence of this transferase, Gal cannot enter the pathway of glycolysis, and it, along with Gal-1-P and its reduction product galactitol, accumulates in blood and tissues. The results are digestive disturbance, failure to thrive, eye cataracts, and mental retardation. The disease is an autosomal-recessive, exhibited by homozygotes only; its frequency is 1/20,000–70,000 live births. The only known cure is complete elimination of galactose-containing foods from the diet.

REFERENCES

Bonnier, G., A. Hansson, and F. Jarl. 1946. Studies in the variation of the calory content of milk. Acta Agric. Suec. 2:159.

Butler, J. E. 1974. Immunoglobulins of the mammary secretions. In Lactation, 3:217. See Larson and Smith 1974.

Davies, D. T., C. Holt, and W. W. Christie. 1983. The composition of milk. In Biochemistry of Lactation, ed. T. B. Mepham. Amsterdam: Elsevier/North-Holland Biomedical.

Ebner, K. E., and F. L. Schanbacher. 1974. Biochemistry of lactose and related compounds. In Lactation, 2:77. See Larson and Smith 1974.

Glass, R. L., and R. Jenness. 1971. Comparative biochemical studies of milk. VI. Constituent fatty acids of milk fats of additional species. Comp. Biochem. Physiol. [B] 38:353.

Glass, R. L., H. A. Troolin, and R. Jenness. 1967. Comparative biochemical studies of milks. IV. Constituent fatty acids of milk fats. Comp. Biochem. Physiol. 22:415.

Hansen, R. G. 1974. Milk in human nutrition. In Lactation, 3:281. See Larson and Smith 1974.

Hartman, A. M., and L. P. Dryden. 1974. The vitamins in milk and milk products. In Fundamentals of Dairy Chemistry, 2d ed., ed. B. H. Webb, A. H. Johnson, and J. A. Alford. Westport, Conn.: Avi.

Jenness, R. 1974. The composition of milk. In Lactation, 3:3. See Larson and Smith 1974.

______. 1979. Comparative aspects of milk proteins. J. Dairy Res. 46:197.

______. 1982. Inter-species comparison of milk proteins. In Developments in Dairy Chemistry, vol. 1, Proteins, ed. P. F. Fox, 87. London and New York: Applied Science.

Kroger, M. 1974. General environmental contaminants occurring in milk. In Lactation, 3:135. See Larson and Smith 1974.

Larson, B. L., and V. R. Smith, eds. 1974. Lactation: A Comprehensive Treatise, vols. 2, 3. New York: Academic.

Lengemann, F. W., R. A. Wentworth, and C. L. Comar. 1974. Physiological and biochemical aspects of the accumulation of contaminant radionuclides in milk. In Lactation, 3:160. See Larson and Smith 1974.

Moore, J. H., and J. A. F. Rook, eds. 1980. Factors affecting the yields and contents of milk constituents of commercial importance. Int. Dairy Fed. Bull. Doc. 125.

Murthy, G. K. 1974. Trace elements in milk. C.R.C. Crit. Rev. Environ. Control 4:1.

Parrish, D. B., G. H. Wise, J. S. Hughes, and F. W. Atkeson. 1948. Properties of the colostrum of the dairy cow. II. Effect of prepartal rations upon the nitrogenous constituents. J. Dairy Sci. 31:889.

______. 1950. Properties of the colostrum of the dairy cow. V. Yield, specific gravity and concentrations of total solids and its various components of colostrum and early milk. J. Dairy Sci. 33:457.

Peaker, M. 1977. The aqueous phase of milk: Ion and water transport. In Comparative Aspects of Lactation. Symposia of the Zoological Society of London, no. 41, ed. M. Peaker, 113. New York: Academic.

Reinart, A., and J. M. Nesbitt. 1956. The composition of milk in Manitoba. Proc. 14th Int. Dairy Congr. 1:946.

Saperstein, S. 1974. Immunological problems of milk feeding. In Lactation, 3:257. See Larson and Smith 1974.

Swaisgood, H. E. 1982. Chemistry of milk protein. In Developments in Dairy Chemistry, vol. 1, Proteins, ed. P. F. Fox, 1. London and New York: Applied Science.

Thompson, M. P., and H. M. Farrell, Jr. 1974. Genetic variants of the milk proteins. In Lactation, 3:109. See Larson and Smith 1974.

Touchberry, R. W. 1974. Environmental and genetic factors in the development and maintenance of lactation. In Lactation, 3:349. See Larson and Smith 1974.

Wilcox, C. J., S. N. Gaunt, and B. R. Farthing. 1971. Genetic interrelationships of milk composition and yield. Northeast, Southeast State Agric. Exp. Stn. Southern Coop. Ser. Bull. 155.

Wolfschoon-Pombo, A., and H. Klostermeyer. 1981. The NPN-fraction of cow milk. I. Amount and composition. Milchwissenschaft 36:598.

CHAPTER 6

MILK COLLECTION

C. WILLIAM HEALD

6.1: INTRODUCTION

Milk secretion proceeds at a variable rate depending on raw product availability and finished product removal. Superimposed on this simplistic input-output relationship is a hormonal control system that orchestrates the flow of milk with parturition and the changing need for nourishment of the offspring. Use of selection and management techniques by humans has the potential to accelerate production of milk.

The nutritional needs of newborns vary with age; initially, these needs are small. As growth proceeds, demand for nourishment increases with increasing body size until the diet is supplemented with foods other than milk. As the newborn becomes independent from its mother's milk supply, it is weaned and the mother's potential to produce milk quickly diminishes, only to be reinitiated after the next pregnancy.

All too often it is forgotten that evolution destined the production of cow's milk for the calf, and only in the last 5,000–7,000 yr has the cow been domesticated and her milk shared with humans. This chapter describes how humans have exerted dominion over *Bos taurus* and points out some voids in our knowledge of milk collection.

6.2: PHYSIOLOGICAL FACTORS AFFECTING MECHANICAL MILKING

6.2-1: Structure and function of the teat. Knowledge of the general structure of the teat and milk cisterns aids understanding of milk removal (Fig. 6.1). Newly formed milk is first collected in the lumen of the alveoli and secretory (terminal) ducts. It then drains into succeedingly larger ducts until it enters the primary ducts attached to the gland cistern, the largest collecting point for milk. Most of the ducts are nonsecretory, and in capacious udders, as much as 40–50% of the milk is stored in the

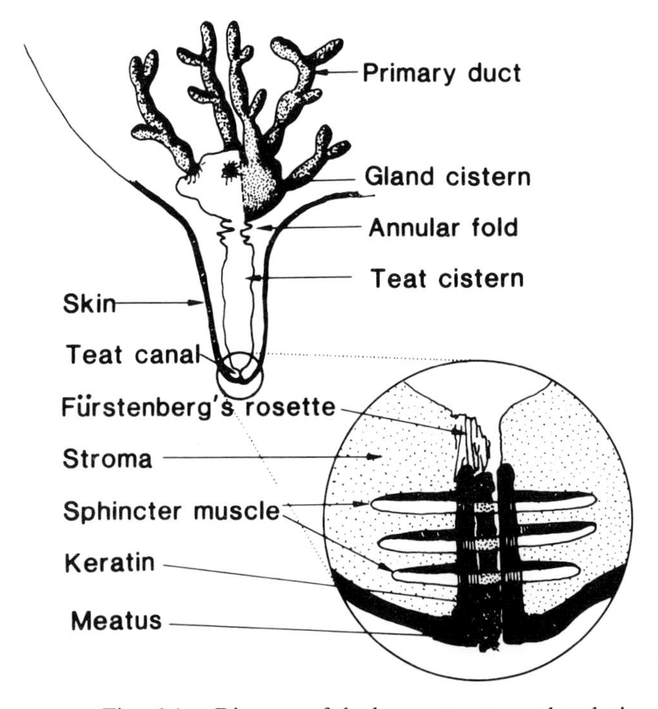

Fig. 6.1. Diagram of the larger structures that drain newly synthesized milk (originates in alveoli and secretory ducts), either into the mouth of a nursing calf or the milking machine.

ducts and cisterns. The gland cistern is attached to the teat cistern, with an annular fold partially separating the two. The teat cisternal milk is prevented from escaping to the outside of the udder by a sphincter muscle, which tightly contracts around the very narrow teat (streak) canal. Another function of the teat canal is to act as a barrier to bacterial penetration (the cause of nearly all mastitis). Evolution has provided the cow with very effective mechanisms to ward off bacterial invasion of the udder. Many of these mechanisms are little understood, but recent research is illuminating their functions. Selection of dairy cattle and use of modern milking practices have neglected defense mechanisms; teats with wide, short teat canals have been found to facilitate rapid milk removal but are more prone to infection.

The epithelium of the gland cistern and, at times, the teat cistern have small patches of secretory alveoli. These misplaced tissues are exceedingly delicate and easily damaged by milking. Traumatized epithelium is believed to be ideal for bacterial colonization, although little evidence exists to demonstrate such.

Recent studies of the epithelial lining of the teat cistern show that certain pathogens stick to dying epithelial cells (Fig. 6.2), identified by their loss of microvilli on the apical surface. Before certain pathogens colonize the teat cistern, they must adhere to the surface of the cistern. Apparently, intact healthy cells are resistant to this adherence.

The skin of the teats of cattle is unique in the absence of hair and glands and is very resistant to tearing, puncture, or abrasions. However, it will succumb to extremes of temperature because of the absence of insulation. The skin, like all skin of the cow, is stratified squamous epithelium covering the outside of the teat, extending up through the teat canal. At the proximal end of the teat canal near the Fürstenberg's rosette, it becomes the more delicate double-layered columnar epithelium of the teat cistern, gland cistern, and ducts, which is very easily damaged.

Between the inner and outer epithelial layers of the teat is a stromal network of connective tissue. Embedded in this stroma are blood vessels, lymphatic vessels, nervous tissue, and muscles. The teat is highly vascularized, but considering the teat is uninsulated, the high degree of vasculariza-

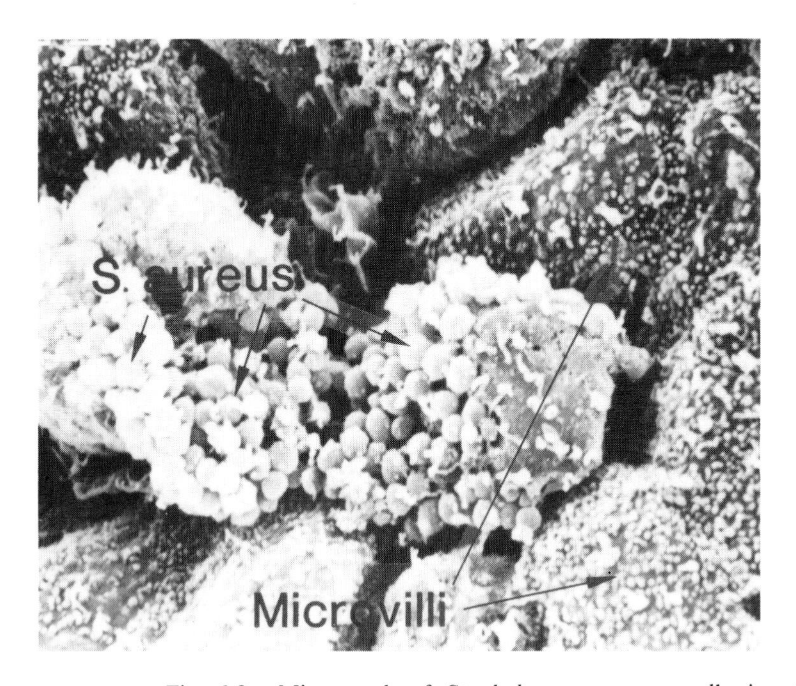

Fig. 6.2. Micrograph of *Staphylococcus aureus* adhering to sloughing (nonmicrovilliated) cells in the teat cistern, as seen using the scanning electron microscope. Microvilliated cells are believed to inhibit bacterial adhesion to the cell surface. ×4,000 magnification. (Provided by M.P. Comalli and R.J. Eberhart)

tion is probably related, in part, to maintenance of normal temperature during exposure to temperature extremes. This high degree of vascularization presents difficulty to the engineer designing milking equipment because the milking machine retards blood flow in the teat and results in vascular congestion and stromal swelling.

6.2-2: Teat orifice, teat canal, and sphincter muscle. All milk must exit the udder through a teat canal 7–16 mm long with a mean diameter of 0.82 mm, and most pathogens that cause mastitis must physically traverse this canal to enter the udder. The lower 2 cm of the teat consists of a complex of tissues designed to act as a valve for milk and a barrier to foreign material. The teat canal portal is closed by a group of circular sphincter muscles surrounding it. The teat is abundantly supplied with nerves, which tend to be more numerous at the proximal end and close to the surface. These nerves sense environmental conditions, aid the timing of milk let-down, and control teat function. Some nerves are sympathetic motor neurons and control the contraction of longitudinal muscles found in the teat wall; a few reach the sphincter muscle.

The nervous response to the milk ejection reflex is divided into two phases. One message is sent to the central nervous system, resulting in the release of oxytocin from the posterior pituitary. Oxytocin initiates the milk ejection cycle by entering the udder via the arterial system, reaching the myoepithelial cells of the alveoli, causing contraction and milk ejection (see Chaps. 1 and 2). This process is frustrated if the teat muscles are not conditioned to facilitate milk flow. Thus, the second phase of milk release is an attenuation of the sphincter tone; the degree of attenuation regulates the milking rate.

The diameter of the teat canal determines the peak rate of milk flow and, probably, ease of bacterial penetration. In general, the larger the diameter, the faster the milk flows. Conversely, the smaller the diameter, the greater the resistance to pathogens.

The terminal end of the teat is exposed to a harsh environment where injury is common and protection is minimal. Human desire to rapidly remove milk through the narrow portal of the teat orifice often unwittingly aggravates the environmental trauma imposed on the teat end. Consequently, the external teat surface often is found to have lesions in which pathogens readily grow and easily spread to milking machines, milkers' hands, washing materials, and other teats. The result is that most cows' udders are frequently challenged by invading organisms, and only the cows with the most effective healthy teat barriers survive long in the herd.

Teats and teat ends vary greatly in shape and size, from cylindrical to funnel shape, with teat ends that are flat, round, or pointed. Pointed teat ends are rare, the slowest milking, and have a high resistance to mastitis; round teat ends are very common, milk more rapidly, and have some resistance to mastitis; flat teat ends are less common, milk most rapidly, and have less resistance to mastitis. Teat length and diameter should be modest to be readily fitted into the teat cup of milking machines. Extremes of length and diameter are prone to machine trauma.

The appearance of teat ends has been an area of great confusion, until recently, when an extensive study was conducted to compare teat-end classifications with percent infections. It was discovered that the perceived ideal teat end was not ideal for mastitis resistance, and the perceived teat-end trauma, due to excessive vacuum and overmilking, was not based on fact (Table 6.1).

The chronic ring is an elevated ring of tissue surrounding the teat orifice (meatus). This ring of tissue, once thought to be undesirable and, when prominent, the result of excessive vacuum and/or overmilking, now appears desirable; it has been found on unmilked heifers and some beef cattle teats, appearing to be a characteristic of high milk production. Further work may show the chronic ring to be part of the teat-end defense mechanism. Table 6.1 further indicates that damage to the teat end facilitates susceptibility to mastitis.

The teat canal is lined with a convoluted epithelium, which provides tissue for expansion of the canal diameter during milking. The lining is coated with a waxy keratin that forms a protective shield during lactation and, in unmilked heifers and dry cows, forms a physical plug, essentially occluding the canal (Fig. 6.3).

During the milking process, the teat canal unfolds peripherally, causing the epithelial lining to thin and encompass a larger bore canal. Because of the physical nature of keratin, it spreads over the surface of the epithelium as the canal dilates, thus forming a bacterial barrier over a greater

Table 6.1. Frequency of teat-end classifications compared to percent infection

Classification	% Infected	No. Teats
Normal (smooth)	30.9	554
Smooth chronic ring		
very mild	24.8	1,177
mild	22.4	1,003
moderate	26.6	312
severe	34.7	72
Rough chronic ring		
very mild	20.8	125
mild	26.1	199
moderate	32.5	151
severe	26.2	80
Acute (ulcer, hemorrhage, or scab)	43.8	16
Traumatized and leakers (tramped or cut)	51.0	293

Source: From Seiber and Farnsworth 1980.

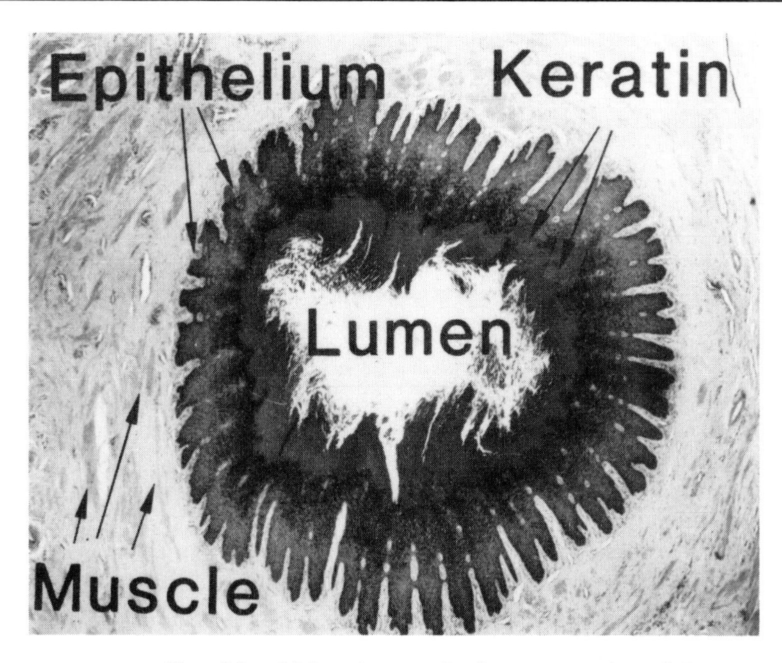

Fig. 6.3. Light micrograph of a cross section of the teat canal showing muscle tissue, keratin, and epithelial lining. ×4,000 magnification. (Provided by M.P. Comalli and R.J. Eberhart)

surface. The milking process washes away part of the keratin layer during the cyclic opening and closing of the teat canal. Further, tissue trauma may cause gaps in this layer, affording areas for bacteria to adhere and colonize. Also, the passage of cannulae, or teat dilators, through the teat canal scrapes away the keratin layer and often traumatizes the delicate epithelial lining.

The keratin has an antibacterial agent that inhibits the growth of pathogens. The origin of the antibacterial activity of keratin is postulated to be the Fürstenberg's rosette, once thought to be a vestigial appendage serving no purpose and, at times, blocking the exit of milk from the gland. Associated with the Fürstenberg's rosette are glandular tissues thought to secrete a protein that could be the bacteriostatic agent. Others believe that the agent is lipid in nature and secreted by the cells making keratin. The teat canal epithelium is actively replicating, evidenced by increased mitoses in the basement membrane and is probably necessary to maintain the keratin within the canal. The epithelial cells also slough into the lumen of the canal where, in conjuction with the other secretions, they form a mucuslike amorphous mass. Peristaltic contractions of the smooth muscle, plus the mucuslike material in the lumen, serve as an expulsion mechanism for bacteria, or other foreign material, entering the canal. The frequency of the peristaltic contractions is proportional to the pressure exerted by the milk in the teat cistern. A decrease in frequency of contractions observed after milking has been suggested as a factor in the increase in susceptibility to infection observed during this period.

The area of antibacterial activity was found to increase in ascending order: keratin, Fürstenberg's rosette, and midstreak canal. The distal teat canal and external surface of the teat had no activity. In proximity to the Fürstenberg's rosette, many cells resembling neutrophils are found in the connective tissue. This is postulated to be a probable source of migrating somatic cells found in the teat canal.

Studies in which pathogens were inoculated 3 mm into the teat canal resulted in more than one-third of the teats becoming infected. The organisms either died within 2–9 milkings or they penetrated the teat cistern, causing infections up to 21 days later. Differences in resistance to colonization exist between cows and quarters within cows. Cows classified as susceptible showed that keratin of the teat canal was thinner, less dense, or detached from the epithelium, and the many faceted defense mechanisms of the teat canal represent the main barrier to infection. Resistance to infection is overcome by removal of keratin (and the associated trauma to ream out the keratin), and full resistance is not reestablished for 2–4 wk after keratin removal. Inoculations 4 mm deep increased the infection rate; inoculations 5 mm deep seemed to exceed the defense mechanisms of the teat canal.

As a cow ages and milk production increases, the teat canal lengthens and dilates. Also, resistance to infection decreases with age until 5 or 6 yr. After this point, only the very resistant cows stay in the herd, and the frequency of infection in older cows appears to fall, probably reflecting the intervention of human selection pressure.

Pathogens that cause mastitis are nonmotile. To gain entrance into the secretory tissue, they must be moved by external physical forces from outside the teat, through the teat canal, teat cistern, gland cistern, ducts, and finally secretory ducts. The first major barrier is the long, narrow teat canal, and two modes of passage are postulated. One is movement by milk traveling back into the gland, caused by vacuum slips and systemic vacuum fluctuations. Once in the teat cistern, retrograde movement of milk is caused by squeezing of the teat during milking, pressure of leg movement, or pressure of the resting body. The second mode is more obscure. Over a period of time, a single bacterium, once too small to be seen, replicates to the point where the colony covers an area often greater than 1 cm in diameter (nearly the length of the streak canal).

The teat canal is often exposed to pathogens during and at the end of milking. However, the majority of new intramammary infections occur as a result of the pathogens entering the teat cistern during the first 10 days of the dry period, 2 wk surrounding parturition, and between milkings. This is frustrating to dairy managers in that the process is little understood, and the prevention of infection is beyond the control of teat dipping, machine pasteurization, and suppression of vacuum fluctuations (including slips). Dry-cow therapy is very helpful during the early dry period, but the other nonmilking times are not well managed and should be the objects of continued research. A clean, dry environment is the best management approach, to date, for the intramilking period. The entry of pathogens is facilitated by injury and local inflammation in and around the teat end, especially if the keratin lining of the teat canal is damaged or the closure of the teat canal by the sphincter muscle is impaired. Mechanical milking should be conducted so that the teat end is uninjured during milking and, if injury does occur, that its healing be aided. New designs of milking equipment must consider the cause of and effect on induced changes to teat-end anatomy and histology, as well as measure the effects on milk yield, milking speed, and infection status.

6.3: MECHANICAL MILKING

The essentials of a milking machine are shown in Figure 6.4. Milk travels from the pulsation chamber to the claw piece, which receives milk from all four teat cups. Milk from the four teats is comingled in the barrel of the claw piece; air is bled into this chamber to displace the mass of milk that must be lifted at any one time in a rising hose or pipe, and to accelerate the movement of milk away from the teat end into a larger vessel, such as a milk bucket, weigh jar, or pipeline. In the larger vessel, the milk and air fractions are separated to favor stable vacuum characteristics. This is accomplished by allowing the slower moving, more dense milk to flow by gravity to the storage tank, or milk receiver. The less dense fraction, air, travels quickly in the space above the milk, and when the flow of air is impeded by the milk, the vacuum drops as the energy of air movement is used to move the more dense milk. Severe fluctuations in the vacuum are associated with increased incidence of mastitis.

The vacuum pump, when applied to a closed system, partially removes the air mass, causing a vacuum. The volume of air so removed is greatly in excess of that necessary to milk and, if applied to the teat end, would cause excessive damage to the delicate tissues of the teat. However, the excessive vacuum is needed to meet the varying load demands found during milking. An example of these demands is two people attaching milking machines at the same time, bleeding in large amounts of air while the vacuum is being used by 2–4 other milking units and milk is being lifted from a cow's teat end to the pipeline. Under these conditions, the remaining machines are

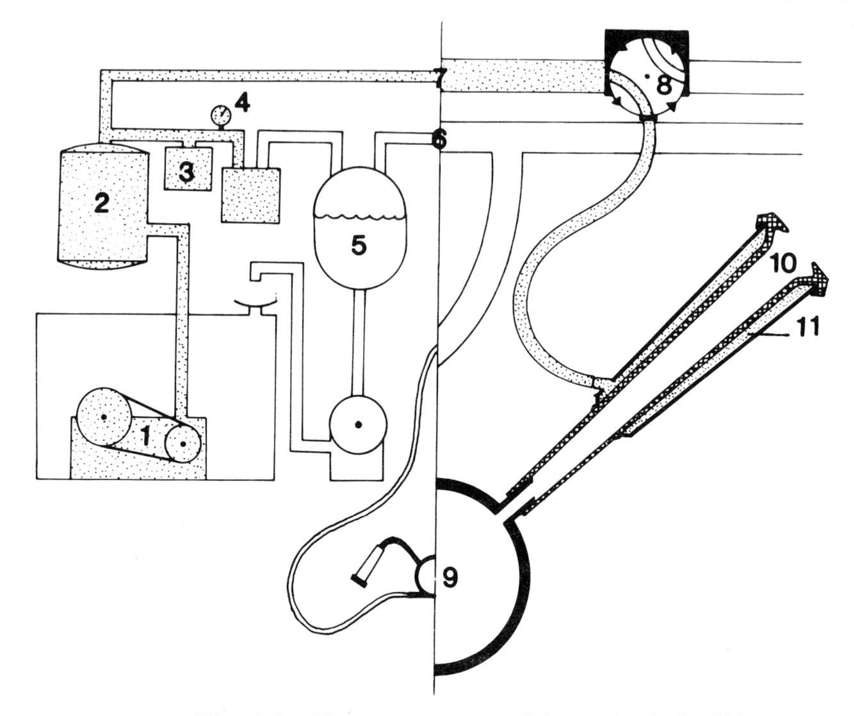

Fig. 6.4. Major components of the mechanical milking system. Vacuum pump (*1*), vacuum reserve tank (*2*), vacuum controller (*3*), vacuum gauge (*4*), milk receiver in pipeline systems, or bucket in bucket systems (*5*), milk line (*6*), vacuum line (*7*), pulsator (*8*), claw with air bleed (*9*), teat cup (*10*), and pulsation chamber (*11*).

expected to operate correctly. To meet the demands of a constant vacuum level over varying conditions, from milking one cow to milking many cows, a device called a vacuum regulator is installed. It senses a predetermined vacuum level, generally 40–50 kPa (kilopascals), and bleeds sufficient air into the vacuum system to lower the partial pressure to maintain this level. During normal operation, the regulator admits large volumes of air into the vacuum system.

Vacuum to the teat-cup pulsation chamber is applied alternately by a valve that opens the chamber to the vacuum supply of 40–50 kPa, followed by admitting atmospheric air. The rate of this alternation is approximately 45–70/min, depending on the design of the equipment. Interest in automatic detachers, positive pressure massages, varying vacuum levels, and automatic backflushing should be directed to other references since they are embellishments to the basic milking machine that relate to labor efficiency problems.

6.3-1: Vacuum level. The pressure due to the weight of air at sea level on the external surface of all things is 30 in. Hg but varies according to the weather or elevation. In general, atmospheric pressure is considered to be approximately 30 in. Hg, 760 mm Hg, or 100 kPa (the preferred unit today). A vacuum pump is used in milking equipment to produce a partial pressure of 50 kPa, which is equal to ½ atmosphere, or 15 in. Hg, in order to draw milk from a cow's teat.

Pressure in a cow's udder shortly after milking is 0.26–0.93 kPa, and pressure rises to 2.63 kPa at 14 hr after the last milking. When the cow is properly stimulated (teats stripped and washed), the pressure often is 5.66 kPa. In most cows, the sphincter muscle, which closes the teat end, is strong enough to retain the milk in the teat. The milking machine applies 37–50 kPa vacuum to the outside of the teat. The difference of 40 kPa vacuum pressure (negative) and 5.66 kPa pressure (positive) is 45.66 kPa. This pressure difference is so great that the sphincter muscle of the cow cannot retain the milk, thus, the milk pushes open the sphincter muscle and enters the milking machine. Hand milking is similar, but instead of the pressure on the outside of the teat being ½ atmosphere, or 50 kPa, it is 1 atmosphere, or 100 kPa. Therefore, the combined internal udder pressure of 5.6 kPa and the closing hand act together to milk the cow. First, the hand closes the top of the teat cistern by squeezing with thumb and forefinger. The remaining fingers and the palm of the hand continue the constriction of the teat, causing the internal pressure of the fluids in the teat to force open the sphincter muscle, and milk escapes. The flow continues until the pressure of the fluids in the teat and the strength of the sphincter are equal; at this point, flow stops. The hand grip is released to allow the teat to fill with milk, and the blood, trapped in the teat tissues, returns to the body. The process of squeezing the teat is repeated throughout the milking process.

During machine milking, as the vacuum is increased, the pressure differential inside and outside the teat becomes greater. In general, as the vacuum is increased, peak milk flow will increase until the diameter of the teat canal is dilated to its maximum and becomes the limiting factor of milk flow. Because of interactions among tissues, fluids, and vacuum, the vacuum can be used to increase milk flow to a point, then the excessive vacuum causes tissue swelling (see 6.3-7) and the need to machine or hand strip cows (6.3-9).

Excessive vacuum, in combination with lighter cluster weights and wide-bore inflations, encourages the teat cup to crawl and results in the teat being pulled into the teat-cup mouthpiece. The annular ring at the distal portion of the gland cistern is then pulled into the teat-cup chamber, restricting milk flow. With the teat cistern closed to milk from the gland, the teat wall thickens, and the vacuum inside the teat cistern approaches the vacuum in the milk hose. Under excessive vacuum, this could lead to rupture of small blood vessels and bruises on the inside teat wall (50 kPa vacuum applied to the human arm will cause bruising). Repeated abuse to this lining results in a buildup of scar tissue, which, over time, can make the cow a slow milker and exaggerate the problems of excessive vacuum, light clusters, and wide-bore mouthpieces.

6.3-2: Double-chamber teat cup. The double-chamber teat cup of mechanical milking machines is designed to simulate the sucking action of the calf. The cup is made of a rigid outer shell with an inner flexible liner, sometimes called an inflation. Between the inner and outer liners is a chamber in which the air is alternately evacuated to approximately 50 kPa (15 in. Hg) and pressurized to atmospheric pressure (approximately 100 kPa, or 30 in. Hg). With the teat inserted into the mouth of the innermost chamber of the teat cup, a second chamber is formed. When partial pressure (vacuum) is applied from the milk hose, this chamber simulates the calf's mouth and tongue. When a calf sucks milk, the mouth chamber is enlarged by dropping the tongue and lower jaw, approximately doubling the mouth chamber size and reducing the atmospheric pressure by approximately one-half. Therefore, the vacuum at the teat end during sucking alternates from atmospheric pressure to something less, which causes the teat end to open and milk to flow. Following sucking, the calf raises the lower jaw and tongue, which causes the teat to be squeezed and flattened. Evidence in goats indicates the milk is removed, not by vacuum in the kid's mouth, but by the clamping of the teat by the foreparts of the mouth, and the pressure of the tongue on the roof of the mouth forces the milk out of the teat. Thus, hand milking would be more comparable to sucking than machine milking.

Machine milking differs in that a constant vacuum is applied to the teat end from the milk hose, while the inflation moves to an expanded position in the teat-cup chamber (Fig. 6.5). At this point, milk flows out of the teat due to the opening of the teat orifice. The vacuum pulling open the inflation comes via the pulsator hose. When the vacuum in the pulsator hose is shut off and atmospheric air is admitted, the stretch of the elastic inflation and the vacuum in the teat chamber cause the inflation to collapse around the teat, squeezing the orifice closed, compressing the teat wall and partially closing the inflation liner below the teat. As a result, milk flow stops, the teat is massaged, blood accumulating in the teat blood vessels is encouraged to return to the udder body, movement of fluids pulled into the tissue spaces from the blood is discouraged, and some milk is returned from the teat cistern to the gland cistern.

There have been many experiments with single-chamber milking clusters and variations on the double-chamber clusters described above, but the

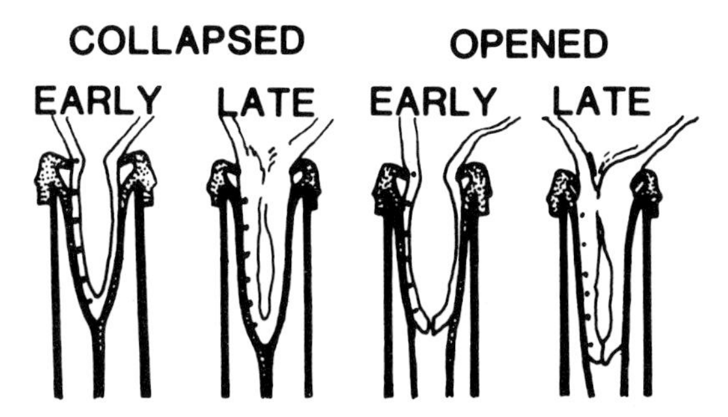

Fig. 6.5. Diagram showing the relationship between the position of the teat end and the liner (inflation) of the teat cup, during the milking process. Observe the depth of teat penetration, thickening of teat wall stroma, and open and closed position of liner as milking process proceeds. (Redrawn from radiograph tracings by Mein, Thiel, and Akan 1973, appearing in Thiel 1974)

conventional double-chamber milking principle prevails as the most successful to date.

6.3-3: Liner characteristics. Much has been stated about the advantages of one liner compared to another, but little research data exist to substantiate the claims. The ideal length, bore, thickness, frictional properties, flexibility coefficients, longevity of inflations, and material compositions have been arrived at by less than ideal comparisons of function. Analytical trials are called for, and the techniques for such trials are being developed.

Some characteristics are generally agreed to be desirable: the barrel geometry is thought to influence milking rate, while the mouthpiece probably affects final milk-out efficiency; inflations that are stretched in the rigid teat-cup shell give noticeably faster milking rates; and soft mouthpieces and narrow-bore inflations seem to favor reduced mastitis, although recent liner design may have overemphasized these two characteristics. Designs that reduce stripping time, fall-offs, air slips, and machine-on times are highly desirable. Inflations should nearly close below the teat end during the massage phase and be comfortable to the cow. Further, good premilking hand stimulation aids yield and persistency in some trials. Inflation designs that demonstrate enhanced tactile stimulation are desirable.

6.3-4: Pulsation rate. Pulsation rate is the number of times the air in the pulsation chamber of the teat cup is evacuated and returned to atmospheric pressure in 1 min. Pulsation rates of 40–160 cycles/min have been studied most frequently; the nursing calf sucks and swallows 80–120 times/min. High pulsation rates at low levels of vacuum have a more

Table 6.2. Comparison of pulsation rate and ratio on percent peak milk flow rate at 50 kPa

Milking:Rest Ratio of Pulsation Cycle	Pulsation Rate/min 40	80	120	160
		(%)		
50	100	108	127	137
67	123	136	142	141
75	134	142	141	140

Source: From Thiel and Dodd 1977

marked effect on increasing the milking rate than at high vacuum levels. As the pulsation rate is increased, milk flow rate increases, but the increase is limited (Table 6.2).

Slow pulsation rates give insufficient massage and are often painful, thus reducing milk ejection. Faster pulsations admit large volumes of air into the milking system and require larger vacuum systems.

6.3-5: Pulsation ratio. Pulsation ratio is the ratio of time that vacuum is applied to the pulsation chamber to the time atmospheric air is admitted to the chamber. Conventional ratios are 50:50, 60:40, and 70:30. The longer the vacuum is applied to the chamber, the longer the teat chamber liner, or inflation, is held open, allowing the pressure differential caused by vacuum to open the teat sphincter. Widening the ratio reduces the amount of time the teat is massaged, or compressed, by the liner. The result is longer milk flow and faster milking rate, accompanied by greater teat swelling and the need for stripping if the ratio is widened excessively.

6.3-6: Cluster weight. Increasing the cluster weight or, with some milking equipment, increasing downward pull of the milking cluster reduces the time spent stripping cows at the end of milking. Clusters vary in weight from 1.4–3.6 kg. By adding 0.5–1.8 kg weight to a conventional cluster, the stripping yields can be decreased from 0.1–0.5 kg. Adding weight to the claw can cause disproportionate amounts of downward pull on the teats, causing the fore teats to milk-out faster than the rear teats. Ideally, weight should be added to each teat cup to provide uniform downward pull to all teats. The danger of adding weight to conventional clusters is an increase in air slipping (air bleeding in around the teat) or cluster fall-off. Both contribute to increased mastitis (see 6.3-8).

6.3-7: Teat congestion. Teat congestion usually occurs in varying degrees with all milking machines, although it is rarely apparent to the operator. Congestion can be truly observed only through radiographs. At the beginning of milking, the teat wall is thin and teat penetration into the teat-cup liner is shallow (Fig. 6.5). During the rest phase, the liner closes beneath the teat and gently pushes inward and upward. At this point, the cistern is full of milk. Although no milk is flowing from the teat, blood in the teat vessels is gently pushed out. As the pulsation cycle continues, the liner is pulled away from the teat end, allowing the vacuum to force open the teat orifice. At the same time, blood is flowing back into the teat vessels, and its return to the body is retarded by the pressure differentials; lymph is inhibited from returning to the body, resulting in a filling of the teat wall (stromal space) with fluid. Accumulation of fluid causes a swelling of the teat wall, but because of the constriction of the teat liner and the rigidity of the teat skin, the teat swells inward.

As milking continues, fluid accumulation in the teat wall progresses until the swelling blocks milk flow. With blockage of the upper teat cistern, the teat sinus experiences the same vacuum level as that found below the teat. At this point, several events can take place. Continued milking beyond this point causes the now dry tissues of the teat cistern to rub against each other with each pulsation cycle. When filled with milk, the pressure holds the teat walls apart and prevents this trauma. Without milk, the collapsed teat walls rub, causing hemorrhages on the cistern wall and forming an ideal environment for bacterial colonization and growth. Second, excessive pulsation cycles to the external teat end can cause lesions, which scab over and are hard to heal with the stretching of the skin during milking. This can be aggravated by harsh teat dips, high vacuum, exposure to extreme cold (frostbite), or sunburn.

6.3-8: Air slips and bacterial transfer. Near the end of milking, vacuum slips are more frequent, particularly if vacuum levels are low or machine stripping is practiced. The air rushing in around the teat causes turbulence below the teat. With the in-rush of air, milk droplets and bacteria can be stripped from the wall of the teat-cup liner. These minute particles are carried by the rushing air to the level of greatest vacuum, which results in a two-way migration of the high-velocity particles. One is out the milk hose toward the vacuum source; another is toward a small reservoir of vacuum, found at the adjacent teat ends where air slips are not occurring, and inside the teats when congestion of teat walls is sufficient to prevent milk flow (Fig. 6.6). This situation is aggravated if the milking machine is taken off under full vacuum. Bacteria moving against the teat end by backward flow of milk droplets are called impacts. The bacteria that are implanted in the teat end by this process are thought to be a common source of new infections. The traumatized tissues of the teat end, streak canal, and internal teat canal wall are easily contaminated with bacteria.

At the end of milking, action of the sphincter muscle is hampered because of exhaustion due to the prolonged dilation of the teat canal and the accumulation of tissue fluids in the teat end. It has been found that many cows do not completely close the teat end for 1 hr after milking, and some cows require 2 hr, or more. During this time, the teat end is vulnerable to bacterial contamination by splashing dirty fluids, dragging teats through mud and manure, or dirty water running down the skin of the flanks and

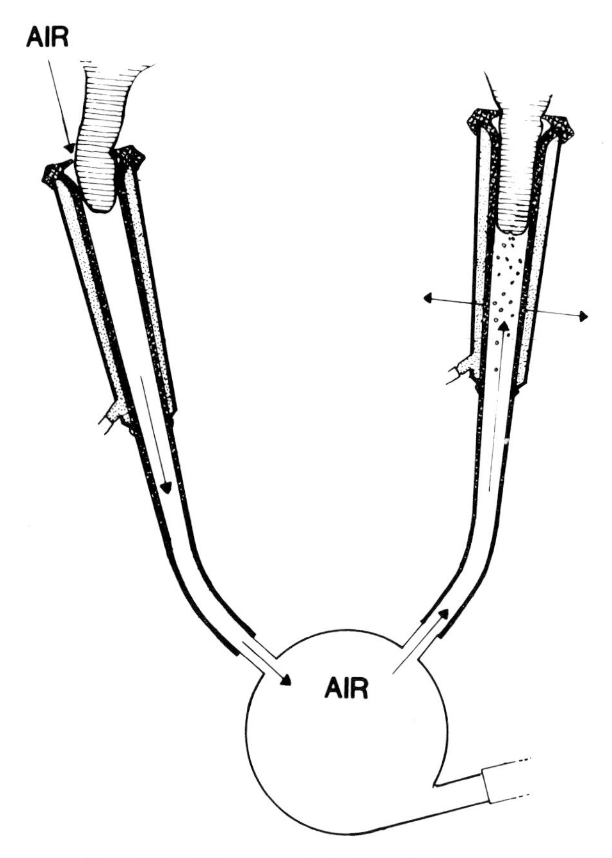

Fig. 6.6. Diagram of air flow during a vacuum slip in a milking machine, often resulting in bacterial contamination of the teat end.

udder. Bacteria that get into the teat orifice by methods of impact or contamination after milking are not dislodged by outward milk flow until the next milking. If the bacteria are not killed or washed away at the end of milking, they remain on the delicate teat tissue for 10–14 hr between milkings, which is sufficient time for bacteria to adhere to and colonize these tissues.

6.3-9: Machine stripping at the end of milking. Machine stripping of teats at the end of milking, that is, the act of pulling downward on the milking cluster with simultaneous hand massage of the udder, is a widely accepted practice. The result is an obvious momentary increase of milk flow in most cows, as seen in a clear hose or claw bowl. A basic rule of good milking is complete removal of all milk present in the udder, since incomplete milking reduces production and persistency and is associated with increased mastitis. In the past, careful studies did not settle the issue of whether to machine strip or not.

New studies show the risk of new infections increases near the end of milking, and sudden changes in vacuum near the teat end lead to droplets of bacteria-laden milk being driven against the teat end. These conditions are most likely to occur with vacuum slips (Fig. 6.6), overmilking, and machine stripping; therefore, the elimination of machine stripping is favored. When 20 cows were studied over an entire lactation, yields increased 431 kg milk and 5 kg fat per lactation when comparing stripping to nonstripping. However, the udder health of stripped cows was much poorer, as indicated by increased WMT (Wisconsin Mastitis Test) scores, and 544 kg more milk was discarded as a result of treatment. Cows were healthier and more milk was sold when machine stripping was not practiced. Further, this group of nonstripped cows was more persistent in their total lactation and had higher flow rates with less exposure to the milking machine.

A frequent testimonial by dairy workers is that automatic milk equipment detachers reduce mastitis. If true, this reduction may be attributed to less overmilking, fewer milk droplet impacts on teat ends, and the elimination of machine stripping. Milk droplet impacts are reduced because automatic detachers remove the milk cluster after the vacuum is released, while many dairy workers remove the cluster under full or partial vacuum conditions.

6.3-10: Electrical sensitivity of dairy cattle. Cows are two to ten times more susceptible to shock than humans, in terms of electrical resistance. Dairy farms were constructed to minimize shock to humans without realizing the sensitivity of cattle to shock, the resultant loss in milk production, and the increased mastitis.

In the current vernacular, this effect results from stray voltage, tingle voltage, transient voltage, or more commonly, neutral-to-ground voltage. The real concern should address the current, or amperage, rather than voltage, which addresses the physiological effect on the cow, not the source of current. This is a relatively new field of study and limited evidence has been reported to aid our understanding.

Cows vary greatly in their sensitivity to electricity, and the pathway through the cow's body affects the sensitivity. Cows appear to be more sensitive when current passes across the mouth to the hooves on wet pavement. Conductivity from the milk hose to teats to hooves appears to be a poor pathway.

Amperages as low as 3 milliamps or voltages as low as 0.7 can result in behavioral responses, such as lifting a foot, moving the mouth, or delaying entry into the milking parlor. In practice, a cow's production of milk is rarely affected until exposure to 5 or more milliamps. Five milliamps can be found with a neutral-to-ground voltage of approximately 1 volt at the entrance transformer. At one time, it was hypothesized that electrical shock reduced oxytocin release at milking or increased epinephrine; epinephrine is an antagonist of oxytocin during milk ejection (see Chap. 2).

Research shows that intermittent currents of 5 milliamps across the cow's body results in decreased milk yield and decreased milking time. At the same time, peripheral concentrations of oxytocin, norepinephrine, epinephrine, and dopamine were not correlated to electrical shocks of 5 milliamps. It was hypothesized that the decrease in milk yield was mediated by neural changes within the mammary gland.

The loss of milk due to neutral-to-ground voltages can be solved by a competent electrician working with the power company. When the neutral-to-ground voltage is reduced to less than ½ volt, most of the milk loss appears to be resolved.

6.3-11: Summation of milking technology. Increasing pulsation rate, pulsation ratio, vacuum level, and cluster weight affect the rate of peak milk flow or stripping milk yield. Each interacts with the other such that there is no equation to describe the ideal combination. Milking equipment companies have established recommendations by empirical evaluation of these factors. Tampering with these parameters of the milking equipment can lead to increased speed of milking, but often the long-term effects are detrimental to udder health and lifetime milk production. If an increase in rate of milking is desired, the use of more machines or automation of the milking operation should be considered. With milking equipment, it is probably better to err toward slower, less harsh procedures and employ more machines, as long as they are removed at the completion of milk flow.

Recommended characteristics for milking equipment today should be pulsation rates of 50–80 cycles/min, favoring the lower of these rates; pulsation ratios of 50:50–70:30; vacuum levels of 43–50 kPa, depending on the amount and distance milk must be lifted; and cluster weights of 1.4–3.6 kg. Vacuum level should be adequate to prevent cluster fall-off but low enough to milk at a reasonable speed without injury to teat ends and internal teat walls. Air slips and machine stripping should be minimized. Teat dipping after milking with an approved product should be used on all cows to reduce new intramammary infections.

6.4: ROLE OF SOMATIC CELL COUNT IN MONITORING UDDER HEALTH

6.4-1: Somatic cell counts. Somatic cells in milk are a mixture of secretory epithelial cells and leukocytes. As the cell count increases dramatically, it generally represents an increase in polymorphonuclear leukocytes, which search out bacteria and their toxins in an effort to protect the udder from damage. Leukocytes are attracted to the site of infection by a process called chemotaxis. The chemical stimuli can be messengers from injured cells, bacterial toxins themselves, or products of an inflammatory reaction (see Chap. 7).

Once the chemical signal for help is released, leukocytes in the vascular system are attracted to the site of infection. Blood flow in the capillaries near the site slows, allowing leukocytes to stick to the blood vessel wall. The leukocytes then move between the cells that form the capillary wall and escape into the tissue spacé surrounding the secretory alveoli, aggregating next to the secretory lining of the alveolar epithelium. At this point, the process of leukocyte migration appears to be impeded. Conventionally, it was thought that leukocytes moved between adjacent secretory cells lining the alveolus, opening the terminal junction between cells and subsequently slipping into the milk space of the alveolar lumen. Contrary to this convention, studies now show that during infections, leukocytes probably do not enter the milk space rapidly until one of the secretory cells dies and sloughs off the basement membrane surrounding the alveolus. The result is a portal for the migration of leukocytes from the tissue space and other blood components into the milk space (Fig. 6.7).

The cause of epithelial cell death is not certain. The loss of one or more secretory cells results in the loss of secretory potential. Evidence suggests that the cells lost in this manner are not replaced in great numbers until the dry period between lactations. Therefore, the measure of somatic cells in milk is an indirect, yet sensitive, method for detecting inflammation of the udder and becomes a tool for estimating the loss of milk production potential due to mastitis.

Somatic cells can be measured using a microscope, but electronic cell counters now count somatic cells automatically and rapidly. Because of the relationship of increased somatic cell counts with mastitis and milk loss, nearly one-half of the dairy workers on Dairy Herd Improvement Association (DHIA) testing programs elect somatic cell data on their cows' monthy records. The dairy workers experience a greatly increased milk yield with low cell count, and processing plants have greater cheese yield with low-cell milks. Therefore, incentive programs are developing to pay dairy workers for low-somatic cell–count milk. Low-cell milk has a higher yield of milk proteins per unit volume then high-cell milks because, as leukocytes enter the milk space, milk protein is replaced by blood proteins that enter milk with the leukocytes. Also, leukocytes are a source of proteolytic and lipolytic enzymes, which can depress the quality or consumer acceptability of dairy products.

Raw data collected for 1 mo in a single state demonstrate the loss in milk yield as somatic cell counts rise (Table 6.3). Because well-managed herds generally have predominantly low cell counts and poorly managed

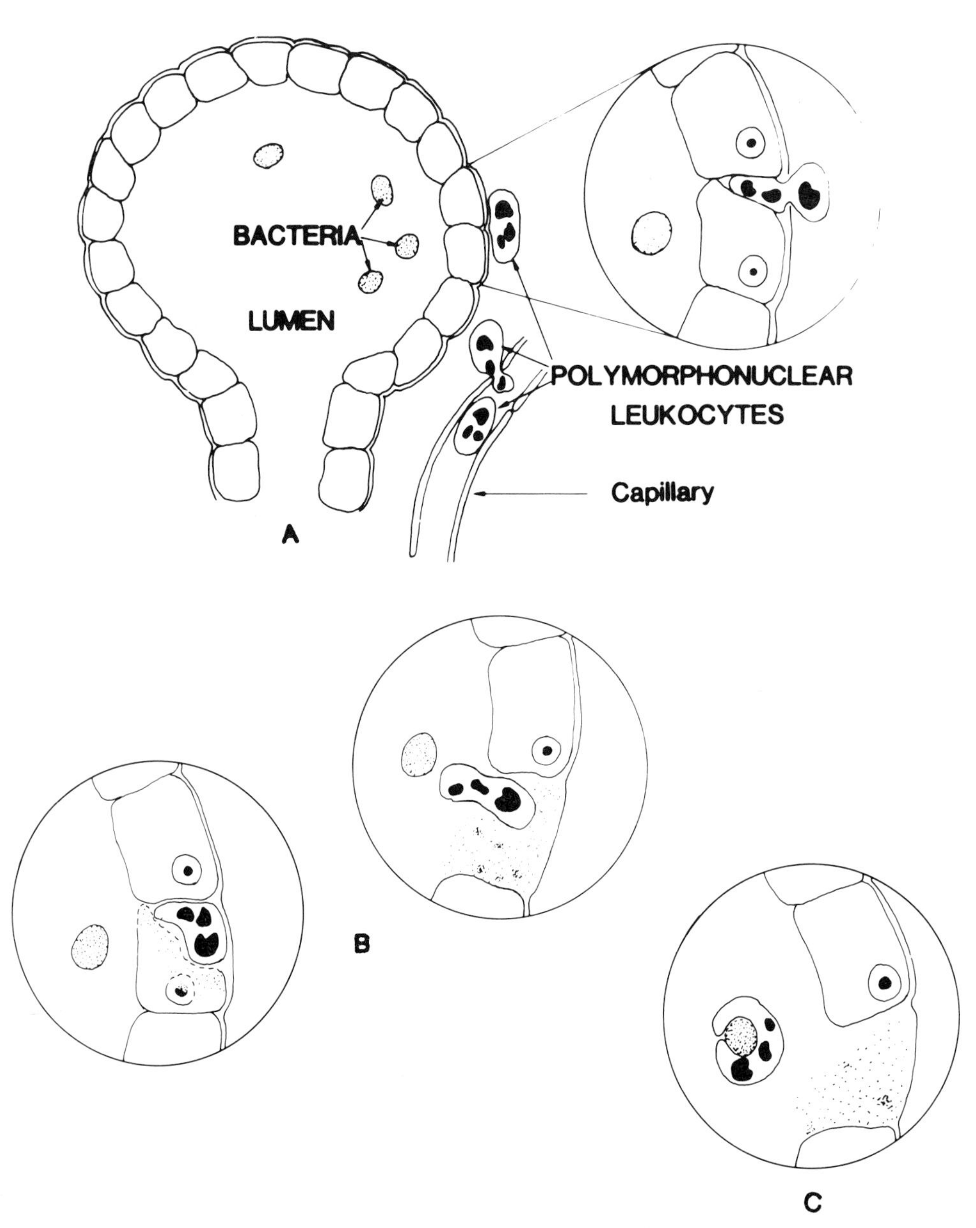

Fig. 6.7. Diagram of the leukocyte response to bacteria and toxins in the alveolar lumen (milk space). (*A*) Leukocyte escapes capillary, aggregates next to alveolar epithelium, and penetrates basement membrane. (*B*) Secretory cell dies and sloughs off, allowing penetration of the lumen. (*C*) Leukocyte engulfs bacterium.

Table 6.3. Electronic somatic cell counts for 139,421 cows compared with the average milk yield for cows in each classification

Somatic Cell Count/ml	Cows	Average Milk Yield
(× *1,000*)	(*%*)	(*kg*)
0–17	4	28.0
18–35	11	26.0
36–70	18	24.5
71–141	22	22.8
142–282	18	21.6
283–565	12	21.0
566–1,130	8	21.2
1,131–2,261	5	21.2
2,262 plus	3	19.5

herds have high cell counts, the raw data must be adjusted for herd effects, in addition to other effects. When this is done on large numbers of cows in various regions of the United States, a general guideline becomes evident. Each time the electronic somatic cell count doubles, milk production is reduced 0.68 kg for the average of all cows. On a lactational basis, the milk loss is 182 kg/lactation. The milk loss for heifers is 50% less than for older cows.

6.4-2: Intramammary devices. An intramammary device (IMD) is a sterile irritant placed in the gland cistern of the cow's udder. One device is made from a solid polyethylene filament (1.6 mm cross section and 12 cm long) that has been modeled into a 2.5 cm diameter coil. Preliminary data show that IMDs stimulate the defense mechanisms, including leukocyte migration into milk, and afford some protection against new intramammary infections caused by certain bacteria. Much controversy surrounds the use of IMDs, due to the lack of sufficient data from long-term experiments with large numbers of cattle, and the use of IMDs in less-than-controlled experiments.

Early studies show that milk production in cows is not improved by the use of IMDs, and, probably, the increased somatic cell content of such treated cows may be detrimental to milk production as described in 6.4-1. Under stringently controlled studies, the device appears to have some promise; new materials and geometry of the devices are being studied.

6.5: TEAT DIPPING

Dipping teats in antiseptic solutions immediately after milking provides some protection to the teat by reducing the number of viable bacteria that survive on the teat end during the postmilking period. Teat dipping with approved products reduces new intramammary infections 50%. The dip coats the skin and drains toward the teat end, leaving a film that aids healing of teat lesions, reduces the source of mastitis-causing bacteria, and provides a protective droplet of antiseptic material on the teat end until the sphincter muscle has a chance to recover from milking exhaustion and close sufficiently to provide its natural barrier to bacterial penetration.

6.6: MILKING METHODS AND RATE OF MILK SECRETION

6.6-1: Secretion rate. Milk precursors are released from the capillary blood and pass into the space between the capillary and the alveolus. The epithelial cell transports these nutrients into the cell (some arrive passively) for milk manufacture. As the precursors are assembled into milk components, they are transported away from the cellular region closest to the capillary source and toward the milk collecting and storage area. The skim milk or solids-not-fat fraction plus water (aqueous phase) is released from the Golgi vesicles. The fat portion is pushed against the apical, or luminal, membrane and extruded out of the cell. Both of these secretory processes are aided by a little-understood intracellular skeletal and contractile system consisting of microfilaments and tubules (see Chap. 4).

The period immediately after milking or nursing, characterized by low intraalveolar pressure, facilitates the transport of newly synthesized milk into the alveolar lumen. As secretion continues between milkings, back pressure is exerted on the secretory process by the alveolar luminal contents. At some point, the luminal pressure exceeds the force of secretion as the alveolar enlargement reaches its limit. It is presumed that the distention pressure of the lumen exceeds the strength of secretory mechanisms needed to push the newly formed milk out of the cell. In turn, the buildup of newly formed milk in the cell retards the uptake of milk precursors, by chemical feedback mechanisms or physical factors, or both. The physical factors are a result of the distended alveoli partially displacing all other intramammary compartments, including the blood vessels. With restricted blood flow, less oxygen is available for metabolism, fewer nutrients are available for milk production, less hormone is available to drive the synthetic apparatus, removal of waste products of synthesis is retarded, oxytocin is restricted from stimulating the myoepithelial cells, and fewer leukocytes are available to ward off infections.

Figure 6.8 shows the relationship between the secretion rate of milk in cows over extended milking periods with increasing udder pressure. These data show that, after 10 hr, the average secretion rate begins to decrease and secretion stops after 35 hr. The hydrostatic pressure measured in the teat cistern increases in three phases. Within 1 hr after the last milking, pressure rapidly increases to approximately 8 mm Hg, believed to be caused by residual milk moving into the cistern from the alveoli and small ducts. The second, slower phase could be an accumulation of newly synthesized milk that is released into the duct system from the alveolar lumens as they

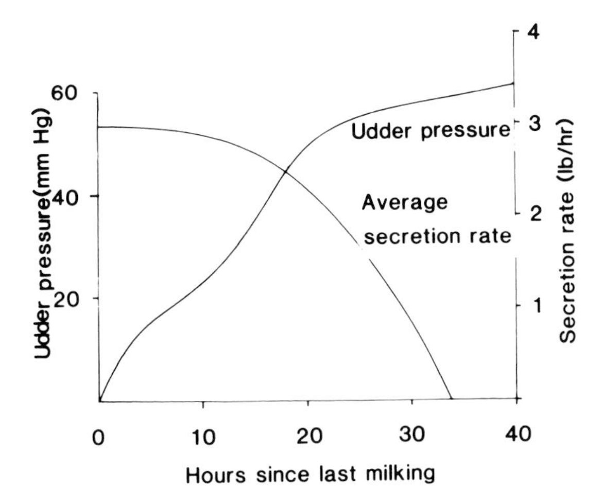

Fig. 6.8. Relationship of udder pressure to secretion rates of dairy cows over a 40-hr period. (From Schmidt 1971)

begin to accumulate milk. The third phase is marked by an accelerated pressure increase and probably represents overfilling of alveoli, ducts, and gland cistern.

The increase in pressure per unit of secreted milk is an individually inherited characteristic. The absolute increase in udder pressure is similar for high- and low-yielding cows, making the increase in pressure per unit of newly formed milk smaller for high-producing cows. In addition to production, the rate of increase in pressure per unit of newly formed milk is lower in high-yielding cows, older cows, in early lactation, in hind quarters, and following the long night interval compared with the shorter day interval.

6.6-2: Variation in milk component secretion. The role of the milking interval on milk production and components is not easily understood, in part, due to the presence of residual milk in the udder (see 6.6-3). In cows that averaged 35 lb production daily, had the residual milk removed after each milking, and were milked at intervals of 4, 8, 12, 16, 20, and 24 hr, the secretion rate of milk and solids-not-fat did not fall until after 16 hr. When the cows, unmilked for 4, 8, 12, 16, 20, and 24 hr in previous intervals, were switched to an 8-hr interval, little effect was found until the cows had experienced a 20- or 24-hr previous milking interval. Intervals at the various milkings longer than 16 hr caused fat percentage to increase and fat yields to fall. Milk yield and solids-not-fat fell markedly after 16-hr intervals. The production drop from an 8-hr interval to 24 hr was 25%.

When comparing these results with those in Table 6.4, one must remember that residual milk was removed after each milking, thus increasing

Table 6.4. Relationship of milking interval to lactation yields

Interval (hr)	No. of Cows	Record Length (days)	Milk (kg)	Fat (kg)	Fat (%)
12–12	35	305	6,242	236	3.8
14–10	35	305	6,222	243	3.9
16– 8	35	305	6,161	238	3.9
12.5–11.5	82	266	4,910	186	3.8
14.5– 9.5	82	266	4,800	181	3.8

Source: From Schmidt and Trimberger 1963; Ormiston et al. 1967.

the storage reserve of the udder and reducing the carry-over effects of residual milk. With low milk production, milking interval has less effect on daily milk yield, but at higher levels of production stress, milking interval appears to have more effect. Table 6.4 demonstrates the effect of equal and unequal milking intervals; there is a small nonsignificant decrease in yield and no consistent trend in the fat test.

The role of unequal milking interval may be of more concern in dairy records programs, where milking weight is used to assist in management decision-making and breeding. Although it has been difficult to demonstrate a beneficial effect, the equal milking interval is widely adopted by U.S. dairy workers. However, regular milking intervals have some effect on production, as demonstrated in three-times-a-day milking herds. Cows milked at 8-hr intervals, compared with 6, 7, and 11 hr, produced 3.9% more milk and 5.2% more fat.

In adjusting daily milk yields to estimate lactation yields in DHIA record systems when milk weights and fat percentages were measured for 1 milking/mo (alternating sampling in the morning one month and in the evening the next month), the predominating factor affecting true milk yield and component percentage was the milking interval. Factors determined for these corrections appear in Tables 6.5 and 6.6

6.6-3: Residual milk, available milk, and cow preparation. Residual milk is the amount of milk left in the udder after a complete milking;

Table 6.5. Factors for estimating DHIA sample-day yield from evening or morning milking in the alternate AM/PM testing program

Daytime Interval (hr)	PM Factor		Nightime Interval (hr)	AM Factor	
	Milk yield	Fat yield		Milk yield	Fat yield
9.0	2.58	2.19	15.0	1.63	1.84
9.5	2.49	2.17	14.5	1.67	1.85
10.0	2.40	2.16	14.0	1.72	1.86
10.5	2.31	2.14	13.5	1.77	1.88
11.0	2.21	2.10	13.0	1.82	1.91
11.5	2.12	2.05	12.5	1.89	1.95
12.0	2.03	2.00	12.0	1.97	2.00
12.5	1.94	1.94	11.5	2.06	2.06
13.0	1.86	1.89	11.0	2.17	2.13

Source: From Shook, Jensen, and Dickinson 1980.

Table 6.6. Daily fat test as a percentage of evening or morning fat at various milking intervals.

Daytime Interval	Daily Test / PM test	Nighttime Interval	Daily Test / AM test
(hr)	(%)	*(hr)*	(%)
9.0	84.9	15.0	112.7
9.5	87.4	14.5	110.7
10.0	90.1	14.0	108.6
10.5	92.7	13.5	106.4
11.0	95.0	13.0	104.6
11.5	96.9	12.5	102.9
12.0	98.6	12.0	101.4
12.5	100.0	11.5	100.0
13.0	101.7	11.0	98.1

Source: From Shook, Jensen, and Dickinson 1980.
Note: Values are based on the adjustment factors in Table 6.5.

10–20% of the cow's total daily production is left in the udder as residual milk. This unrecovered milk can be measured by giving the cow oxytocin and, one minute later, milking the cow again. Part of the residual milk can never be harvested by practical milking procedures, but another fraction can be harvested if the amount of residual milk is large due to poor milking procedures and is referred to as available milk. Available milk reflects how well the cow was stimulated for milking. If a cow is not well trained and well prepared for milking, the available milk unharvested will be great.

If a cow has a large amount of available milk residing in the alveoli and upper ducts, she has less space to hold newly manufactured milk, so her instantaneous milk production decreases earlier in the between-milking interval. The final outcome is reduced daily milk production, reduced lactation production, and fewer days in milk. Large amounts of residual milk also reduce fat tests.

The quantity of available milk is decreased in machine milking by training the cow to let down her milk in the absence of the calf and to let the machine take all the milk twice a day. The success of the dairy worker is only part of the process. To encourage let-down, a cow should be introduced to the milking area twice a day for a number of days before parturition. Threatening, frightening, and strange experiences in the milking area should be avoided. A regular routine should be established: strong stimuli to induce milk ejection should be given at the appropriate time to achieve the highest level of oxytocin release; the cow should be made comfortable in the milking stall; several streams of milk should be forced from each of the cow's teats (there is no stronger stimuli to induce milk ejection than removal of milk); wash the teats with uncontaminated materials, such as single-service towels dipped in sanitizer solution, using a strong stripping action in the process; dry the teats thoroughly. Comparison of the level of oxytocin measured in the blood of cows properly prepared and in those unstimulated is in Figure 6.9.

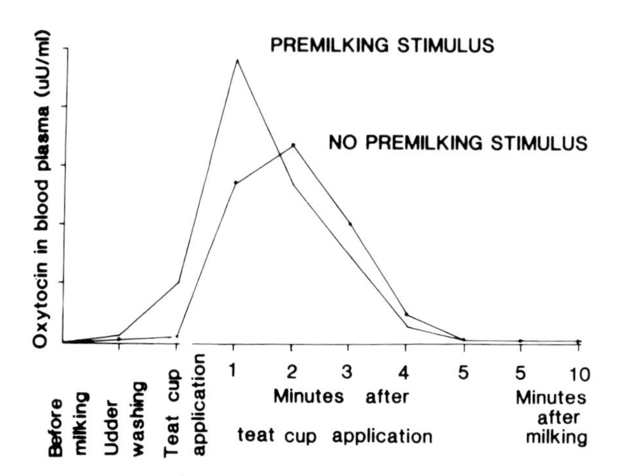

Fig. 6.9. Blood plasma oxytocin activity of Holstein cows before, during, and after milking, when milked with and without a premilking stimulus. This demonstrates the effect of strong premilking stimulation on speed and concentration of blood oxytocin activity and its importance in good milking management practices. (Redrawn from Momongan and Schmidt 1970, as presented in Schmidt 1971)

Premilking preparation should not be rushed. From the start of stripping until the end of washing should be at least 25 sec (many dairy workers spend 10 sec or less). If all is well, a copious flow of milk should start within 60–90 sec after starting the preparation and should peak within 2 min of applying the milking machine. Generally, the machine is removed after 4–6 min; however, cows vary in their response. The response is greatly affected by level of milk production, peak milk flow of each cow, diameter of the teat canal, success of milking preparation, and type of milking equipment used.

The milk ejection process was developed for feeding the calf, and humans have changed the biology of milk ejection very little in selecting for higher milk yield. To recover maximum production, the principles of good milking machine management must be tailored after the biology of the cow, rather than extending machine time and increasing detrimental machine effects.

6.6-4: Diurnal trends in fat content. Milk has two phases: aqueous and lipid. Compared to the aqueous phase of milk, milk lipid has a lower specific gravity; thus, milk lipid rises. This is often overlooked in this age of homogenized milk. This phase difference in milk accounts, in part, for the variation in fat content as it leaves the udder. First-drawn milk may be only 1-2% fat, whereas, at the end, fat precentages between 5–10% are common. Residual milk can be as high as 20% fat.

Fat droplets pass less readily from the udder than the aqueous phase because they rise from the gland cistern to upper ducts and because they rise in the alveoli (Fig. 6.10).

As the alveoli collapse under the forces of the myoepithelium, the phases separate as the milk enters the ducts until the myoepithelium contraction reduces the volume of the alveolar lumen to the point that the fat is expelled from the lumen. Some fat remains in the upper alveolar lumen with residual milk, but only newly released fat remains in the lower alveolar residual milk. Variable amounts of fat remain in the lateral alveoli, depending on the completion of milking. The lower alveolus probably lost much of its fat to the duct before milk ejection occurred. In addition to the fat rising, fat droplets may pass more slowly though portals in the alveoli due to their size and viscosity, the cream fraction being more viscous than skim milk.

As a general rule, residual milk is a percentage of milk yield and is drastically affected by completeness of milk ejection, resulting in variations even within individuals. Therefore, the apparent differences reported in day-to-day variation in fat content of individual cows is a result of chance variations in the completeness of milk ejection from one milking to another. The diurnal variation in fat content at AM and PM milkings is a result of carry-over effects of residual milk; the greater the cow's production, the wider the variation in fat percentage found in first- and last-drawn milk. Milk drawn with the shortest previous milking interval will have the highest fat content because the high-fat milk remaining from the previous milking is diluted less by the milk produced in the shorter milking interval. The variation in fat percentage from one milking to another for an individ-

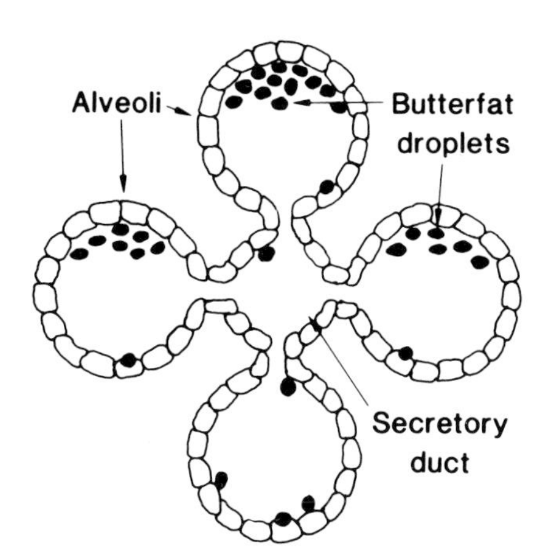

Fig. 6.10. Idealized alveolus showing the phase separation of butterfat from the aqueous in the gland.

ual cow is probably the best indicator of completeness of milk ejection and removal of available milk. A reduction in residual milk results in higher daily yield except in the first part of lactation, when only a higher fat content in the milk could be demonstrated. In heifers, the influence of a better milking routine on yield is limited.

Time delays between udder preparation and milking result in higher residual milk, lower peak flow rates, and low milk and fat yields (Table 6.7). The removal of residual milk itself has a profound effect on the subsequent secretion rate, and the concentration of butterfat appears to be one of the factors regulating total fat secreted. During involution, the buildup of long-chain, unesterified fatty acids, such as oleic acid, in the secretory cell causes uncoupling of oxidative phosphorylation of mammary gland mitochondria. A similar feedback mechanism could be in effect with the buildup of butterfat resulting from residual milk.

6.6-5: Frequency of milking. The more frequently cows are milked each day, the more milk is produced. Milking twice a day yields at least 40% more milk than once a day, three times a day may yield 5–20% increase over twice-a-day milking, and four times a day may yield an additional 5–10%. Thus, the response diminishes with increasing frequency. An adequate physiological explanation is not known, and the effect is certainly multifaceted. Increased milking is generally associated with increased feeding frequency. Assuming the milking equipment is in good working order, teat ends are exposed to less machine trauma at each milking, teat ends are washed and dipped more frequently, and diseased cows are found sooner. The dairy manager interested in more frequent milking is interested in greater production per cow and is likely to be a better manager because of added motivation.

Speculation on the physiological factors that contribute to increased production are (1) less intramammary pressure generated with frequent milking, (2) increased stimulation of hormone activity favorable for milk production, and (3) less negative feedback on the secretory cell synthetic machinery due to the buildup of milk components.

The lifetime effects of three-times-a-day milking have not been

Table 6.7. Comparison of milk production of identical twins milked at different intervals after preparation

	Delay after Preparation	
Production	1 min	5 min
Milk (kg/day)	14.56	12.54[a]
Butterfat (%)	3.87	3.93
Butterfat yield (g/day)	563	493
Residual milk plus hand stripping (%)	11.2	24.8
Fat in residual milk (%)	10.1	12.3[a]
Peak flow rate (kg/min)	2.81	2.56[a]

Source: Adapted from Brandsma 1978.
[a]$P < 0.05$.

measured, although many high-producing herds have been milked three times a day for more than 3 yr. Most herds milked three times a day are milked for temporary economic reasons, and the requirement of additional labor for three-times-a-day milking results in a return to twice-a-day milking in most situations. As time goes on, some herds milked three times a day for 2–3 yr experience less effect from the extra milking. Signs of management failures, such as increased calving intervals, are manifested. Only the exceptionally well managed herds experience the benefits of three-times-a-day milking over extended periods of time.

The DHIAs have relied on factors to correct records on three-times-a-day milked cows to a comparable two-times-a-day record. The formula is $2 \times \text{record} = 3 \times \text{record}/(1 + \text{age factor})$. The relative increase based on the age factor is 0.20 for 2-yr olds, 0.17 for 3-yr olds, and 0.15 for 4 yr and over. Thus, DHIA acknowledges a 15–20% increase in production of three times a day over twice a day, with the most benefit attributed to younger animals.

6.7: TERMINATION OF LACTATION

Most dairy advisors agree that lactation should be terminated when milk production falls below 9 kg/day or 60 days before the next expected parturition, whichever comes first. Also, all quarters of all cows should be treated with an approved dry-cow intramammary antibiotic infusion. The wide use of antibiotics is troublesome to most dairy advisors, but research data continue to support the economics of this practice, as well as the efficacy. Underlining the issue is the fact that nearly one-fifth of new intramammary infections occur during the first 1–2 wk of the dry period. The dry-cow therapy product, formulated to be much stronger than the lactational therapy product, is formulated to remain in the udder for 3–4 wk. Consequently, the dry-cow infusion antibiotic is very effective in preventing most new infections that occur during the early udder involution and in eliminating most chronic infections that resist treatment during lactation.

The greatest controversy concerns how to force a cow to involute her mammary tissue. Some support "skip" milking, where the cow is milked once a day for at least three days. Opponents favor abrupt cessation of milking and, for very high producers, eliminating feed or water for several days to reduce milk production before the abrupt cessation. The use of dry-cow therapy after the last milking appears to mask any benefit of one procedure over the other.

One certainty is that as production drops toward the end of lactation, the frequency of elevated somatic cell count increases. It is becoming widely accepted that a somatic cell count greater than 200,000 has an important impact on milk yield. As more research is being reported on somatic cell counts and the relationship to milk production, many researchers are beginning to think that a somatic cell count of 200,000 is too high as an indication of infection and that this number should be lowered. Research shows that, as the cell count increases in some cows near the end of lactation, the frequency of bacterial isolation from these cows increases, indicating a higher level of infection as milk yield falls. The increase in infection is probably related to milking management.

6.7-1: Length of dry period. The data supporting the recommended length of dry period for cows are very repeatable. Most point to an ideal dry period length of 40–70 days. When comparing average herdmate difference data for over ¼ million cows for 1 yr, the Southern Regional Records Processing Center confirms earlier research (Table 6.8).

Once it was thought that cows needed a dry period to restore nutritional reserves, but this was disproven when cows had one udder half milked and one udder half unmilked during the period prior to the next parturition. Results showed the unmilked half produced markedly more milk than the milked half in the subsequent lactations (presumably the halves were exposed to the same hormones and nutrients). Today, the favored hypothesis is that the involutionary process replaces the old worn-out cells from the previous lactation with new cells for the subsequent lactation. The extent of the cell replacement is not well established.

6.7-2: Prepartum milking. Aside from the period 1–2 wk into the dry period, the time of next greatest susceptibility to new intramammary infections is during the two weeks surrounding parturition. During these periods, the intragland defense mechanisms are least able to ward off infections but probably more important is the patency of the teat canal. Normally, the canal is sealed with a keratin plug during the dry period. With cessation of milking, the canal is not washed twice daily with the flow of milk and the keratin lining thickens, eventually occluding the canal (Fig. 6.11). During the buildup of colostrum and milk at lactogenesis, it is conceivable that the keratin seal could be flawed if not washed away. Furthermore, there may be an interaction with teat edema that could hamper the

Table 6.8. Effect of days dry on production in the subsequent lactation for 281,816 cows

Days Dry	Cows (%)	Av. Herdmate Difference for Milk (kg)
5–20	2.9	−585
21–30	3.7	−286
31–40	6.5	−71
41–50	12.3	+86
51–60	21.5	+135
61–70	20.3	+142
71–80	9.4	+72
81–90	6.0	+29
90	17.4	−49

Source: From Butcher 1974.

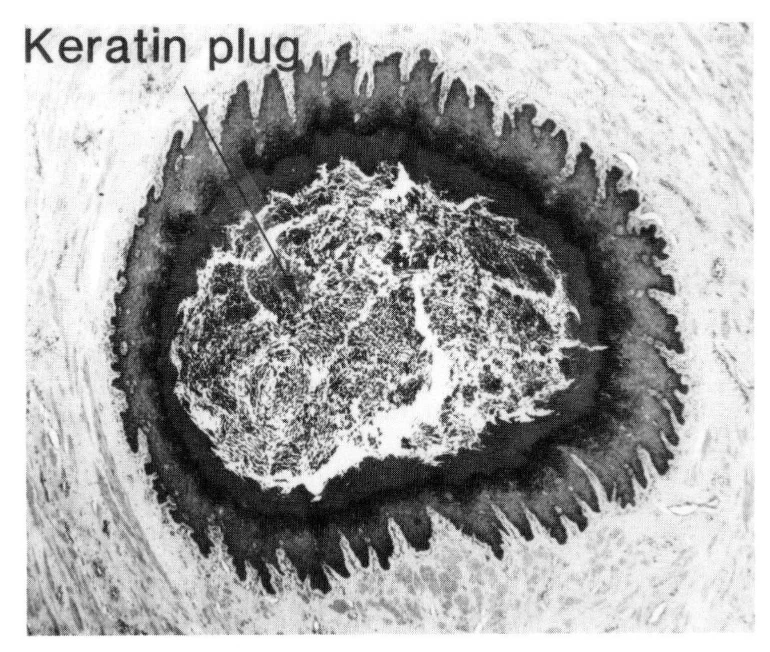

Fig. 6.11. Micrograph demonstrating the sealing of the teat canal 16 days after involution. ×4,000 magnification. (Provided by M.P. Comalli and R.J. Eberhart)

contraction of the sphincter muscle. Milking the gland lessens the clinical symptoms of edema, reduces intramammary pressure, and washes the teat canal of bacteria and toxins. Prepartum milking of the gland should be considered under these conditions, since most studies show little or no detrimental effect. Conversely, most studies show that production peaks earlier, frequency of ketosis and milk fever is not affected, and the stress of first milking is not combined with the stress of parturition if cows are milked prepartum. Remember, immunoglobulins of colostrum are removed during the first milking and should be saved and fed to the calf.

The defense mechanisms of the dry gland and the periparturient udder will be areas of intensive research in the future as scientists try to understand the susceptibility of the udder to new infections during this period of high risk.

REFERENCES

Brandsma, S. 1978. Institut voor Veeteeltkundig Onderzock "Schoonoord," Zeist. NMC Proceeding, The Netherlands.

Butcher, Kenneth R. 1974. Effect of days dry on production in the subsequent

lactation. Dairy Herd Improvement Record Briefs of the Southern Region Processing Center Extension Newsletter 10.
Logan, T. R., D. V. Armstrong, and R. A. Selley. n.d. Three times a day milking. Western Reg. Ext. Publ. Tucson: Univ. of Arizona Press.
Ormiston, E. E., S. L. Spahr, R. W. Touchberry, and J. L. Albright. 1967. Effects of milking at unequal intervals for a complete lactation on milk yield and composition. J. Dairy Sci. 50:1597.
Proceedings of the Annual Meeting of National Mastitis Council, Inc. 1976–1983. Washington, D. C.: National Mastitis Council.
Schalm, O. W., E. J. Carroll, and N. C. Jain. 1971. Bovine Mastitis. Philadelphia: Lea & Febiger.
Schmidt, G. H. 1971. Biology of Lactation. San Francisco: W. H. Freeman.
Schmidt, G. H., and G. W. Trimberger. 1963. Effect of unequal milking intervals on lactation milk, milk fat, and total solids production of cows. J. Dairy Sci. 46:19.
Seiber, R. L., and R. J. Farnsworth. 1980. The etiology of bovine teat end lesions. In Proceedings of 19th Annual Meeting National Mastitis Council, Inc., 5. Washington, D.C.: National Mastitis Council.
Shook, G. E., E. L. Jensen, and F. N. Dickinson. 1980. Factors for estimating sample-day yield in AM/PM sampling plans. USDA, Dairy Herd Improvement Letter 56(4):25.
Thiel, C. C. 1974. Mechanics of the action of the milking machine cluster. Bienn. Rev. Natl. Inst. Res. Dairying. Shinfield, Reading, Eng.
Thiel, C. C., and F. H. Dodd, eds. 1977. Machine Milking. Shinfield, Reading, Eng.: Natl. Inst. Res. Dairying.

CHAPTER 7

MASTITIS AND THE IMMUNE SYSTEM OF THE MAMMARY GLAND

ALBERT J. GUIDRY

7.1: INTRODUCTION

The mammary gland serves two functions: provision of nutrition and passive immunity to the offspring. Nutrition of the offspring has been recognized as a major function since the beginning of history. Only during the past century has the transfer of immunity via the mammary gland been recognized. Only during the past decade have physiologists and immunologists begun to understand the basic mechanisms of synthesis, transfer, and function of the various components of the immune system. A great deal of this understanding is the result of basic and applied research on passive immunity in the bovine neonate and the function of the immune system in defense against infection of the bovine mammary gland.

7.2: FUNCTIONS OF THE MAMMARY GLAND

7.2-1: Nutrition. Although species within the mammalian class vary in the length of the suckling period and the extent to which suckling is supplemented by other forms of nutrition, by definition, the newborn mammal is dependent on the mammary gland for postnatal nutrition (see 5.4-1). However, in humans a great deal of research has been directed toward developing substitutes for mother's milk to free the mother from the "burden" of nursing. Emphasis has been placed on the nutritional completeness, digestibility, and allergenic properties of these substitutes (see 5.4-2). In developed countries, where diseases have been controlled by sani-

Chapter 7 was prepared by Albert J. Guidry as an employee of the federal government.

tation, immunization, and antibiotics, substitutes for mother's milk (infant formulas) have worked quite well. However, as the feeding of infant formulas spread to developing countries, where sanitation, immunization, and antibiotic prophylaxis and therapy are not commonly practiced, infant mortality rose to alarming proportions. It was discovered that systemic immunity, which in humans is passed to the offspring in utero (Figure 7.1), did not protect the unsuckled young against enteric infections; antibodies to the indigenous gut-associated pathogens were also needed in the lumen of the newborn's digestive tract to protect it until its own gut-associated immune system began to function (see 5.4-1).

Similarly, as dairy workers began to remove calves from their dams shortly after birth to improve production and facilitate management practices, there was a concomitant increase in enteric infections, as well as other

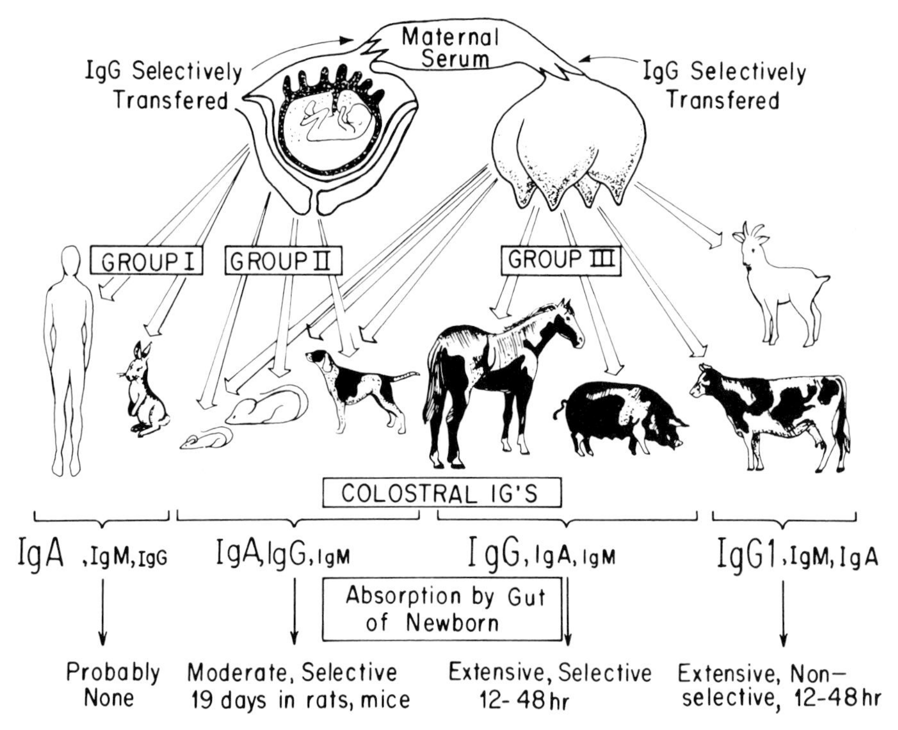

Fig. 7.1. The transfer of maternal Ig (universal carrier of passive immunity in all species) to offspring in representative species. Transfer in Group I is in utero, via colostrum in Group III, and mixed in Group II. The relative concentration of Ig in colostrum is depicted by the size of the Ig designation. Relative absorption and timing of absorption by the newborn gut are also shown. (From Butler 1974)

diseases in the calves. As with humans, enteric infections were prevalent regardless of the supplemental diet, which often included antibiotics. Unlike humans, however, the bovine does not receive antibodies from the dam in utero but is dependent on colostrum for both systemic and gut-associated passive immunity.

These observations renewed interest in the transfer of immunity from dam to offspring. Also, it was observed that the components of the immune system responsible for the transfer of immunity to the young may serve to protect the mammary gland of the dam against bacterial infection. Because this chapter is devoted primarily to mastitis, immune defense of the mammary gland will be emphasized.

7.2-2: Transfer of immunity. Prior to birth, the fetus is in a sterile environment. Since the fetal immune system has not been exposed to the microbial challenge it will receive in its external environment, the neonate is dependent on a passive transfer of resistance to microbial infection from the dam. Elements of this resistance include antibodies, leukocytes, lysozyme, complement, and lactoferrin, each containing antimicrobial capabilities. Experiments conducted to test the relative importance of these parameters showed that animals reared normally on colostrum and milk from unimmunized dams readily succumbed to infection when exposed to the homologous pathogen, indicating nonspecific factors in mammary secretions alone are ineffective and specific antibodies must be available.

Prior to discussing the transfer of immunity, one needs to have a basic understanding of the major components of the immune system. The mammalian immune system is a dual system (cellular and humoral), each of which responds specifically to stimulation by foreign substances (e.g., bacteria, toxins, viruses, allografts, tumors).

7.2-2a: Cell-mediated immunity. The cell-mediated immune system (CMI) is mediated by T-lymphocytes that originate in the bone marrow and differentiate in the thymus, therefore, the term T-lymphocyte. T-lymphocytes respond to stimulation by foreign substances by producing memory cells, cytotoxic T-lymphocytes (killer cells), and T-lymphocytes that synthesize and secrete biologically active proteins known as lymphokines. The killer cells bind to target cells and kill them directly or indirectly by the elaboration of cytotoxin. They may also bind via antibody, killing by way of antibody-dependent cytotoxicity.

Some of the effector properties of lymphokines are shown in Table 7.1. Most of these mechanisms have been demonstrated in vitro using homogeneous cell preparations. Though their significance in vivo is not totally understood, in vitro studies have greatly increased our understanding of the importance of lymphokines to the mammalian immune-defense system. T-lymphocytes also produce interferons, which stimulate the production of antiviral proteins, both in the cells in which they are produced and in those

Table 7.1. Effector function, by cell type, of T-lymphocyte lymphokines

- Macrophages
  - migration inhibition
  - migration stimulation
  - aggregation
  - stimulate adherence to peritoneal mucosa
  - chemotaxis
- Neutrophils
  - chemotaxis
  - inhibition
- Lymphocytes
  - mitogenesis
- Lymphocytes (*cont.*)
  - enhance antibody production
  - inhibit antibody production
- Eosinophils
  - chemotaxis
  - migration stimulation
- Basophils
  - chemotaxis
- Other cell types
  - cytotoxic effect
  - growth inhibition

to which they are exposed, and transfer factor, which is capable of transferring delayed hypersensitivity to specific antigens from one animal to another.

The CMI response is particularly sensitive to exposure to fungi, parasites, intracellular viral infections, cancer cells, and foreign tissues. Bacterial antigens elicit a specific CMI response in the mammary gland of bovines, resulting in the production of lymphokines; this in turn results in an increase in neutrophils in the gland upon subsequent exposure of the gland to the homologous antigen. This influx of neutrophils could have a significant impact on the resistance of the mammary gland to invading pathogens (see 7.5-3).

Transfer of CMI from dam to offspring has been demonstrated and suggests a passage of either T-lymphocytes or transfer factor or both through the neonatal gut. The significance of this transfer to the defense of the neonate has not been determined.

7.2-2b: Humoral immunity. Humoral immunity is a function of antibodies, which are products of B-lymphocytes or plasma cells; plasma cells evolve from B-lymphocytes following stimulation with antigen. The antibodies produced are glycoproteins (immunoglobulins) that bind specifically to antigen and initiate various responses that result in antigen neutralization and/or elimination from the body. Effector mechanisms of the humoral immune system are fewer and more clearly understood than those of the CMI. The humoral immune system is most effectively directed toward the killing of bacteria and neutralization of their toxins. Because bacteria and their toxins are the major causative agents in mastitis, the humoral immune system will be discussed in considerable detail.

There are five major classes (isotypes) of immunoglobulins (Igs): IgA, IgG, IgM, IgD, and IgE. In those species examined thus far, except for human colostrum and milk and porcine milk, IgG is the predominant class of Ig (Table 7.2). The basic structure of all Igs, similar to IgG, is composed of two identical light chains (23,000 MW) and two identical heavy chains (53,000 MW) of amino acids. The four chains are joined together by disulfide bonds (Figure 7.2) The complete molecule has a molecular weight of approximately 180,000 and a sedimentation constant of 7S. Each segment (domain) of the light and heavy chain (V_L, C_L, V_H, $C_{H_{1,2,3}}$) is composed of 110 amino acids (AA). The hinge portion of the molecule allows for flexibility in the polypeptide chains during antigen-antibody reactions. The AA sequences of the N-terminal domain of both V_H and V_L varies extensively from polypeptide to polypeptide and is consequently designated the variable region. This variation results in a three dimensional structure that gives molecular complementarity between antibody and antigen. The complementary region (the antigen-binding site) is responsible for antibody specificity for the antigen. Each Ig molecule has at least two identical antigen-binding sites that allow antibodies to cross link antigens. Binding of the antibody to antigen molecules on the surface of foreign substances, such as bacteria, increases the ability of polymorphonuclear neutrophils (PMNs) and macrophages to ingest (phagocytose) and destroy invading pathogens. The process of preparing foreign substances for ingestion by phagocytes is called opsonization.

The constant regions (C_L and $C_{H_{1,2,3}}$) and the degree of disulfide binding are identical for all Igs of a given class or subclass. These regions are responsible for the effector functions characteristic of each class and subclass of Ig (i.e., complement activation, cell-associated antibody-dependent cytoxicity, etc.).

Enzyme degradation and functional analysis of the resulting fragments have contributed to a better understanding of the functions of the various regions of the Ig molecule. Papain cleaves Ig near the hinge portion of the molecule, yielding three distinct fragements: two Fab and one Fc polypeptide (Fig. 7.2). The Fab fragments are composed of light chains (V_L, C_L) bound to corresponding regions on the heavy chains (V_H, C_{H_1}) via disulfide

Table 7.2. Concentration and relative percentage of immunoglobulins in the serum and mammary secretions of three representative species

Species	Immuno-globulin	Concentration (mg/ml)			% Total Immunoglobulins		
		Serum	Colostrum	Milk	Serum	Colostrum	Milk
Human	IgG	12.1	0.43	0.04	78	2	3
	IgA	2.5	17.35	1.00	16	90	87
	IgM	0.93	1.59	0.10	6	8	10
	FSC		2.09	+			
Porcine	IgG	21.5	58.7	3.0	89	80	29
	IgA	1.8	10.7	7.7	7	14	70
	IgM	1.1	3.2	0.3	4	6	1
Bovine	IgG_1	11.0	47.6	0.59	50	81	73
	IgG_2	7.9	2.9	0.2	36	5	2.5
	IgA	0.5	3.9	0.14	2	7	18
	IgM	2.6	4.2	0.05	12	7	6.5
	FSC		0.5	0.06			

Source: From Butler 1973.

bonds. The Fc fragment, however, only consists of constant heavy chains bound to each other via disulfide bonds.

Bovine IgG can be further divided into subclasses (IgG_1 and IgG_2) according to antigenicity and electrophoretic mobility. These subclasses have different biological functions (opsonization, cytolysis) and heritabilities, which may be linked to disease resistance. IgG transport and effector mechanisms will be discussed in more detail in 7.5-4a.

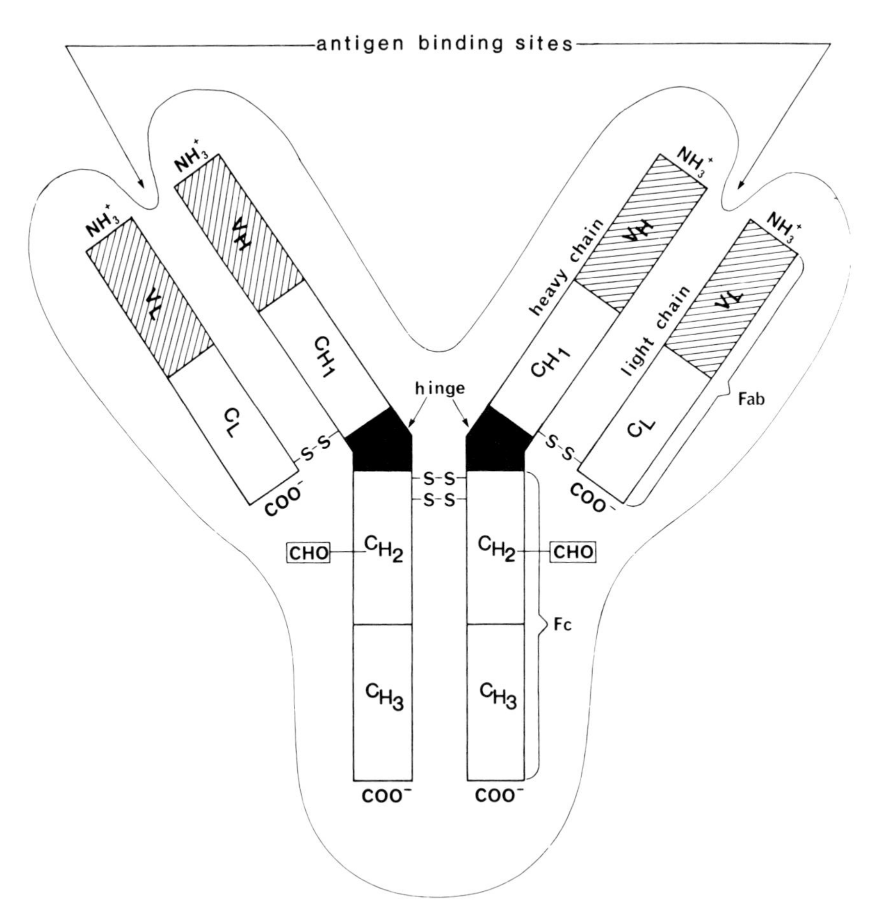

Fig. 7.2. Schematic diagram of a 7S (sedimentation constant) Ig molecule depicting two heavy and two light chains joined by disulfide bonds (*s-s*). *V* = variable region; *C* = constant region; *L* = light chain; *H* = heavy chain; *1, 2,* and *3* subscripts refer to the three constant regions of the heavy chains; *CHO* refers to the carbohydrate moiety; *Fab* refers to the antigen-specific portion of the Ig molecule; *Fc* refers to the cell-binding effector portion of the Ig molecule.

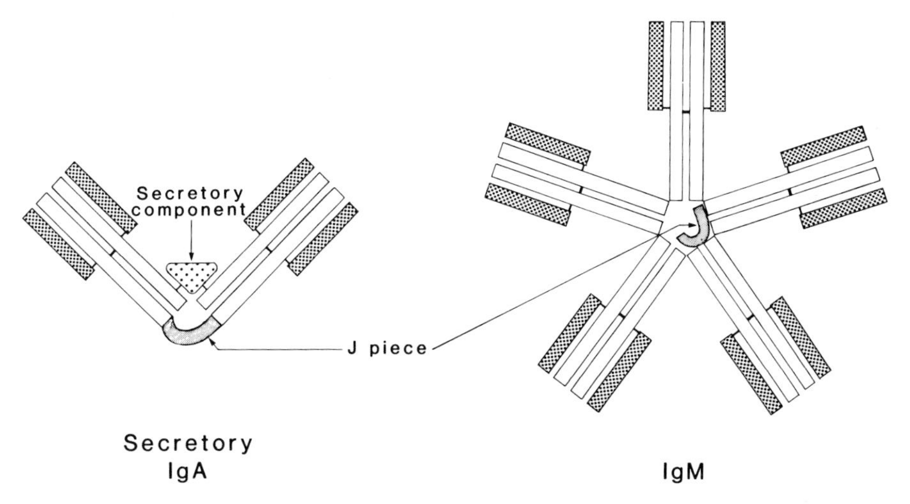

Fig. 7.3. Schematic diagram of secretory IgA and IgM.

The basic structure of monomeric IgA and IgM is similar to IgG except for the addition of a C-terminal octadecapeptide (C_{H_x}) to the heavy chains. The C_{H_x} domain is the binding site of the J chain and possibly the transmembrane protein, commonly referred to as secretory component (SC).

IgA is a carbohydrate-rich Ig that occurs as a monomer or dimer of two 7S molecules joined by the J chain (Fig. 7.3). The dimer, plus J chain (15,000 MW), has a 380,000 MW and a sedimentation constant of 9S.

Except for the ruminant mammary gland secretions, IgA is the major Ig in the external secretions of the body in most species (Table 7.2). Dimeric IgA is secreted by plasma cells; in the submucosa of the respiratory, intestinal, and urinary tracts; and in the interstitial spaces adjacent to the epithelium of exocrine glands (mammary gland), as a dimer bound to the J chain. The SC is synthesized in epithelial cells of glandular acini and mucous membranes and is bound to IgA as it passes through the epithelial cells to the external mucosal surface. Binding of IgA to SC is an integral part of the transcellular transport mechanism. The source of IgA in the ruminant mammary gland is not clear. Some say it is produced by local plasma cells, while others say it is transported from serum. Though the sparsity of IgA-plasma cells in the bovine mammary gland suggests that serum transport is quantitatively the most significant route, some estimate that 54% of the IgA in colostrum and 98% of the IgA in milk is synthesized locally. Also, local and parenteral stimulation of the bovine mammary gland has been shown to increase the local synthesis and secretion of IgA.

Binding sites for SC have been identified on the mucosal surface of the respiratory, intestinal, and urogenital tracts, but not on the apical surface of the mammary epithelium. SC protects IgA from proteolytic enzyme degradation in the gut. IgA does not bind complement nor act as an opsonin in phagocytosis. It can agglutinate particulate antigens and neutralize viruses and viral and bacterial enzymes. The mode of protection of mucous membranes is thought to be the prevention of adherence of bacteria and viruses to the mucous membranes. Another unique property of the secretory IgA system is that antigenic stimulation of the gut results in specific IgA antibodies in the above-mentioned secretory tissues. This gut–secretory gland relationship is particularly important to the monogastric neonate. Specific IgA antibodies in colostrum and milk afford passive protection against intestinal pathogens, common to the environment of the dam and offspring, until the neonate can develop an active gut-associated immune system. Ruminants, which require an active flora in the rumen, are deficient in both colostral and milk IgA. If IgA were present in high concentrations in ruminant colostrum and milk, it could interfere with the development of the ruminant digestive flora of the neonate (Table 7.2).

IgM (900,000 MW) consists of five 7S subunits, similar to monomeric IgG (Fig. 7.3), linked in a circular fashion by disulfide bonds and the J chain. Although IgM antibodies are produced in much smaller quantities than IgG, they are considerably more efficient at complement fixation, opsonization, agglutination, and neutralization of viruses. Because of its large size, IgM is primarily restricted to the intravascular space. However, IgM binds SC similarly to IgA and has been shown to be present in increased amounts in secretory tissues in persons with IgA deficiency. IgM-producing plasma cells have also been identified in the bovine mammary gland, and it is estimated that they contribute 33% of the IgM present in milk. IgM-producing plasma cells also respond to local and parenteral stimulation. The relative importance of IgM in the secretory immune system is not clearly understood.

IgM is of special importance in the primary immune response. When an animal is exposed to an antigen for the first time, the synthesis of IgM antibodies far exceeds that of IgG. This synthesis, however, is transient, and IgG soon becomes the dominant antibody. Upon subsequent exposure to the same antigen, IgM production is similar to the primary response. IgG, however, is synthesized much more rapidly and in two to three magnitudes greater concentration than during the primary response.

IgE is similar to the Y-shaped IgG molecule except that there is an additional segment in the area of the hinge, resulting in 190,000 MW. IgE is bound to basophils in the circulation and mast cells in the tissues, which could account for its presence in extremely low quantities in serum and other body fluids. Upon subsequent exposure to antigen, IgE causes a degranulation of these cells with a release of histamine, resulting in a hypersensitivity (allergic) reaction. IgE has been identified in humans, sheep, cattle, and dogs.

IgD is a 7S Ig that has been identified only in the human and murine species; no specific function has been ascribed to IgD.

7.2-2c: Species differences: intrauterine vs. postnatal. IgG has been defined as the universal carrier of passive immunity because it is selectively transferred to the offspring in utero in group I animals (human, rabbit), via colostrum in group III animals (horse, swine, cow, and goat), and both in utero and via colostrum in group II animals. These groups also differ in the relative concentrations of IgA, IgG, and IgM in colostrum. Where IgG is transferred totally in utero (group I), IgA is the predominent Ig in colostrum (Fig. 7.1) and milk (Table 7.2), with no Ig absorption in the gut. Where IgG is transferred via the mammary gland, IgG is the dominant Ig class, and the gut is permeable to Ig absorption during the colostral phase of lactation. Also, in the nonruminant animals of group III (horse, swine), IgA becomes the dominant Ig in lacteal secretions following closure of the gut to Ig absorption. Whether for protection of the gut or for systemic immunity or both, transfer of immunity via the mammary gland is important to the well-being of the neonate in all mammalian species.

Although a great deal has been learned about the immunology of the mammary gland from a study of passive immunity of the neonate, an equal or perhaps greater knowledge of the subject has evolved from studies on the immune defense of the bovine mammary gland against mastitis pathogens.

7.3: MASTITIS

Mastitis (from the Greek *mastos* – breast and *itis* – inflammation) is a general term used to refer to any inflammation of the mammary gland. Mastitis may be noninfectious, resulting from physical injury to the gland, or infectious, caused by microbial pathogens. In the bovine, noninfectious mastitis is rare and usually transient but may cause the gland to be more vulnerable to microbial infection (teat and udder lesions). More than 99% of all intramammary infections are caused by bacteria. Infections caused by algae and yeasts are not common but can cause individual cow and herd problems; these will be discussed in some detail later. Viral mastitis is extremely rare.

The interior environment of the mammary gland is most favorable for the growth and multiplication of bacteria, which enter through the streak canal (see 6.2-2). Only rarely have cases been reported in which bovine mastitis was associated with the entry of bacteria from the circulation. By-products of bacterial growth and metabolism are chemotactic for PMNs and result in an influx of PMNs. The PMNs phagocytose and destroy the bacteria, resulting in breakdown products of both bacteria and leukocytes (see 7.5-3). These breakdown products also serve as chemotactic agents to increase the influx of PMNs, causing an inflammatory response.

Inflammation is characterized by gross swelling, heat, redness, pain, and disturbed function, which is characterized by a decrease in production and change in milk composition (see 4.10-2 and 5.2-1d). Where these signs are accompanied by the systemic signs (fever, depression, shivering, loss of appetite, and rapid loss of weight), the mastitic condition is classified as *peracute;* with lesser systemic signs (fever and mild depression), it is classified as *acute;* when mammary gland effects are minimal and no systemic signs are visible, it is classified as *subacute;* and *subclinical* mastitis is characterized by changes in milk composition (pH, ion concentration, cell numbers) in the absence of gross signs of inflammation. These changes in composition are commonly used for diagnosis (see 7.7-2). An inflammatory process that exists for months and may continue from one lactation to another is referred to as *chronic* mastitis. Chronic mastitis, for the most part, exists as subclinical but may exhibit periodic flare-ups to subacute or acute, which last for short periods of time to days. Microbial infections, with no signs of mastitis, are referred to as latent infections. It is estimated that, in herds without effective mastitis control programs, 50% of the cows are infected in 50% of the quarters and three of every four cows are infected for 75% of their lactation life. It is also estimated that 95–98% of these infections are subclinical. Combined estimates of the direct losses due to mastitis in the United States are presented in Table 7.3.

The common mammary pathogens are streptococci, staphylococci, and coliforms. Staphylococci and streptococci are the most common mastitis-causing pathogens, accounting for more than 90% of all mastitis infections; however, coliforms are the major cause of mastitis in some herds. The percentages presented herein are meant to be used in a relative fashion for comparing the different pathogens and for large differences in the relative precentage of the organisms that exist due to geographical area and individual herd management.

7.3-1: Gram-positive cocci. Of the genus *Streptococcus, Str. agalactiae, Str. dysgalactiae,* and *Str. uberis* are the most frequently reported.

Str. agalactiae was a major cause of mastitis prior to the advent of antibiotics. However, because it is an obligate pathogen and is susceptible to antibiotics, complete eradication can be effected in well-managed herds. *Str. agalactiae* is not an active tissue invader but readily adheres to the epithelial surface of the cisterns and large ducts. The waste products of growth and multiplication cause an influx of serum proteins and PMNs, which results in the formation of fibrin clots that block the ducts and prevent drainage of that area of the gland. The accumulation of bacterial

Table 7.3. Combined estimates of direct mastitis losses per cow per year corrected to 1979 prices ($14/cwt)

Loss Basis	Decreased Yield	Discarded Milk	Replacement Cost	Decreased Sale Value	Drug Therapy	Veterinary Services	Labor	Total
Per Cow ($)	118.30	23.66	16.38	10.92	7.28	3.64	1.82	182.00
Total for USA ($ millions)	1,301.43	260.29	180.20	120.13	80.09	40.04	20.02	2,002.20
Percent of Total	65	13	9	6	4	2	1	100

Source: From Jasper et al. 1982.

wastes intensifies the inflammatory response, resulting in necrosis of the secretory tissue and, consequently, decreased milk production (agalactia).

Str. uberis is not an obligate udder pathogen but is ubiquitous in the environment of the cow, having been recovered from the soil and bedding. *Str. uberis* has been isolated from the skin of the belly, udder and teats, lips, nostrils, and vagina. Since isolation from the rectum has been infrequent, feces is not thought to be an important vector in the spread of this organism. Mastitis caused by *Str. uberis* is usually subclinical, often transitory, not contagious, and normally does not spread from cow to cow during milking. Clinical cases, which can be acute and chronic, are usually sporadic and associated with teat injury or faulty milking equipment. This bacterium is the most frequent cause of new infections during the dry period. New infection rate has been shown to be seasonal, with the highest infection rate occurring in winter. This coincides with the fact that *Str. uberis* is resistant to cold temperatures.

Str. dysgalactiae also is not an obligate pathogen. It is present and survives a long time in the environment. Considerable strain variation in virulence exists, which has been attributed to variation in its adherence to epithelial surfaces. It has been recovered from normal and inflamed bovine uteri, vaginas, tonsils, skin lesions, and aborted fetuses. *Str. dysgalactiae* mammary infections often follow teat injury. The frequency, severity, and course of infections range from infrequent, mild, and temporary to relatively high frequency, acute, and prolonged in a given herd; the latter extreme is relatively rare. Affected quarters may be partially or completely destroyed.

Str. zooepidemicus, Str. pyogenes (of human origin), and Lancefield groups G and L streptococci have been reported as causing individual cow or isolated herd problems. In *Str. agalactiae*–free herds, enterococci have been reported as being responsible for 25% of the streptococcal infections. Enterococci produce severe, acute mastitis that is difficult to treat with antibiotics. However, spontaneous cures are commonplace, and with proper management, most herds seldom experience clinical mastitis due to this organism.

In herds that are cleared of *Str. agalactiae*, staphylococci become increasingly prominent; *Staphylococcus aureus* and *S. epidermidis* are the two major types associated with mastitis. *S. aureus* causes a form of mastitis that is mainly subclinical and chronic but may cause peracute mastitis, which can lead to gangrene. *S. aureus* has the capacity to adhere to and penetrate epithelial tissue, producing deep-seated foci of infection (abscesses) that become walled off by antibiotic-impermeable scar tissue, thus creating a chronic situation with periodic flare-ups. The production of hyaluronidase, a tissue-solubilizing enzyme, by *S. aureus* is thought to be responsible for its tissue-penetrating capability. *S. aureus* also produces toxic products that enhance its pathogenicity, including coagulase and alpha-, beta-, gamma-, and delta-toxins. Coagulase reacts with the products of inflammation to form fibrinlike clots, which inhibit leukocyte mobility, thus decreasing the effectiveness of the phagocytic defense mechanism. The presence of coagulase activity is used as a criterion for identifying *S. aureus*.

All of the toxins appear to act on cell membranes. Alpha-toxin is the most tissue damaging of the four toxins, primarily because it causes vasoconstriction, which leads to local anemia and necrosis. However, beta- and delta-toxins are irritating, especially when both are present. Beta-toxin is the predominant toxin secreted by *S. aureus* of animal origin.

Leukocidin is another cytotoxic substance produced by *S. aureus* that is specific for leukocytes. It has a cytolytic effect on both PMNs and macrophages, severely interfering with phagocytosis, one of the host's most effective defense mechanisms. Interestingly, this mechanism appears to be strain and host specific. For example, leukocidin from human strains of *S. aureus* has no effect on bovine leukocytes and vice versa.

S. aureus possesses structural characteristics that contribute to its pathogenicity. Peptidoglycan, the major structural component of the cell wall of *S. aureus,* has been shown to cause a delayed hypersensitivity, typical of a CMI response. Hypersensitivity to peptidoglycan can cause periodic flare-ups in chronic cases of subclinical *S. aureus* mastitis, resulting in considerable tissue damage. Another cell wall component contributing to the virulence of *S. aureus* is teichoic acid. In vivo, teichoic acid can be converted to teichuronic acid, which the CMI and humoral immune systems may not recognize. A third cell wall component present in varying degees on most *S. aureus* is Protein A. Protein A binds IgG via the Fc portion of the Ig molecule, thus inhibiting phagocytosis by blocking the PMN-binding sites on the Ig. However, this is not thought to be a significant virulence factor in bovine *S. aureus* infections because bovine Igs bind very poorly to Protein A.

Under certain conditions, *S. aureus* produces capsules that cover the cell-wall antigens and inhibit opsonization by complement and antibodies to cell wall components. Until recently it was thought that less than 5% of all *S. aureus* possessed a capsule. However, when grown in vivo, recent evidence has shown that the majority of *S. aureus* develop a capsule or pseudocapsule that appears to be closely related to the slime layer or clumping factor, which has been shown to impart virulence to *S. aureus*.

The virulence of each strain of *S. aureus* varies tremendously. *S. aureus* also has the ability to mutate and form new strains, with coincidental gain or loss of one or more virulence factors. The appearance of antibiotic-resistant strains of *S. aureus* is a classical example of natural selection for genetic resistance. Though the mechanism(s) of antibiotic resistance is not clearly understood, the use of suboptimal doses of antibiotics has been shown to promote growth of the more resistant strains.

Coagulase-negative *S. epidermidis* (*S. albus*) traditionally has been considered nonpathogenic but is becoming recognized as a common cause of disease in both humans and animals. Much of the confusion has been the result of the transient, subclinical nature of *S. epidermidis* infections. Studies involving frequent sampling have revealed that 75% or more of bovine mammary quarters that become infected with *S. epidermidis* heal spontaneously. The seemingly low pathogenicity and transient nature of *S. epidermidis* infections as compared to *S. aureus* have been attributed to a number of physiological differences between the two organisms.

S. epidermidis produces epsilon-hemolysin, which is thought to be identical with the delta-hemolysin of *S. aureus* but does not produce coagulase or hyaluronidase.

Structurally, *S. epidermidis* is similar to *S. aureus*. However, there are differences, some of which have been related to pathogenicity. For example, *S. epidermidis* is Protein A negative, thus eliminating the potential for inhibition of opsonization. *S. epidermidis* teichoic acid contains glycerol, whereas *S. aureus* contains ribitol, which has been associated with increased pathogenicity. The peptidoglycan moiety of *S. epidermidis* possesses less complete cross linking, which decreases the stability of the cell wall.

However, it is likely that no single factor is responsible for the pathogenic differences of the two species of staphylococci, since mutant strains of *S. aureus* exhibiting one or more of the above deficiencies have failed to exhibit corresponding decreases in pathogenicity.

7.3-2: Gram-negative rods. In the preceding paragraphs, we discussed the gram-positive cocci, which represent 95% of the mastitis-causing pathogens. The major portion of the remaining 5% of mastitis has been attributed to a group of lactose-fermenting gram-negative rods of the family *Enterobacteriaceae: Escherichia coli, Klebsiella,* and *Enterobacter* (formerly *Aerobacter*). *E. coli* and *Enterobacter* possess flagella, but *Klebsiella* does not. These bacteria synthesize and secrete an iron-binding compound (enterochelin), which promotes the absorption of iron by these bacteria. Variants of each possess a capsule. Collectively, they are referred to as coliforms because they inhabit the intestinal tracts of humans and other animals without causing disease. Most intramammary infections caused by these organisms are transient, less than 7 days, but in some instances may be chronic. Severity of inflammation may range from subacute to acute.

Experimental infections with *Klebsiella* have shown that within several hours after the inoculation of small numbers of this bacterium, bacterial counts increased rapidly. Phagocytosis of the *Klebsiella* by PMNs results in the release of endotoxin, which results in further diapedesis of PMNs, udder swelling, fever, depression, and anorexia. The systemic signs are believed to be due to the absorption of endotoxin. A systemic leukopenia develops, which cannot be attributed solely to movement of PMNs into the mammary gland because there is a concomitant decrease in circulating lymphocytes, monocytes, and eosinophils. Similar results are obtained following the intravenous injection of endotoxin, indicating a direct cytolytic effect of endotoxin on circulating leukocytes. It is generally agreed that the systemic symptoms associated with acute coliform infections are referable to toxemia and not to bacteremia. Some cows return to normal milk production, while others must be culled for agalactia. Still others may die from the infection.

The transient nature of coliform infections results in an underestimation of the incidence of infection in a herd over time; most estimates of mastitis caused by given pathogens are made on one-time herd surveys, causing transient infections to be underestimated. In some herds, coliforms may become the dominant cause of clinical mastitis. Investigators have reported a herd where 80% of all cases of clinical mastitis were caused by coliforms. Such reports suggest that these organisms are highly contagious. However, in some herds, there were as many coliform serotypes as there were infections, indicating that transmission from one quarter or one cow to another was uncommon. It is generally agreed that coliform organisms causing mastitis are contracted from either the bedding, teat-cup liners, or excess udder wash water carrying the organisms to the teat end. Both *Klebsiella* and *E. coli* have been associated with sawdust bedding (see 7.4-3). Most surveys indicate that *E. coli* is the coliform most prevalent in barnyard environments and the most frequent cause of coliform mastitis.

Antibiotics, traditionally used for the treatment of mastitis, have been directed against gram-postive organisms and are, for the most part, ineffective against coliforms. Improved management practices involving housing, bedding, sanitary practices, milking management, water supply, and manure disposal, appear to be the most efficacious approach to prevention of coliform mastitis.

The last organism we will consider under the gram-negative rods is *Pseudomonas aeruginosa*. Though the occurrence of *Ps. aeruginosa* is usually sporadic, it can be a serious herd problem. It can produce disease in virtually all animal species, including humans. Resistance to treatment gives *Ps. aeruginosa* an importance not correlated with incidence, which is less than 1% in most herd reports. It is ubiquitous in nature and its nutrient requirements are minimal. *Ps. aeruginosa* infections usually occur after injury or as secondary infections to other infectious diseases. Outbreaks of mastitis caused by this organism have been attributed to poor sanitation in the milking parlor, direct inoculation of the organism into the gland via intramammary infusion of contaminated antibiotic preparations, and to contaminated water. Mastitis due to *Ps. aeruginosa* may be chronic, subacute, acute local, or acute systemic, with periodic flare-ups occurring at intervals of a few days to weeks. During acute infections, milk may acquire a bluish tinge and, in severe cases, may have a grapelike odor. Chronic infections may clear up spontaneously or persist indefinitely. The animal may develop septicemia, which leads to localization of the organism in other tissues and death. Pathogenicity has been attributed to extracellular products, such as proteases, lecithinase, and a beta-hemolytic toxin, which are toxic to cells, and an extracellular slime that inhibits phagocytosis. Specific antibiotic treatment is often unsatisfactory, even though in vitro tests show sensitivity to the antibiotics. *Ps. aeruginosa* also is resistant to the teat dips used for postmilking sanitation. An additional complication arises from the fact that antibiotics and teat dips, shown to reduce the prevalence of *Corynebacterium bovis* (see 7.3-3) and coagulase-negative micrococci, may leave the udder more susceptible to *Ps. aeruginosa*. Immunization with isolates from cases of mastitis have been ineffective, for the most part, in either preventing or reducing the severity of infection by *Ps. aeruginosa*.

7.3-3: Gram-positive rods. *C. bovis* are nonencapsulated, contain no flagella, inhabit the streak canal, and are seldom found beyond Fürstenberg's rosette. They result in slightly elevated milk leukocyte counts of approximately $1.5-3.0 \times 10^5$ cells/ml (normal $= 0.5 - 1.0 \times 10^5$ cells/ml); however, strict foremilk from *C. bovis*–infected quarters may be three to four times higher. This may account for the resistance to challenge with pathogenic bacteria that has been demonstrated in *C. bovis*–infected quarters.

C. bovis is one of the bacteria most frequently isolated from bovine milk samples. One field study on 2,772 quarter milk samples from 14 farms reported that 31% of the samples contained *C. bovis*. However, only 1.6% of the *C. bovis*–infected quarters showed signs of clinical mastitis. Individual herd estimates from other studies report herds with *C. bovis* in more than 90% of all quarters. There are no reported cases of severe mastitis caused by *C. bovis;* therefore, *C. bovis* is not regarded as a major mastitis pathogen.

C. pyogenes causes a severe, acute mastitis in cattle, yet it has been isolated from genital tract, mouth, and nasal mucus of clinically normal cattle. Mastitis caused by this pathogen is more frequent in heifers and dry cows but seldom appears in the lactating gland. Also, unlike other mastitis-causing pathogens, there are reported incidences of *C. pyogenes* entering the mammary gland from the bloodstream. Early treatment with antibiotics may eliminate the infection but is ineffective in the later stages.

7.3-4: Yeasts. The most common yeast causing severe bovine mastitis is *Cryptococcus neoformans.* It is an encapsulated, nonspore-forming organism that is highly resistant to antibiotic therapy. *C. neoformans* causes a severe, chronic mastitis, usually confined to the udder and supramammary lymph nodes and results in permanent udder damage. Cases with elevated systemic temperature and anorexia are not uncommon.

Candida is another yeastlike species that has been associated with bovine mastitis. Clinical signs vary greatly and are not diagnostic. The majority of cases are mild and spontaneous cures frequently occur. Secretion usually returns to normal within 1–2 wk.

7.3-5: Mycoplasma. Mycoplasmas have been incriminated as important primary and secondary pathogens in a wide variety of diseases in humans and animals. Mycoplasmas are the smallest free-living microorganisms. Unlike true bacteria, they lack a cell wall and therefore are pleomorphic, due to the effects of their environment. Mycoplasma mastitis has been diagnosed in many parts of the world since the initial reported incident in England in 1960. Most infections have been due to the species now known as *Mycoplasma bovis.* Other species include ST-6, *M. canadensis, M. bovigenitalium, M. alkalescens, M. arginini,* and *M. bovirhinis.* Clinical signs include (1) severe purulent mastitis that resists treatment but shows little systemic effect, (2) involvement of more than one quarter, often all four, (3) marked loss in production, and (4) tannish milk with sandy or flaky sediments becoming watery or serous with time. *M. bovis* has been recovered from lymph nodes, uteri, lungs, kidneys, spleens, synovial fluids, amniotic fluids, eyes, and blood.

Though no reliable treatment is known, control of the spread of infection in the herd by early diagnosis, culling, and sanitation are highly effective in stopping herd infection.

7.3-6: *Prototheca.* *Prototheca* are achloric algae that are oval to spherical, large and variable in size (6–17 μ), have thick cellulose walls, and reproduce by internal cleavage of endospores, which are released by rupture of the mother cell. On blood agar, they form white, waxy, yeastlike colonies. Since *Prototheca* was first recognized as the causative organism in a case of mastitis in 1952, it has been observed with increasing frequency. Part of the increase in frequency is due to improved diagnostic methods that differentiate *Prototheca* from yeasts.

Because of unsuccessful attempts to infect laboratory animals and the association of protothecosis with concurrent infections, trauma, or debilitation, it has been recognized as a pathogen of low virulence. Quarters can be chronically infected for months with secretions appearing normal. However, clinically infected quarters become hard, and the secretions are watery and contain large clots. Extensive necrosis can develop, resulting in complete destruction of the entire quarter. *Prototheca* is highly refractory to therapy and culling is recommended in most cases.

7.4: ENVIRONMENTAL FACTORS AFFECTING MASTITIS

Thus far, we have seen that mastitis is a very complex disease caused by numerous pathogens of differing virulence, invasiveness, and modes of pathogenicity. Many questions regarding the environmental effects on the complex host-parasite interactions in mastitis remain unanswered because the carefully controlled experiments necessary to minimize the many variables are difficult and costly. Nearly every factor of environment and management has been mentioned as a possible contributor to the mastitis problem. For purposes of experimentation and management, these factors have been grouped into the following categories.

7.4-1: Nutritional factors. Heavy feeding for increased milk production has been associated with clinical mastitis in cows with subclinical or latent infections. For example, heavy concentrate feeding or the feeding of a particular concentrate, such as cottonseed meal, has been implicated. Forages high in estrogen, whether fresh or ensiled, have been associated with an increase in clinical mastitis. Studies designed to determine the physiological mechanism involved have not been conclusive. However, one such study did show estrogen to have an inhibitory effect on the bactericidal properties of PMNs, the mammary gland's second line of defense against invading pathogens (see 7.5-3). There is no good evidence showing that a particular mineral, vitamin, or feed additive increases resistance to mastitis.

7.4-2: Housing. Housing factors that affect udder and teat trauma, cow comfort, and sanitation have been associated with an increased incidence of mastitis. Teats being stepped on is the primary cause of teat trauma. Adequate space for resting and freedom of movement on rising help prevent teat and udder injury. Cows in uncrowded housing with soft bedding have been shown to have a lower incidence of mastitis. Overcrowding induces problems of sanitation, availability of nutrients, and the possibility of stress. Crowding, coupled with behavioral dominance, can cause subordinate animals to be stressed to the point of developing clinical mastitis in subclinical cases. Adequate housing includes (1) light, airy buildings free of drafts; (2) adequately sized stalls; (3) ample dry bedding; (4) daily removal of manure; and (5) exercise lots free of wire, stones, and sharp objects.

7.4-3: Bedding. Bedding can have a profound influence on the type, as well as the incidence, of bacterial infection. Sawdust bedding, so commonly used thoughout the dairy industry, is an excellent habitat for coliforms. *E. coli,* the dominant organism of bovine feces, grows extremely well in warm, damp sawdust. *Klebsiella,* which is present in virtually all sawdust as it leaves the mill, also finds damp sawdust a favorable habitat. *Ps. aeruginosa*, which commonly contaminates the water supply, grows quite well in damp bedding but does not survive in a dry environment for extended periods. Since control measures that are effective against streptococci and staphylococci are not particularly effective against coliforms, it is imperative that management practices reduce the level of environmental coliforms wherever possible. Keeping the bedding area dry and free of feces has been shown to be effective in reducing new coliform infection rates.

7.4-4: Milking machines. Poor milking machine design and operation has been incriminated as an important vector for the transmission of mastitis pathogens and can have profound detrimental effects on the anatomy and physiology of the teat (see 6.2), which could increase susceptibility to infection. However, controlled studies have been unable to conclusively link milking machine design and operation to the incidence of new infections. Nevertheless, modern milking machine design and recommended milking machine management have been directed toward removing these potential problems (see 6.3).

7.4-5: Weather. The direct effects of seasonal changes are difficult to assess because changes in weather are accompanied by changes in a multiplicity of other environmental factors. These changes may include management factors, such as a change from indoor housing to pasture, seasonal calving, occurrence of peak lactation relative to weather, or a shift in demand for labor. Moisture and temperature have a profound effect on the quantity and quality of forage, which could increase susceptibility to mastitis (see 7.4-1). Moisture and temperature also increase the populations of both the mastitis-causing pathogens and the insect vectors that help transmit them. In most areas of the United States, the greatest incidence of clinical mastitis occurs in the summer. Though most of this increase has been attributed to an increase in the bacteria and insect populations, some of the increase in clinical mastitis has been attributed to direct stress of temperature on subclinical cases.

7.5: DEFENSE SYSTEM

The mammary gland is protected by a complex system of primary and secondary defense mechanisms, including anatomical, chemical, cellular, and immunological mechanisms. The primary defense mechanisms are those mechanisms that prevent entry of pathogens into the mammary gland and are associated with the streak canal. The secondary defense mechanisms are a complex system of chemical, cellular, and immunological mechanisms, located within the mammary gland.

7.5-1: Streak canal. Bacteria must pass through the streak canal to enter the mammary gland. Therefore, changes in the anatomy and physiology of the streak canal, which occur during the various stages of the lactation cycle and as a result of mechanical milking, hand milking, and suckling, greatly influence susceptibility to mastitis (see 6.2).

7.5-2: Chemical defenses. Chemical defenses, as used in this section, refer to those defenses that are neither cellular nor immunological but may interact with either.

7.5-2a: Lactoferrin. Virulence of pathogenic bacteria has been associated with their ability to obtain iron from the environment for respiratory enzyme kinetics. Conversely, the ability of the host to restrict bacterial iron uptake has been associated with host resistance to these pathogens. Apolactoferrin, the iron-deficient form of lactoferrin, is an iron-binding glycoprotein present in mammary secretory cells, mammary secretions, and in PMN granules (see 5.2-3b). It reversibly binds two ferric ions with the incorporation of two molecules of HCO_3. Lactoferrin is 20–30% saturated with iron in vivo. Bacterial growth is restricted by the ability of bacteria to compete for the protein-bound iron. *E. coli,* for example, synthesizes iron-chelating compounds, enterochelins, that have association constants similar to lactoferrin. Also, citrate, which competes with lactoferrin for iron, forms a citrate-iron complex that is available to bacteria for growth. The citrate:lactoferrin ratio in mammary gland secretions varies with stage of lactation cycle, which could influence the growth of pathogens, making the animal more vulnerable (see 7.6). Conversely, bicarbonate increases the iron-binding capacity of lactoferrin, which can reverse the effect of citrate. Therefore, during the inflammatory response, serum bicarbonate transudates into milk, increasing the iron-binding capacity of milk lactoferrin. Its protective value at this stage of the infection process is questionable, but this reversal of the citrate-iron binding by bicarbonate may serve as a protective mechanism in the neonatal gut, which has a high bicarbonate concentration. It also has been shown that lactoferrin, in conjunction with specific antibody, can have a powerful inhibitory effect on *E. coli* through antibody interference with enterochelin production.

7.5-2b: Lysozyme. Lysozyme (*N*-acetyl muramylhydrolase) lyses bacteria by hydrolyzing the beta-linkage between muramic acid and *N*-acetylglucosamine of bacterial cell wall peptidoglycan. Depending on the organism and the conditions under which it was studied, lysozyme has been shown to (1) independently lyse bacteria after they have been killed, (2) lyse bacteria in the presence of complement, (3) kill bacteria in the presence of complement and antibody, (4) stimulate the opsonic activity of IgM, and (5) increase the bactericidal activity of IgM plus complement. Though the concentration of lysozyme is extremely low in both bovine milk and bovine

PMNs, additional studies are needed to determine if the synergistic effects mentioned above affect its importance as a mammary gland defense mechanism.

7.5-2c: Lactoperoxidase-thiocyanate-H_2O_2. The lactoperoxidase-thiocyanate-H_2O_2 (LP) system has been shown to inhibit gram-positive bacteria and to be bactericidal for certain gram-negative bacteria, such as *Ps. aeruginosa* and *E. coli.* Milk LP has been shown to be inhibitory to bacterial growth by modifying the sulfhydryl groups in the bacterial cell membrane, which are responsible for glucose transport. Since H_2O_2 is not present in milk, the importance of the LP system to the protection of the mammary gland is questionable. However, H_2O_2 is found in saliva and may be of protective value in the neonate.

7.5-3: Leukocyte phagocytosis. Phagocytosis is the process of recognition, ingestion, and digestion of foreign particles (bacteria, necrotic tissue, tumor cells) by phagocytic cells. PMNs and macrophages, the principal phagocytes, constitute 80–90% of the cells found in milk. The milk of uninfected ruminant mammary glands contains an average of 50,000–200,000 of these cells/ml. However, because these cells have reduced phagocytic and bactericidal capabilities when present in milk, more than 500,000 cells/ml are needed to protect the mammary gland against bacterial infection. This level may ultimately be reached after the entry of a few pathogenic bacteria into the mammary gland; however, a 24 hr lapse is generally required before these concentrations accumulate in the milk. Some bacteria (i.e., *E. coli*) cause a much more rapid response. The time lapse allows sufficient time for the bacteria to become established. Macrophages do not appear until 7–10 days postinfection to clean up the debris left by the PMNs. Studies with neutropenic cows have clearly shown that the PMNs are essential for defense against invading pathogens.

The decreased killing capacity of milk PMNs, compared to blood PMNs, has been attributed to (1) 38% less glycogen in milk PMNs, (2) deficiency of opsonins and complement in milk, (3) coating of the surface of PMN with casein, (4) loss of PMN pseudopods due to ingestion of fat, and (5) a decrease in the supply of hydrolytic enzymes within the PMNs following the ingestion of fat and casein.

In vitro phagocytosis studies have shown a threefold difference among cows in the ability of milk to support phagocytosis and a twofold difference in the ability of milk PMNs to phagocytose. These studies also showed a negative correlation between the presence of clinical mastitis and the ability of milk to support phagocytosis. A more detailed discussion concerning the ability of milk to support phagocytosis will be presented in 7.5-4.

The above-mentioned deficiences of both milk PMNs and the ability of milk to support phagocytosis are consistent with the observed requirement of high cell counts in milk to protect the mammary gland against invading pathogens. However, because the concentration of leukocytes is used to assess milk quality, the practice of maintaining a high concentration of PMNs in the gland is not desirable unless they can be restricted to fractions other than the primary (bulk) milk of the mammary gland, such as in foremilk and/or in strippings. This would present the effective high concentration of PMNs necessary for defense against invading pathogens in the teat cistern prior to milking, as well as at the time the cow leaves the milking parlor.

Another way in which effective leukocyte numbers could be made available in sufficient numbers to prevent infection would be to decrease the magnititude of the signal and/or response time needed to trigger an influx of PMNs and opsonins from the circulatory system. Methods of effecting an increase in PMN mobilization will be discussed in 7.6.

7.5-4: Immunological defense mechanisms. Both humoral and CMI systems were discussed in some detail under transfer of immunity (see 7.2-2). This section is concerned primarily with their function in defense of the mammary gland.

7.5-4a: Humoral immune system. The antibodies of the humoral immune system of the mammary gland serve as opsonins for PMNs and macrophages, toxin neutralizers, and as bactericidins. Killing and/or removing organisms from the gland are paramount to preventing infection, whereas neutralization of toxins decreases the severity of an established infection.

Bacterial killing is effected by either direct lysis via antibody, antibody plus complement, or complement plus lysozyme or phagocytosis via antibody (with or without complement) serving as an opsonin and/or an enhancer of the intracellular kill. Direct lysis of bacteria is considered to be of minor importance because it is confined primarily to gram-negative organisms of low virulence. Phagocytosis of invading pathogens is the major defense mechanism preventing establishment of intramammary infection.

Milk PMNs are less phagocytic than blood PMNs, and milk is less efficient in supporting phagocytosis than serum (see 7.5-3), due to a deficiency in opsonins and complement. Numerous attempts have been made to increase specific opsonins in milk via various modes of immunization. These studies have had limited success, mainly because of the superficial approach used to characterize the immune response. Some of the reasons for this approach were due to an eagerness to find a means of immunizing cows against mastitis, a lack of understanding of the bovine immune system, and inadequate methods of measuring various aspects of the immune response. However, as more in-depth techniques have become available for studying both the humoral and CMI systems, our knowledge of the bovine immune system has increased. The following is a brief summary of the current knowledge of the humoral immune system relative to defense of the bovine mammary gland.

Until recently, opsonic activity was attributed to IgG, with no reference to the relative opsonic activity of IgG subclasses. It has recently been shown that bacteria that have been opsonized with IgG_2, but not IgG_1, enhance bovine PMN phagocytosis, whereas both IgG_1 and IgG_2 enhance phagocytosis by macrophages. Also, IgG_2 has been shown to bind to PMNs (cytophilic) in serum and milk, thus being piggybacked on the PMNs during diapedesis into the milk. Because macrophages are the predominant cell type in uninflamed lacteal secretions and IgG_1 is the predominant Ig, it has been suggested that IgG_1 is more important to the defense of the mammary gland in the early stages of infection, and the importance of IgG_2 increases as PMNs enter the gland during inflammation.

Receptors for IgM have been demonstrated on bovine blood and milk PMNs, but not on macrophages. In the past, many workers have overlooked the opsonic nature of IgM because of its strict requirement for complement, without which IgM has no opsonic activity. However, with complement, it is 500–1,000 times more opsonic than IgG. Also, with complement, IgM has been shown to kill *M. bovis.* Although the concentration of complement in milk is only 2% of that present in blood, complement passes from serum to milk during inflammation, which would increase its effectiveness in the inflamed gland. Therefore, IgM could be an important opsonin in an inflammatory situation.

The major function of IgA appears to be the prevention of bacterial adherence to epithelial surfaces, thereby preventing colonization, subsequent penetration, and establishment in the tissues (see 7.2-2b). This function has been associated with the ability of IgA to bind to receptors on the mucous membranes (lungs and intestine). The antiadherence function of IgA has been shown to be protective against enteric infections in the neonate. However, since the mammary gland lacks a mucous layer, this mechanism is not considered a viable defense mechanism against mastitis-causing pathogens. It also has been shown that IgA is neither bacteriolytic nor opsonic and, under certain circumstances, may even suppress IgG opsonization by competing for, or steric hindrance of, the same binding sites on the PMNs. It has been suggested that IgA may function by (1) agglutinating bacteria, thus facilitating their removal during milking, (2) preventing bacterial multiplication, or (3) neutralizing bacterial toxins.

For a complete appreciation of the role of Igs in defense of the mammary gland, we need to have an understanding of their relative concentrations in mammary secretions and of their synthesis and transport into these secretions. Table 7.2 shows the relative concentrations of the various Igs in serum, colostrum, and milk. The predominance of IgG_1 over IgA in ruminant lacteal secretions suggests that, in ruminants, IgG_1 may perform functions mediated by IgA in other species. Experimental observations that support this hypothesis include (1) ruminants immunized parenterally with *Rotavirus* show high titers of protective IgG antibodies in colostrum and milk, (2) high titers of enteric–organism specific IgG_1 in bovine colostrum are analogous to the enteric–organism specific IgA found in the lacteal secretions of group I animals (Fig. 7.1), (3) IgG_1 is resistant to proteolysis, (4) IgG_1 neutralizes viruses and prevents bacterial adhesion, and (5) IgG_1 is not opsonic for PMNs. Unlike IgA, the predominance of IgG_1 over IgG_2 in ruminant lacteal secretions is due to a selective transport mechanism at the secretory cell level, not to local synthesis.

The synthesis and transport mechanisms for IgG_2 are not as clearly defined. Mechanisms that have been identified include (1) transudation via a breakdown in the tight junctions between epithelial cells, (2) transcellular movement via active transport, (3) piggybacking PMNs during diapedesis, and (4) local synthesis. One report attributed 49% of the IgG_2 present in milk to local synthesis.

The information above and in 7.2-2b on the humoral immune system of the ruminant mammary gland is sketchy; however, it serves as a basis for research that will eventually present the entire picture.

7.5-4b: Cell-mediated immune system. Since most of the CMI data has come from in vitro studies, the significance of these findings to in vivo CMI is not clear (see 7.2-2a). Also studies that have been conducted have used human and laboratory models. Recently, CMI studies with bovines have opened the door to research on CMI in the mastitis complex. Results of these studies show that 73% of bovine peripheral blood lymphocytes are T-lymphocytes and 27% are B-lymphocytes, which are comparable to the data on blood lymphocytes in humans (70-80% T-lymphocytes, 14–17% B-lymphocytes) and in the mouse (70–75% T-lymphocytes, 15% B-lymphocytes). Percentages of T- and B-lymphocytes in bovine milk were 31–65% and 22-42%, respectively.

There are also data from studies on the effector function of T-lymphocytes in the bovine mammary gland in response to intramammary infusion of heterologous protein and bacterial antigens in naive and parenterally immunized cows. Though response varied with antigen, mode of immunization, and antigenic challenge (intramammary infusion), leukocyte counts in the milk increased 100–1,000 times in immunized cows following infusion of homologous antigen. Lymphocytes isolated from the vaccinated cows are responsive to challenge with homologous antigens in vitro. Supernatant fluids from in vitro lymphocyte cultures, stimulated with the respective antigens, demonstrated macrophage migration inhibitory and chemotactic activity, clearly demonstrating an active CMI system that could be stimulated to respond to bacterial challenge. A great deal needs to be learned concerning effector functions and antigens, adjuvants, modes of immunization, and timing of immunizations to determine the efficacy of stimulating CMI for protection against pathogens invading the mammary gland.

7.6: TIMING OF NEW INFECTIONS

A new infection is defined as the appearance of bacteria in a quarter previously diagnosed as bacteria free. Infection of the mammary gland can occur at any time; however, the greatest incidence of new infections has been shown to occur during the dry period and the first 3 mo of lactation.

Most new infections occur during the first 2 wk of the dry period and 1 wk prior to and 1 wk after calving. Infection rate during the first 2 wk of the dry period is higher than any other period during the entire lactation cycle, and many of these infections persist into the next lactation. The factors affecting susceptibility during the dry period have not been studied extensively. However, sufficient observations on various parameters that could affect susceptibility have been made to allow some speculation.

Drying-off terminates twice-a-day flushing of the streak canal and teat dipping, two processes that tend to rid the teat orifice and streak canal of organisms capable of penetrating the streak canal. Also, at this point, the gland is still secreting; pressure buildup tends to distend the teat and open the streak canal, increasing accessibility to such pathogens (see 6.7). Pathogens entering the mammary gland in the early dry period find the intramammary defense mechanisms weakened in several areas. The concentration of leukocytes is lower than that considered necessary for effective defense against invading pathogens. Also, during the first 10 days to 2 wk of the dry period, the gland rapidly changes from a highly secretory organ to one that is relatively dormant, involving biochemical changes that could affect susceptibility. For example, the citrate:lactoferrin ratio is very high, resulting in an increased proportion of iron bound to citrate rather than to lactoferrin, thus increasing the availability of iron needed for bacterial growth. This ratio decreases as involution progresses but returns to similar high levels peripartum. Also, the concentration of cystine, which has been shown to inhibit the LP system (see 7.5-2c), increases tenfold during the period of involution.

It has been shown that shortening the involution period, via the infusion of either colchicine or endotoxin, reduced new infections during this period 50%, suggesting that shortening the involution period decreases the length of this highly vulnerable period. The decrease in susceptibility of the involuted gland has been attributed to (1) a decrease in pressure in the gland, (2) sealing of the teat end with the mucous keratin plug, (3) an increase in PMNs, (4) a decrease in the citrate:lactoferrin ratio, and (5) a decrease in cystine.

At the end of the dry period, as the gland returns to its secretory status in preparation for parturition, the above-mentioned parameters are again reversed to a similar status as that observed during the early dry period. These changes are associated with an increase in susceptibility during the peripartum period.

All of the above references to infections are assuming natural or simulated natural infections with the organisms having to penetrate the streak canal. To study the intramammary defenses independent of the streak canal, a study was conducted where *Str. uberis* was introduced into the lactiferous sinus at weekly intervals during the dry period. Infection rate increased from 12% the first week of drying-off to 80% during the third week of the dry period. During the last half of the dry period, 100% of all inoculated quarters became infected, suggesting that the streak canal and teat cistern play a major role in resistance of the involuted gland. Conclusions concerning the importance of the citrate:lactoferrin ratio cannot be drawn from this study because *Str. uberis* has a low requirement for iron. Consequently, fluctuations in the citrate:lactoferrin ratio would have little effect on the growth of this organism. Also, coincident to the period of increasing susceptibility to *Str. uberis* is the phenomenon of increasing viscosity of lacteal secretions from the beginning of the dry period to about day 21, which could have an inhibitory effect on the movement of PMNs, resulting in a decrease in phagocytosis.

Parturition and the physiological stresses associated with it can cause subclinical cases of mastitis to become clinical. The actual infection in many cases may have occurred during the dry period. Following parturition during the colostral phase, still another set of conditions exists that could contribute to increased susceptibility. The gland continues to be distended due to a conversion from colostrum formation to copious milk synthesis and secretion. This translates to a distention of the papillary duct and an overall stress on the udder and the rest of the cow; heavy milk synthesis and secretion continue throughout the first 3 mo of lactation, the citrate:lactoferrin ratio is high, the PMN-macrophage population is low, and the viscosity is high. Also, during the first day postpartum, the population of leukocytes consists primarily of macrophages, which are less efficient than PMNs in phagocytosing and destroying bacteria.

Definitive studies to identify the factors responsible for decreased resistance to infection observed during these periods remain to be done. However, the information currently available can and does serve as a guide for prophylaxis, diagnosis, and therapy of mastitis, as well as for the design of future studies in these areas.

7.7: MASTITIS CONTROL

From the preceding discussion, it is evident that while a great deal remains to be learned about the mastitis complex, a great deal is known concerning the major pathogens involved, anatomical and physiological defense mechanisms, and factors in the environment that affect both pathogen and host. Using this information, researchers, veterinarians, and extension personnel have formulated programs in the areas of prevention, diagnosis, and therapy that can significantly reduce both the incidence and severity of mastitis. A brief discussion of each of these applied areas will help clarify the current status of mastitis control.

7.7-1: Prevention. Mastitis prevention is best thought of as a herd problem rather than an individual cow problem. Keeping in mind the environmental factors affecting mastitis (see 7.4), its prevention needs only the use of a common sense approach.

Since 45–55% of all new infections occurring during lactation are the result of cross infection of quarters within or between cows, a major emphasis should be placed on sanitation in all aspects of the milking procedure. Correct design, installation, and use of a functionally sound milking system is an essential part of mastitis prevention and should include (1) rountine checking of vacuum stability; (2) scheduled replacement of teat liners; (3) sanitation of the teat cups between cows; (4) washing and drying of teats with individual wipes prior to placement of the milking machine (extensive washing of the animal just prior to milking should be avoided to prevent drainage water, contaminated by organisms on the body surface, from contaminating the teat); (5) dipping teats in a germicidal teat dip after each milking; and (6) milking of cows, known to be infected, last. All of these procedures should become routine, without losing sight of the importance of each to the prevention of new infections.

Housing should provide adequate space for resting and freedom of movement, avoiding teat and udder injury, and avoiding physical and psychological stress. Barns, corrals, and pastures should be free of obstacles that could cause teat and udder injury, bedding should be kept dry, and manure removed daily.

At the beginning of the dry period, all quarters should be treated with a high-persistency antibiotic preparation. With products presently available, new infections during the dry period can be decreased by 50–75%. Also, 40–90% (depending on the pathogen) of existing infections can be eliminated via dry-cow therapy.

7.7-2: Diagnosis. From the preceding discussion, it would appear that prevention of new infections would effectively decrease the incidence of mastitis. However, since 45–55% of all new infections result from cross infections, subclinical and clinical cases occurring during lactation must be identified and treated to remove these reservoirs of contamination.

Tests for mastitis are based on examination of the udder and the milk. Visual examination of the udder for signs of injury, redness, and swelling, and palpation for signs of hardness should be done at each milking. Examination of the milk with a strip cup and routine measurement of milk production are effective in clinical cases. Diagnosis of subclinical mastitis requires chemical, cultural, and microscopic testing of the milk. The chemical changes associated with mastitis include increases in pH, Na^+, Cl^-, conductivity, serum albumin, and various enzymes and decreases in K^+, lactose, and citrate. The decreases in lactose and citrate are the result of a decrease in synthesis and transport by the secretory cells. The dynamics of the changes in the other elements are the result of a breakdown in the tight junctions between the secretory cells and the concentration gradients of these elements that exist between tissue fluids and milk. Leukocytes that enter the gland during inflammation also enter the milk by passage between the secretory cells.

Milk leukocyte counts are determined, either microscopically or by an electronic cell counter, or they may be estimated via several chemical techniques. Estimates of leukocytes using the chemical techniques are based on the degree of gel formation in a sample of milk following the addition of an anionic detergent. The gel formed is the result of a reaction of the detergent with leukocyte nuclear proteins. Milk cell counts are commonly referred to as somatic cell counts because they include all types of leukocytes, as well as epithelial cells. However, very early in the inflammatory response, neutrophils become the predominant cell type.

Any one or combination of the above measures could serve as a means of identifying quarters with subclinical mastitis. However, because state milk quality-control programs use the number of leukocytes in milk as a measure for the acceptance of bulk tank milk, attention has been focused on milk leukocytes as an indicator of mastitis. Leukocyte counts in excess of 2.0×10^5 cells/ml in an individual cow sample are considered suspect and warrant individual quarter sampling and testing by one of the chemical methods mentioned earlier. Quarters identified as positive should be tested for the presence of specific pathogens; bacteriological testing is seldom done except in problem herds, due to the cost involved.

Conductivity as an indicator of subclinical mastitis, though not in commerical use to any extent at the present time, is gaining recognition as a practical method for routine monitoring of individual quarters. Conductivity has been shown to be as sensitive as leukocyte counts in identifying subclinical mastitis and has the additional advantage of being adaptable to in-line monitoring of milk from individual quarters.

7.7-3: Therapy. Most mastitis therapy is administered by the dairy workers in the milking parlor. Diagnosis is usually limited to the visual observation and palpation of the udder and the appearance of foremilk in the strip cup. Tests with the California Mastitis Test (CMT) paddle are used only in questionable cases. Only in chronic cases, or where systemic signs are observed, is the veterinarian called for further diagnosis and treatment. Broad spectrum antibiotics (Table 7.4) are used to treat all subclinical and clinical cases except in instances where a particular pathogen has been identified.

The treatment most frequently recommended is an intramammary infusion of antibiotic, using a single-dose disposable syringe and cannula to

Table 7.4. Route of administration and specificity of antimicrobial drugs

State of Lactation	Antimicrobial Drug	Spectrum of Activity	Principal Organisms
	Intramammary Infusion		
Lactating only	Cephapirin	G+ or G−, slt	PR staphylococci
	Procaine penicillin	G+	Streptococci
	Penicillin and novobiocin	G+ or G−, slt	PR staphylococci
	Hetacillin[a]	G+,G−	G− rods and cocci
	Novobiocin[a]	G+ or G−, ltd	PR staphylococci
	Cloxacillin[a]	G+	PR staphylococci
Lactating and dry	Erythromycin	G+	PR staphylococci
	Furaltadone	G+, G−	G+ cocci and coliforms
	Oxytetracycline	G+, G−	G+, G− in general
Dry only	Benzathine cloxacillin[a]	G+	PR staphylococci and streptococci
	Cephapirin benzathine	G+ or G−, slt	PR staphylococci and streptococci
	Nitrofurazone	G+, G−	G+ cocci and coliforms
	Novobiocin	G+ or G−, ltd	PR staphylococci and *Proteus*
	Injectable		
Lactating only	Penicillin and dihydrostreptomycin	G+, G−	G− rods and streptococci
	Ampicillin	G+, G−	G− rods and cocci
	Erythromycin	G+	PR staphylococci
	Procaine penicillin G	G+	
	Procaine penicillin G and dihydrostreptomycin[b]	G+, G−	G− rods and streptococci
Dry only	Sulfadimethoxine	G+, G−	PR staphylococci and streptococci
	Sulfamethazine	G+, G−	PR staphylococci and streptococci
	Tylosin	G+ or G−, slt	Mycoplasma
	Oxytetracycline	G+, G−	

Note: PR = Penicillin resistant; G+ = Gram positive; G− = Gram negative; slt = slight; ltd = limited.

[a]These drugs to be used by or on the order of a licensed veterinarian.

[b]Combination to be used by or on the order of a licensed veterinarian.

avoid cross infection. A minimum of three (preferably four) infusions are given after consecutive milkings; suboptimal treatment leads to the development of resistant strains of bacteria (see 7.3-1).

The effectiveness of antibiotic therapy is dependent on getting the antibiotic to the site of infection at therapeutic levels for sufficient time to kill the invading pathogen. Factors that influence this objective are (1) stage of lactation and level of production (dilution factor); (2) treatment of infected quarter after each milking; (3) fibrous tissue or edema of involved quarter, which inhibits distribution; and (4) physical and chemical properties of the antibiotic and its vehicle. Systemic antibiotic is recommended where intramammary infusion is inappropriate due to any of the above circumstances. In more advanced cases, frequent milking-out (2-hr intervals) is recommended to remove toxins and other waste products of inflammation. Where coliform mastitis is suspected, early detection and both intramammary and systemic antibiotic therapy are recommended.

When a cow shows signs of systemic disease (high temperature, depression, anorexia), the veterinarian should be consulted for further diagnosis and treatment. The additional cost of treatment and the prognosis should be weighed against the animal's future potential for milk production and breeding. In severe cases, such as peracute toxic mastitis, treatment may include (1) oxytocin to facilitate milk-out, (2) intravenous electrolyte solutions to reestablish fluid and electrolyte balance, (3) glucose to combat hypoglycemia, (4) antiprostaglandins and corticosteroids to reduce inflammation, (5) systemic antibiotics, and (6) calcium to combat hypocalcemia.

7.8: SUMMARY AND CONCLUSIONS

In herds where improved hygiene, teat dipping, dry-cow therapy, and close observation of individual cows have been practiced, the incidence of mastitis has been reduced 50–75%, suggesting that the "key" to the mastitis problem has been found. However, as these methods of control have gained acceptance, it has been found that nature changes the "locks." For example, with the advent of antibiotics, the number of *Str. agalactiae*–free herds increased, but a concomitant increase in *S. aureus* infections was observed. Similarly, there are herds where neither of these organisms are encountered with any frequency, but they experience frequent coliform or mycoplasma infections. This suggests the trend is toward antibiotic-resistant organisms that are both difficult to diagnose (mycoplasma) and highly pathogenic (coliforms). It also indicates that, at best, antibiotics can only be considered a stopgap means of mastitis control. For as long as antibiotics command the major role in either prophylaxis or therapy, we will continue to have the problem of the development of resistant strains. With such widespread use of antibiotics, the awesome possibility of the development of pathogens resistant to all antibiotics and chemicals exists. Antibiotic and chemical contamination of the food supply also remains a problem (see 4.9-8).

What then is the solution to mastitis control? The answer to this question depends on development of a thorough understanding of the pathogens, the host defense mechanisms, and the pathogen/host interaction under the various environmental situations encountered in the dairy industry. This understanding can only be obtained through intensive basic research on the anatomy, physiology, and biochemistry of both pathogen and host, and their interaction, as encountered under herd management conditions. A brief discussion of some potential areas of research seems an appropriate conclusion.

Research currently underway suggests that streak canal penetrability, as it affects morphology, sphincter muscle function, and the keratin and mucuslike secretion of the epithelium relative to bacterial invasion, warrant additional study.

Some of the many important questions concerning the second-line defense mechanisms within the mammary gland that remain unanswered are (1) the nature and origin of the chemotactic factors that stimulate movement of PMNs and macrophages into lacteal secretions; (2) factors limiting effective opsonization of bacteria in lacteal secretions (Ig, complement, lactoferrin); (3) inhibitors of phagocytosis in lacteal secretions (fat, casein); (4) mode of passage of PMNs and macrophages through the secretory epithelium (intracellular vs. intercellular) and its effect on subsequent phagocytic ability of these cells; (5) means of increasing the phagocyte population in the foremilk, independent of the primary milk; and (6) means of increasing the sensitivity of the chemotactic response to foreign antigens. Studies on factors affecting PMN and macrophage movement into lacteal secretions and their phagocytic and bactericidal properties are currently underway but need expanding. This research is focused on identifying the factors responsible for the decreased effectiveness of milk PMNs, as compared to blood PMNs, and means of increasing their numbers in milk to compensate for their decreased efficiency without affecting milk quality. One such approach has been the placement of a plastic loop in the gland cistern, which increases the neutrophil count in the foremilk to protective levels, while maintaining a low cell count in the total milk from the gland. Another novel approach to increasing the effectiveness of the PMN defense system has been to establish a subclinical infection with either *C. bovis* or *S. epidermidis,* since it has been shown that quarters infected with these organisms tend to be resistant to infection with the more pathogenic organisms (see 7.3-3). This increase in resistance is thought to be due to a lymphokine-mediated increase in both speed and magnitude of diapedesis of PMNs into the gland upon subsequent exposure to pathogens. Most of the above-mentioned studies have been conducted during normal lactation, with little attention given to the dry period and early lactation (periods with the highest rate of new infections) (see 7.6).

It is evident that a great deal is known about the mammalian humoral immune system (see 7.2-2b). However, it is also evident that application of this knowledge to the mammary gland has been limited (see 7.5-4a). Research on the humoral immune system of the mammary gland is needed to determine (1) the functional nature of Ig classes and subclasses in lacteal secretions (opsonic, cytolytic, antiadherence, agglutination); (2) the relative importance of local vs. systemic synthesis of Igs to their availability and protective function in lacteal secretions; (3) the mode of transport of Igs across the secretory epithelium of the mammary gland; and (4) modes of immunization (i.e., antigens, adjuvants, route) to enhance the protective antibodies in lacteal secretions. Both local and systemic immunization have proven effective in increasing specific antibodies in lacteal secretions. The most elusive area of the immunization protocol has been that of determining the optimum composition of the antigen to obtain protective antibodies. Additional research is needed to determine the importance of bacterial cell wall and capsular antigens and their relative occurrence in mastitis-causing pathogens.

Though an active CMI system has been demonstrated in the mammary gland (see 7.7-2a), no research has been reported correlating CMI function with effective defense of the mammary gland. Research in this area could lead to modes of immunization with bacterial antigens that would increase the sensitivity of the CMI system to subsequent exposure to homologous bacteria, resulting in the production of lymphokines, which could contribute to the defense of the mammary gland in numerous ways (Table 7-1).

More in-depth studies are needed on the biochemistry, physiology, and epidemiology of mastitis-causing pathogens, as affected by the environment (climate, bedding, pasture, milk). Studies of the mechanisms involved in the development of antibiotic-resistant strains are also needed. With an in-depth knowledge of the dynamics of the immunologically important bacterial antigens, more effective immunization programs can be devised and tested for their efficacy in enhancing resistance to mastitis and for conveying passive immunity to mammalian neonates.

With the widespread use of artificial insemination, it would seem that considerable progress could be made by selecting for sires with daughters of known mastitis resistance. However, before selecting for mastitis resistance, a clearly defined trait(s) and its heritability must be determined. The complexity of the mastitis defense system and the limited knowledge currently available on specific components of that system, discussed in this chapter, suggest that selection for mastitis resistance must await additional research on basic defense mechanisms.

Not withstanding positive results from all of the research mentioned above, research on milking machines will be needed to determine those characteristics of design and function that affect the transfer of bacteria into the udder: (1) inflation design and formulation; (2) claw design (individual quarter vs. common milk collection and the effects on cross-contamination of quarters); (3) sanitation of teat cups and claw; (4) automated alternatives to teat dipping; (5) alternative systems of pulsation, i.e., positive pulsation vs. no pulsation; and (6) vacuum stability.

Because early diagnosis is advantageous to effective therapy, no discussion of mastitis research would be complete without mentioning the need for improved diagnostic methods. In-line methods for identifying cows with subclinical mastitis, as well as improved on-the-farm methods of rapidly identifying the causative organism, would greatly facilitate the rapid implementation of the appropriate therapy.

Knowledge obtained from the above-mentioned areas of research should lead to a decrease in both incidence and severity of mastitis, decreased use of antibiotics, and an increase in effectiveness of passive immunity.

REFERENCES

Bellanti, J. H. 1978. Immunology II. Philadelphia: Saunders.

Butler, J. E. 1973. Synthesis and distribution of immunoglobulins. J. Am. Med. Assoc. 163:795.

______. 1974. Immunoglobulins of the mammary secretion. In Lactation, 3:244. See Larson and Smith 1974.

______, ed. 1981. The Ruminant Immune System. New York: Plenum.

______. 1983. Ovine immunoglobulins: An augmented review. Vet. Immunol. Immunopathol. 4:43.

Cohen, J. O., ed. 1972. The Staphylococci. New York: Wiley-Interscience.

Colloquium on Bovine Mastistis. 1977. J. Am. Med. Assoc. 170(10)pt.2.

Davis, B. D., R. Dulbecco, H. N. Eisen, H. S. Ginsberg, W. B. Wood, and M. McCarthy, eds. 1973. Microbiology. New York: Harper & Row.

Dodd, F. H., T. K. Griffin, and R. G. Kingwill, eds. 1975. Proceedings of the International Dairy Federation Seminar on Mastitis Control. Reading Univ., Shinfield, Reading, Eng.

Jasper, D. E., J. S. McDonald, R. D. Mochrie, W. N. Philpot, R. J. Farnsworth, and S. B. Spencer. 1982. Bovine mastitis research: Needs, funding, and sources of support. In Proceedings of 21st Annual Meeting of National Mastitis Council, Inc., Louisville, Ky., 184–93. Washington, D. C.: National Mastitis Council.

Larson, B. L., ed. 1978. Lactation: A Comprehensive Treatise, vol. 4. New York: Academic.

Larson, B. L., and V. R. Smith, eds. 1974. Lactation: A Comprehensive Treatise, vols. 2, 3. New York: Academic.

McFeely, R. A., G. E. Morse, and E. I. Williams. 1970. Proceedings of the VI International Conference of Cattle Diseases. American Association of Bovine Practitioners. Stillwater, Okla.: Heritage.

Newby, T. J., C. R. Stokes, and F. J. Bourne. 1982. Immunological activities of milk. Vet. Immunol. Immunopathol. 3:67.

Ogra, P. L., and D. H. Dayton, eds. 1979. Immunology of Breast Milk: A Monograph of the National Insititute of Child Health and Human Development. New York: Raven.

Schalm, O. W., E. J. Carroll, and N. C. Jain. 1971. Bovine Mastitis. Philadelphia: Lea & Febiger.

Tizard, I. R. 1977. An Introduction to Veterinary Immunology. Philadelphia: Saunders.

Woolcock, J. B. 1979. Bacterial Infection and Immunity in Domestic Animals. New York: Elsevier/North-Holland.

INDEX